Study Guide
TO ACCOMPANY

THIRD EDITION

Fundamentals of Nursing

CONCEPTS, PROCESS, AND PRACTICE

Kathleen G. Hoover, RN, MSN
Assistant Professor
Barnes College
St. Louis, Missouri

Printed in the United States of America

Copyright © 1993 by

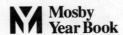 Mosby
Year Book

St. Louis Baltimore Boston Chicago London Philadelphia Sydney Toronto

Preface

Students are continually challenged to apply theoretical concepts to clinical practice. The volume and complexity of information that must be mastered to administer safe, competent care may often seem overwhelming. A *Study Guide to Accompany Fundamentals of Nursing* has been developed to provide students with strategies to assist in learning and to reinforce essential theoretical concepts, skills, and techniques basic to nursing practice.

This study guide consists of 48 chapters that correspond to the chapters in the text *Fundamentals of Nursing: Concepts, Process, and Practice*. Study guide chapters include prerequisite reading, learning objectives, review of key concepts from the text, critical thinking and experiential exercises, skill and technique activities, and a brief annotated reading list. An answer key for self-study questions is given at the end of the text.

Before beginning the study guide activities in a chapter, it is strongly recommended that students complete the "Prerequisite Reading" of the corresponding chapter in the *Fundamentals* text and review the "Objectives." Each chapter includes a "Review of Key Concepts." This section explores major concepts presented in the *Fundamentals* text through the use of a variety of objective questions. Students have the opportunity to reinforce and validate their understanding of fundamental concepts of nursing practice through true-false, matching, multiple-choice, fill-in, listing, and short-answer questions. Students should use their own paper for all sections that need answers. The section entitled "Answers to Review of Key Concepts" at the end of the book provides students with immediate feedback regarding their attainment of the learning objectives.

The "Critical Thinking and Experiential Exercises" may be used to reinforce concepts presented in the corresponding chapter of the text. These have been structured to allow students to initiate activities independently or to be incorporated by instructors into their teaching plans. The "Skill and Technique Activities" include suggestions for exercises that facilitate student practice of the technical skills described in the text. The nature of the activities in these sections prohibits providing an answer key. Although the general information needed to complete segments of these exercises may be found in the *Fundamentals* text, optimal learning will occur through interaction with peers and feedback from instructors.

The "Additional Readings" identify selected resources that may be particularly useful to the beginning nursing student. These readings expand content presented in the chapter to reinforce major themes and concepts. The annotated format is intended to present information that may stimulate interest and provide direction for further reading and study.

Although students may engage in a variety of learning experiences, content mastery rarely occurs without dedicated independent study. It is hoped that the learning activities presented in this study guide will facilitate this process.

We would like to express sincere appreciation to Patricia A. Castaldi, RN, BSN, MSN, Program Director of the School of Nursing, Elizabeth General Medical Center, Elizabeth, New Jersey, for reviewing this text. Her contributions, suggestions, and promptness were a valuable addition in the development of this publication.

Contents

Chapter 1
The Profession of Nursing

PREREQUISITE READING

Chapter 1, pp. 1 to 35

OBJECTIVES

Mastery of content in this chapter will enable the student to:

- Define selected terms related to the nursing profession.
- Discuss the historical development of the nursing profession.
- Discuss the modern definitions, philosophies, and theories of nursing practice.
- Describe educational programs for becoming a registered nurse.
- Describe practice settings for nurses.
- Describe the roles and functions of a nurse.
- List the five characteristics of a profession and discuss how nursing demonstrates these characteristics.
- Discuss the influence of social and economic changes on nursing practice.
- Discuss the influence of nursing on political issues and health care policy.

REVIEW OF KEY CONCEPTS

1. Define nursing according to the American Nurses Association (ANA), the Canadian Nurses Association (CNA), or the International Council of Nurses (ICN).
2. The profession of nursing was founded by Florence Nightingale. (True or false?)
3. Throughout history men and women have practiced nursing. (True or false?)
4. Entry of women into nursing was due to:
   a. improved social position of Roman women.
   b. Christian teachings of equality of men and women.
   c. the Christian mandate to care for those in distress.
   d. all of the above.
5. Match the person with the appropriate contribution to nursing practice and health care.

Person

a. Florence Nightingale ___4___

b. Clara Barton ___6___

c. Mary Adelaide Nutting _____

d. Mary Agnes Snively _____

e. Isabel Hampton Robb _____

f. Mary Brewster/Lillian Ward ___5___

Contribution

1. Initiated affiliation of nursing education with universities
2. Founded the Canadian National Association of Trained Nurses, later named the Canadian Nurses Association
3. Founded the Nurses' Association of Alumni of the United States and Canada, later named the American Nurses Association
4. Established the first organized program for nursing education
5. Expanded the nursing role in the community setting
6. Founded the American Red Cross
6. The survey of nursing education advocating financial support to university schools is the ___Goldmaric REPORT___.
7. The study clarifying nursing roles and responsibilities in relation to other health care professions is the _____.
8. List at least seven common goals of theoretical nursing models.

   a.

   b.

   c.

   d.

   e.

   f.

   g.
9. Match the nurse theorist with the appropriate nursing model description.

Theorist

a. Levine ___5___

b. Johnson ___7___

   c. Rogers __6__

   d. Orem __3__

   e. King __4__

   f. Henderson __8__

   g. Neuman __2__

   h. Roy __1__

   i. Watson __10__

   j. Nightingale __9__

Model

1. An adaptation model that contends that the need for nursing care arises when the client cannot adapt to internal or external demands. Nursing care focuses on assisting the client to adapt.
2. A model that views the person as an open system interacting with stressors. Nurses assist individuals, families, and groups to attain and maintain an optimal level of wellness.
3. A model based on the self-care deficit theory, in which the need for nursing arises when the client is unable to fulfill own needs. The goal of nursing is directed toward helping the client attain self-care.
4. A model that defines nursing as a dynamic, interpersonal process between the nurse, client, and health care system. The goal of nursing is to use communication in helping the client to adapt to the environment.
5. An adaptation model that views the human as an integrated whole interacting with and adapting to the environment. Nursing focuses on conservation activities aimed at optimal use of the client's resources.
6. The unitary man theory that views the client as continually changing and coexisting with the environment. The goal of nursing is to maintain and promote health, prevent illness, and care for and rehabilitate the ill and disabled throughout the "humanistic science of nursing."
7. A model that focuses on the client's adaptation to illness and the effect of stressors on this process. Adaptation is based on basic needs in seven behavior categories. The goal of nursing is to reduce stress so that the client can move more easily through the recovery process.
8. A theory involving basic needs of the whole person. It views nursing as assisting individuals, ill or well, in the performance of activities contributing to health or its recovery and doing so in a manner that helps the client gain independence.
9. A model directed toward facilitating the body's reparative processes through manipulation of the client's environment.
10. A theory involving the philosophy and science of caring. It views caring as an interpersonal process comprising interventions that result in meeting human needs.
11. In the table below, compare the three most common programs by which an individual can become a registered nurse.

	Length of Program	Educational Institution	Degree Granted	Program Focus
Associate degree program				
Diploma program				
Baccalaureate program				

11. RN licensure for practice requires completion of a prescribed course of study from an approved program and satisfactory performance on a written licensure examination. (True or false?)
12. According to the ANA, what is the purpose of graduate nursing education?
13. Identify at least three goals of continuing education in nursing.

   a.

   b.

   c.

14. Selected states require nurses to take continuing education courses for license renewal. (True or false?)
15. Define in-service education.
16. A mechanism for career mobility that seeks to promote nurses based on their clinical competencies rather than education and seniority within an institution is called a _____
17. Describe how each of the following influences nursing practice:
   a. Standards of nursing practice
   b. Nurse practice acts
   c. Practice settings
18. Most nurses are employed in hospitals. (True or false?)
19. Identify three factors contributing to rising hospital acuity rates.

   a.

   b.

   c.

20. Identify three factors that have contributed to the growth of long-term care facilities.

   a.

   b.

   c.

21. Identify four major health-related activities of community-based agencies.
    a.
    b.
    c.
    d.
22. Briefly describe the nursing role in each community-based setting:
    a. Community health centers
    b. Schools
    c. Occupational health
    d. Home health care agencies
23. Identify the role or function that the nurse fulfills in each of the following situations:
    a. The nurse feeds a client breakfast. _____
    b. The nurse answers a client's questions about discharge medications. _____
    c. The nurse writes out an organizational plan for the day. _____
    d. The nurse provides emotional support to a client who is crying. _____
    e. The nurse teaches a client how to walk with crutches. _____
    f. The nurse tests the temperature of a baby's bath water to prevent burns. _____
    g. The nurse delays the client's lunch to allow an extended nap after a painful procedure. _____

24. The role central to all other nursing roles is _____.

25. Match the career role (employment position) with the most appropriate description of its work-related activities.

Career role

    a. Nurse educator _____
    b. Clinical nurse specialist _____
    c. Nurse practitioner _____
    d. Certified nurse-midwife _____
    e. Nurse anesthetist _____
    f. Nurse administrator _____
    g. Nurse researcher _____

Work-related activities

1. Manages client care and delivery of nursing services within a health care agency
2. Provides independent care for women during normal pregnancy, labor, and delivery, as well as some routine gynecological services
3. Teaches nursing students; provides in-service education or patient teaching
4. Provides primary health care to clients, usually in outpatient, ambulatory, and community-based settings
5. Administers surgical anesthesia under the supervision of a physician
6. Investigates problems to improve nursing care and to define and expand the scope of nursing practice
7. Functions as a clinician, educator, manager, consultant, and researcher within a specific practice area.

26. Fill in the role of each health care team member based on the descriptions provided.
    a. An individual licensed to make a medial diagnosis and treat clients is a _____
    b. An individual trained in certain aspects of medical practice who provides support to physicians is a _____
    c. An individual licensed to assist in the examination, testing, and treatment of physically disabled or handicapped people through use of exercise and other treatment modalities is a _____
    d. An individual licensed or certified to develop and use adaptive devices that help chronically ill or handicapped clients carry out activities of daily living is an _____
    e. An individual licensed to deliver treatments to improve clients' ventilatory function or oxygenation is a _____
    f. An individual licensed to formulate and dispense medications is a _____
    g. An individual trained to counsel clients and their families is a _____
    h. An individual trained to offer spiritual support and guidance to clients and their families is a _____
27. List the five primary characteristics of a profession as described by Etzioni and briefly correlate these characteristics to nursing.
    a.
    b.
    c.
    d.
    e.
28. Name the following professional organizations and identify the major objectives of each.
    a. ANA
    b. CNA

  c. NLN
  d. ICN
  e. NSNA
  f. CSNA

29. Identify four societal changes influencing current nursing practice.

  a.

  b.

  c.

  d.

30. Identify three ways in which nurses may become more politically influential.

  a.

  b.

  c.

31. Briefly describe. *Nursing's Agenda for Health Care Reform.* (ANA, 1991).

CRITICAL THINKING AND EXPERIENTIAL EXERCISES

1. Societal effect on nursing/nursing effect on society
   a. Identify a period in history and discuss how events and societal characteristics of that time influenced nursing practice.
   b. Identify a current nursing leader/educator and describe how the individual has influenced nursing and/or society.
2. Conceptual models
   a. Review the conceptual model of your nursing curriculum.
   b. Identify the theorist or theorists whose goals of nursing and frameworks for practice most closely correlate with your program.
3. Nursing theories
   a. Select a nursing theorist. Review the literature for an article detailing that theory. Describe how the theory correlates or conflicts with your beliefs about nursing.
4. Definition of nursing
   a. Formulate your personal definition of nursing. Compare your definition with the 1973 ICN definition and the 1965 and 1980 ANA definitions.
5. Nurse practice legislation
   a. Review and discuss the major points of the nurse practice act for your state or province.
6. Employment opportunities
   a. Review the newspapers for advertisements of nursing positions. Identify the career roles, employment opportunities, and recommended position requirements.
7. Current issues having an impact on practice
   a. Review the daily or weekend newspaper. Identify issues that may have an impact on nursing prac-

tice and those that may be influenced by professional nurses.
8. Professional organizations
   a. Contact the student nurses association in your area to learn more about its activities and membership policies.
9. Standards of practice
   a. Observe nurses in clinical practice. Compare their activities to the ANA *Standards of Nursing Practice* or the CNA *Standards for Nursing Practice.*
10. Roles and functions of the nurse.
    a. Observe nurses in clinical practice. Identify their activities as they relate to roles and functions of the nurse. If possible, describe how these roles and functions are influenced by the health care setting.
11. Roles of health care team members
    a. Care for, interview, or review the medical record of a hospitalized client. Identify health care team members coming in contact with the client and describe their roles in providing care.

ADDITIONAL READINGS

DeLoughery G, editor: *Issues and trends in nursing*, St Louis, 1991, Mosby–Year Book.
 Provides a survey of current issues and trends in nursing practice. Appropriate reading for students and practitioners.
Donahue MP: *Nursing: the finest art, an illustrated history*, St Louis, 1985, Mosby–Year Book.
 A richly illustrated, well-referenced historical compendium of the art and science of nursing.
Fawcett J: *Analysis and evaluation of conceptual models of nursing*, ed 2, Philadelphia, 1989, Davis.
 Presents major conceptual models of nursing with analysis of their applicability to practice.
Hinshaw AS: Nursing science: the challenge to develop knowledge, *Nurs Sci Q* 2(4):162, 1990.
 Explores issues surrounding nursing theory development as they relate to advancing practice.
Huey, FL: Looking at ladders, *Am J Nurs* 82:1520, 1982.
 Defines the concept of clinical ladders as a mechanism for recognition and reward of nurses electing to remain at the bedside.
Marriner-Tomey A: *Nursing theorists and their work*, ed 2, St Louis, 1989, Mosby–Year Book.
 A presentation and analysis of popular nursing theories.
Mason D, Talbott S, editors: *Political action handbook for nurses*, Menlo Park, Calif, 1985, Addison-Wesley.
 Examines influence of nurses on health care via the political system. Demystifies politics in the workplace, government, organization, and community. Encourages nurses to accept their professional role of political activism.
News: North Dakota's high court frees nursing board to enforce its BSN requirement for RN licensure, *Am J Nurs* 87(3):372, 1987.
 Discussion of a 1987 state supreme court decision barring ADN and diploma graduates from the RN licensure examination.

Rogge MM: Nursing and politics: a forgotten legacy, *Nurs Res* 36(1):26, 1987.

Discussion of the political activities of nurses through American history. Highlights nurses' effect in creating health care policy change.

Walker LO: Toward a clearer understanding of the concept of nursing theory, *Nurs Res* 20(5):428, 1971.

Analysis of the concept of nursing theory. Examines conflicting issues between practical and theoretical knowledge, and theory and practice.

Chapter 2
Health and Illness

PREREQUISITE READING

Chapter 2, pp. 36-63

OBJECTIVES

Mastery of content in this chapter will enable the student to:
- Define selected terms related to health and illness.
- Discuss definitions of health and related concepts.
- Discuss each of the following: health-illness continuum model, high-level wellness model, agent-host-environment model, health-belief model, evolutionary-based model, health-promotion model.
- Describe health-promotion and illness-prevention activities.
- List and discuss the three levels of preventive care.
- List and explain four kinds of risk factors.
- Describe variables influencing health beliefs and practices.
- Describe variables influencing illness behavior.
- List and discuss the stages of illness behavior.
- Describe the impact of illness on the client and family.
- Discuss the nurse's role for the client in health and illness.

REVIEW OF KEY CONCEPTS

1. Define health in a way that may be applicable to any client.
2. Define health beliefs.
3. List three positive health behaviors.

   a.

   b.

   c.

4. List three negative health behaviors.

   a.

   b.

   c.

5. Match the health model with the most accurate description.

Model

   a. Health-illness continuum model _____

   b. Health-promotion model _____

   c. Agent-host-environment model _____

   d. Health-belief model _____

   e. Evolutionary-based model _____

   f. High-level wellness model _____

Description

1. Model deriving health outcomes from complex interaction of affective responses in combination with life events, personal adaptive strategies, perception of control over life circumstances, and functional capacity to promote survival and well-being
2. Model viewing health as a dynamic state continually changing as a person adapts to alterations in internal and external environment and illness as an abnormal process diminishing or impairing the person's ability to function in one or more dimensions when compared with previous condition
3. Model predicting a person's response to health and health care by examining personal perception of susceptibility to illness, seriousness of the illness, and benefits of taking action
4. Model explaining why persons engage in health activities by examining cognitive-perceptual factors and other external variables enhancing or diminishing participation in health promotion; health promotion viewed as increasing client's level of well-being and self-actualization
5. Model originating in community health setting, expanded to describe levels of health or illness of an individual or group based on the dynamic relationships among three variables: the person, the environment, and factors leading to illness
6. Model oriented toward maximizing a person's health potential, allowing progression to higher levels of functioning

6. For the past 5 years, Mrs. Jones has been taking medications and following a low-salt diet to control her blood pressure. During this time, she has adhered to her prescribed therapy 90% of the time. Mrs. Jones says that she takes her medicines and stays on her diet because they make her "feel so much better." Which of the four models of health best explains Mrs. Jones' behavior?

   a. Health-illness continuum model

b. Agent-host-environment model
c. High-level wellness model
d. Health-belief model

7. Internal variables influencing health beliefs and practices include:
   a. Family practices and cultural background.
   b. Socioeconomic factors and intellectual background.
   c. Spiritual factors and developmental stage.
   d. Cultural background and perception of functioning.

8. Actions that help a client maintain or enhance present level of health are called _____ .

9. Actions that protect a client from actual or potential threats to health are called _____ .

10. An active health promotion strategy would include:
    a. fluoridating drinking water.
    b. fortifying milk with vitamin D.
    c. working in a smoke-free environment.
    d. beginning a weight-reduction program.

11. The primary goal of a total health program is improvement of a person's physical health. (True or false?)

12. List seven categories of major lifestyle habits important in determining a person's health status.

    a.

    b.

    c.

    d.

    e.

    f.

    g.

13. Match the level of prevention to the nursing activity.

Activity

   a. Bathing a client _____

   b. Teaching a stroke victim ways to check bath water temperature to avoid burns _____

   c. Leading a children's exercise class _____

   d. Administering medications _____

   e. Administering immunizations _____

Level

   1. Primary
   2. Secondary
   3. Tertiary

14. Any variable increasing the vulnerability of an individual or a group to an illness or accident is a (an):
    a. Illness behavior.
    b. Risk factor.

c. Negative health behavior.
d. Lifestyle determinant.

15. For each category, identify at least two risk factors.
    a. Genetic and physiological factors
    b. Age
    c. Environment
    d. Lifestyle

16. Illness is synonymous with disease. (True or false?)

17. Define illness.

18. All of the following characterize illness behavior *except:*
    a. Calling a physician.
    b. Ignoring a physical symptom.
    c. Interpreting physical symptoms.
    d. Withdrawing from work activities.

19. A client's perception of symptoms influences illness behavior. (True or false?)

20. Clients with chronic illness are more likely to seek health care and comply with therapy than clients with acute illness. (True or false?)

21. List at least five determinants influencing illness behavior.

    a.

    b.

    c.

    d.

    e.

22. List and briefly describe the five stages of illness behavior.

    a.

    b.

    c.

    d.

    e.

23. All clients go through each stage of illness behavior. (True or false?)

24. Mr. Green entered a rehabilitation center to learn to care for himself after an automobile accident that has left him partially paralyzed. Mr. Green is very quiet, stays in his room, and avoids interacting with other clients and staff. This behavior is characteristic of which emotional response to illness?
    a. Shock
    b. Anger
    c. Withdrawal
    d. Denial

25. A subjective concept of an individual's physical appearance is the individual's _____ .

26. An individual's mental image of self, including all aspects of personality, is the individual's

_____ .

27. Identify the four factors that influence the reactions of a client and family to a change in body image.

a.

b.

c.

d.

CRITICAL THINKING AND EXPERIENTIAL EXERCISES:

1. Models of health and illness
   a. Identify the health model that most closely corresponds to your beliefs about health and health care.
   b. Discuss the reasons for your selection.
   c. Describe the ways this model influences nursing care.
2. Risk factors and health promotion
   a. Perform a self-assessment or interview a peer to elicit information about the presence of risk factors in each major category. Formulate realistic related actions to prevent illness and promote health.

	Risk factors	Actions
Genetic and physiological		
Age		
Environment		
Lifestyle		

3. Stress assessment
   a. After a client care experience or interaction, use the Hospital Stress Rating Scale (Volicer, 1974) in your text to determine actual and potential stressors experienced by the client. Discuss your findings and propose ways that the nurse might assist in reducing the client's stress and its potential complications.

4. Illness behavior
   During a client care experience or interaction:
   a. Identify the client's stage of illness behavior.
   b. Describe client behaviors reflecting this stage of illness.
   c. Identify the client's or family's behavioral or emotional response to illness.

ADDITIONAL READINGS

Edelman C, Mandle CL: *Health promotion throughout the life span,* ed 2, St Louis, 1990, Mosby–Year Book.
   Examines health promotion activities from a developmental perspective.
Muhlenkamp AF, Styles JA: Self-esteem, social support and positive health practices, *Nurs Res* 35:334, 1986.
   Attempts to identify relationships among perceived social support, self-esteem, and positive health practices in a small sample of adults.
Pender NJ: A conceptual model for preventive health behavior, *Nurs Outlook* 23:385,1975.
   Describes personal, interpersonal, and situational factors motivating persons toward preventive health actions. Discusses the nursing role in influencing client motivation.
Pender NJ, Pender AR: Attitudes, subjective norms and intentions to engage in health behaviors, *Nurs Res* 35:15, 1986.
   Explores influence of intent on health behaviors in areas of exercise, weight control, and stress management.
Pollock SE: Human responses to chronic illness: physiological and psychosocial adaptation, *Nurs Res* 35:90, 1986.
   Identifies factors promoting adaptation to chronic illness. Differentiates physiological and psychosocial adaptation and the influence of "hardiness characteristics" in selected chronic illness states.
Spector, RE: *Cultural diversity in health and illness,* ed 3, Norwalk, Conn, 1991, Appleton & Lange.
   Describes the impact of cultures on health promotion and illness behaviors.
Volicer BJ: Patient's perceptions of stressful events associated with hospitalization, *Nurs Res* 23:235, 1974.
   Gives results of patients' responses to a survey regarding stress-producing events associated with hospitalization. Emphasizes the high level of psychosocial stress experienced and ranks events according to perceived level of stress.

Chapter 3
The Health Care Delivery System

PREREQUISITE READING
Chapter 3, pp. 64 to 93

OBJECTIVES
Mastery of content in this chapter will enable the student to:
- Define selected terms related to the health care delivery system.
- Discuss major events in the evolution of the health care delivery system.
- Describe society's influence on the health care delivery system.
- Discuss factors influencing entry into the system.
- Describe the six types of health care agencies.
- Discuss the client's right to health care and describe client rights within the health care delivery system.
- Compare the various methods for financing health care.
- Explain the advantages and disadvantages of a prospective reimbursement system.
- Describe the problems of the health care delivery system.
- Explain solutions for each problem of the health care delivery system.

REVIEW OF KEY CONCEPTS
1. Third-party payment for financing health care was introduced in the 1920s because:
   a. affluent people could not afford quality health care.
   b. middle class people could afford only home care.
   c. hospitals were successfully supported by patient payment.
   d. hospitals were experiencing financial losses.
2. The U.S. government program providing medical and hospital insurance for persons who are disabled or over age 65 is _____ .
3. The U.S. government program providing a joint federal and state health insurance program for low-income persons is _____ .
4. Canadian provincial governments offer medical care plans that are more inclusive than those available in the United States. (True or false?)
5. The federal law allowing nurse practitioners to deliver primary health care in underserved areas is the:
   a. Rural Health Clinics Act.
   b. Hill-Burton Act.
   c. National Health Planning and Resources Development Act.
   d. Social Security Amendment Act of 1972.
6. The prospective payment plan for health care represents:
   a. the merger of national and private insurance programs to reduce client costs.
   b. a method for controlling local and regional hospital expansion.
   c. fixed payments to hospitals based on diagnostic categories.
   d. payments to hospitals based on costs incurred by each client.
7. State the two major issues associated with today's health care system.
   a.
   b.
8. Health promotion activities are designed to help clients:
   a. reduce the costs of health care.
   b. maintain maximal function.
   c. promote habits related to good health.
   d. all of the above.
9. Illness prevention activities are designed to help clients:
   a. reduce risk factors.
   b. promote habits related to good health.
   c. manage stress.
   d. identify disease symptoms.
10. Traditionally, the most commonly used services of the health care delivery system have included:
    a. rehabilitation and nursing home care.
    b. illness diagnosis and treatment.
    c. illness prevention.
    d. health promotion.
11. Define rehabilitation.
12. Rehabilitation services begin:
    a. when the client enters the health care system.

b. after the client requests rehabilitation services.
c. after the client's physical condition stabilizes.
d. when the client is discharged from the hospital.
13. Match the health care agency with the most appropriate description.

Agency

    a. Outpatient _____

    b. Community-based _____

    c. Volunteer _____

    d. Support group _____

    e. Institution _____

    f. Hospice _____

    g. Government _____

Description

    1. Clinics, hospitals, and other health care services supported by local, state, provincial, or national taxes
    2. Settings that include physician's offices, clinics, or urgent-care centers
    3. Family-centered care system focusing on maintenance of comfort and a satisfactory lifestyle for clients in the terminal phase of illness
    4. Settings in which clients are admitted and remain for diagnosis, treatment, or rehabilitation
    5. National or community not-for-profit groups established to meet specific client needs
    6. Agencies providing health care to clients in their neighborhoods
    7. Organized groups providing self-help services by focusing on shared experiences, problem solving, and emotional support
14. Describe the major services provided by each type of health care agency.
    a. Residential/retirement community
    b. Day care center
    c. Crisis intervention center
    d. Intermediate care/skilled-care facility
    e. Long-term care facility/nursing home
15. In Canada, insured health care services must be available to:
    a. residents.
    b. members of the military service.
    c. inmates of federal prisons.
    d. all of the above.
16. Identify the five major factors influencing the health care delivery system over the past decade.

    a.

    b.

    c.

    d.

    e.

17. Briefly describe three reasons for rising health care costs.

    a.

    b.

    c.

18. The Patient's Bill of Rights, developed by the American Hospital Association, is a legally binding document. (True or false?)
19. The legal permission obtained from the client before an invasive procedure, administration of experimental medication, or involvement in research is _____.
20. Match the major methods for financing health care services with the description provided.

Insurance

    a. Private insurance plan _____

    b. Health maintenance organization _____

    c. Preferred provider organization _____

    d. Long-term insurance plan _____

    e. Government insurance plan _____

Description

    1. Program to deliver care based on prepaid fees with emphasis on health promotion and illness prevention
    2. Program to supplement Medicare, in varying amounts, for extended care costs
    3. Contractual agreement, usually between a group of physicians and a hospital, to provide comprehensive health services at a discount to companies under contract
    4. Traditional approach to health care financing obtained by the individual (or through a group plan) that is retrospective fee for service (third-party reimbursement)
    5. System supported by state, provincial, or federal programs, significantly affected by political and economic trends
21. Briefly discuss four major problems with the present health care system in the United States.

    a.

    b.

    c.

    d.

22. Briefly describe four possible solutions for the current problems in the health care system.

    a.

    b.

    c.

    d.

CRITICAL THINKING AND EXPERIENTIAL EXERCISES

1. Current health care issues
   a. Review local or national news publications for information about the health care system. Discuss the immediate and long-term ramifications of the issues described.
2. Nurses' position on current health care issues
   a. Contact your professional nursing organization for information concerning positions on pending health care legislation and other health care issues.
3. Representatives' position on current health care issues
   a. Contact your government representative and request information about his or her position on pending health care legislation. Write to your government representative to give your position on pending health care legislation or other health care issues.
4. Patient's Bill of Rights
   a. Review the Patient's Bill of Rights (see Chapter 14). Summarize the rights of clients in the health-care system and identify ways nurses can actively assist in protecting the client's rights.
5. Informed consent
   a. Examine your institution's consent form and compare it to the criteria described in your text. In what ways does it meet the stated criteria? In what ways does it meet or not meet the needs of the client?
6. Health insurance plans
   a. Review your (or your family's) health insurance plan. Identify the type of plan and its major benefits and limitations.
7. Health care cost
   a. Contact the client accounts or billing department of your institution to determine typical costs incurred during hospitalization. Determine whether nursing costs or the percentage of cost related to nursing care is specified in the client's bill.
8. Health care cost containment
   a. Interview a staff nurse and a nursing manager about ways in which nursing is attempting to control health care costs in the agency.
   b. Observe activities in a health care agency for a few hours. Identify activities that help to control the cost of health care. Identify activities that inhibit cost control and propose actions to minimize these problems.
9. Community health care agencies
   a. Select a local geographical area or community.
   b. Survey the area to determine agencies offering health care and the nature of their services.
   c. Talk to nurses employed by the health care agencies to determine their role in providing care.
   d. Talk to staff and clients to identify factors that tend to facilitate or limit client access to care in the setting.

ADDITIONAL READINGS

American Nurses Association: *Nursing's agenda for health care reform,* Kansas City, Mo, 1991, The Association.
   Details the ANA proposal for improved quality and access to health care for the United States. All health care professionals should be familiar with the strategies presented in this important document.
Cohen SS: The politics of Medicaid 1980-1989, *Nurs Outlook* 38(5):229, 1990.
   Reviews the Medicaid program in the context of the political system in the past decade. Suggests that child health advocates must remain vigilant if Medicaid is to continue to help women, infants, and children in need.
Harrington C: Policy options for a national health care plan, *Nurs Outlook* 38(5):223, 1990.
   Presents current proposals for national health care reform in three major categories: incremental expansion of public programs, mandatory requirements for employers, and comprehensive national plans for health care. Intended to help nurses understand the implications of major programs for professional practice and the nation's health.
Maraldo PJ, Solomon SB: Nursing's window of opportunity, *Image J Nurs Sch* 19:83, 1987.
   Explores the current crisis in health care as the opportunity for nursing to provide workable solutions, further legitimizing the role of nurses and actualizing the profession's potential. Directs nurses to remove economic and policital barriers to nursing practice, increase professional preparation at a master's degree level, and implement strategies to enable nurses to compete with other health care providers.

Chapter 4
Culture, Ethnicity, and Nursing

PREREQUISITE READING
Chapter 4, pp. 94 to 117

OBJECTIVES
Mastery of content in this chapter will enable the student to:
- Define selected terms related to culture and ethnicity.
- Explain the need for a nurse's self-evaluation when providing care to clients from other sociocultural backgrounds.
- Describe heritage-consistent and heritage-inconsistent attributes.
- Describe the relationship of sociocultural background to health and illness beliefs and practices.
- Describe cultural phenomena—environmental control, biological variations, social organization, communication, space, and time—that apply to culturally sensitive nursing practice.
- Compare concepts of traditional and modern health and illness beliefs and practices.
- List traditional health and illness beliefs and practices of Asian, African, Native, Spanish, and European Americans.
- Perform a cultural assessment using the heritage consistency assessment tool.
- Discuss several ways in which planning and implementation of nursing interventions can be adapted to a client's ethnicity.

REVIEW OF KEY CONCEPTS
1. Define transcultural communication.
2. The nurse facilitates transcultural communication

   through identification of _____ .

3. In the next century, "average" American residents will no longer include:
   a. European Americans.
   b. African Americans.
   c. Asian Americans.
   d. Native Americans.
4. The client's responses to health and illness are culture specific, based on experience and perception. (True or false?)
5. Compare the melting pot theory to the heritage-consistency theory.
6. A person's lifestyle may simultaneously reflect heritage-consistent and heritage-inconsistent characteristics. (True or false?)
7. Nonphysical traits, such as values, beliefs, attitudes, and customs shared by a group of people and passed from generation to generation are that

   group's _____ .
8. A cultural group's sense of identification associated with common social and cultural heritage is

   called _____ .
9. A belief in a divine or superhuman power (or powers) to be obeyed and worshiped as the creator and ruler

   of the universe is a _____ .
10. Compare heritage-consistent attributes with heritage-inconsistent attributes in each of the designated areas in the table below.
11. List and briefly describe the six phenomena differentiating cultural groups.

    a.

	Heritage Consistent	Heritage Inconsistent
a. Location of childhood development		
b. Visits to a country or neighborhood of origin		
c. Location of family home		
d. Extended family relationships		
e. Name		
f. Education		
g. Knowledge of culture and language		
h. Participation in traditional religious or cultural activities		
i. Individual's personal philosophy		

b.

c.

d.

e.

f.

12. Describe the four zones that make up an individual's personal space.

a.

b.

c.

d.

13. Define traditional epidemiology.
14. The most important factor in providing nursing care to clients in a specific ethnic group is:
   a. communication.
   b. time orientation.
   c. biological variation.
   d. environmental control.
15. The use of objects, substances, and religious practices to prevent or treat illness is known as _____ .
16. Compare the traditional healer with the modern physician.
17. Characteristic beliefs of a cultural group are held by each person in the group. (True or false?)
18. Match the common traits with the characteristic ethnic group.

Traits
   a. View health as a result of good luck; reward from God for good behavior; balance of hot and cold, wet and dry _____
   b. Have traditional remedies that include Sloan's Liniment and Father John's Medicine _____
   c. View illness as an imbalance between yin (negative energy) and yang (positive energy) _____
   d. Believe that health reflects the ability to live in harmony with nature, and the ability to survive under extreme difficulty _____
   e. Have traditional remedies that include bangles, talismans, and asafetida (incense of the devil) _____
   f. Define health as the ability to do activities of daily living or a state of physical and emotional well-being _____
   g. Believe that illness is prevented by maintaining harmony with body, mind, and spirit and by avoiding factors leading to disharmony _____

   h. Have traditional remedies that include burning novena candles, manzanilla tea, anis seeds, and amulets _____
   i. View life as a process and health as harmony with nature _____
   j. Have traditional remedies that include acupuncture, moxibustion, and ginseng root _____

Ethnic group
   1. Native Americans
   2. Asian Americans
   3. Spanish Americans
   4. African Americans
   5. European Americans
19. Before effectively caring for a client from an ethnic group, the nurse must first:
   a. study the ethnic culture.
   b. determine personal cultural beliefs and values.
   c. work with an ethnic folk healer.
   d. minimize transcultural communication.
20. It is appropriate to include the client's cultural beliefs and practices in planning and providing the client's nursing care. (True or false?)

CRITICAL THINKING AND EXPERIENTIAL EXERCISES

1. Cultural assessment
   a. Conduct a cultural assessment on yourself, a peer, or relative using the heritage assessment tool (pp. 112-113 in your text).
   b. Where would you place the individual on the heritage-consistency continuum? Why?
   c. How would your findings influence planned nursing care (for example, alternative approaches to care provision)?
2. Acculturation
   Care for a client in any health care setting
   a. Identify the client's cultural group.
   b. Describe the traditional definitions of health and illness, beliefs about the causes of illness, methods of prevention, and illness remedies associated with the identified cultural group.
   c. Compare the client's beliefs and practices with traditional and dominant cultural beliefs and practices.
   d. Identify specific nursing actions to promote individualized, culturally sensitive care to the client.
3. Clinical situation: heritage consistency
   Mrs. Antonio and Mrs. Totino are both of Italian descent. Mrs. Antonio, a recent immigrant, is a 62-year-old widow. She is living with her daughter, son-in-law, and their three school-age children. Mrs. Antonio speaks little English because all her family members and close relatives speak Italian. She lives in an area of the city almost entirely populated by families of the same ethnic origin. Mrs. Antonio

attends the local church, which continues to offer a weekly Mass in Italian.

Mrs. Totino is 50 years old. She and her husband have three children. Two are attending a university and living at home. The eldest is married, has three small children, and lives in a different part of the same city. Mrs. Totino speaks fluent English and Italian. She is active in a local church group and is a volunteer at a local nursing home.

a. Both women are admitted to the hospital with arthritis-related problems. Would you expect these two individuals to react in the same way to hospitalization? Support your answer by considering each of the variables influencing heritage consistency.

4. Clinical situation: ethnicity and culture

Mrs. Sanchez, a 38-year-old Spanish American, is admitted to the hospital with the diagnosis of menorrhagia (excessive bleeding during menstruation). She is scheduled for several diagnostic tests and possible surgery to remove her uterus. Mrs. Sanchez speaks very little English. Mr. Sanchez's work takes him away from home for several weeks at a time, so he is not able to visit his wife at the hospital. Mrs. Sanchez seems very tense. This is the first time she has ever been hospitalized.

a. Discuss how Mrs. Sanchez's ethnicity may influence her perception of her current illness and cooperation with hospital care givers.

b. Discuss ways to bridge the existing language barrier.

c. Identify ways the nurse can provide culturally sensitive care to Mrs. Sanchez.

ADDITIONAL READINGS

Boyle JS, Andrews MM: *Transcultural concepts in nursing care,* Glenview, Ill, 1989, Scott, Foresman.

Presents transcultural concepts through an integrated approach. Explores theories and foundations of transcultural care. Discusses each phase of the life span and special topics, including chronic illness, critical care, pain, mental health, nutrition, and religion from the transcultural perspective.

Rempusheski V: The role of ethnicity in elder care, *Nurs Clin North Am* 24(3):717, 1989.

Examines concepts of ethnicity within the context of elder care. Addresses issues in assessment of ethnicity and methods for incorporating ethicity into the plan for improved client care.

Spector RE: *Cultural diversity in health and illness,* ed 3, Norwalk, Conn, 1991, Appleton & Lange.

Explores traditional and modern health care practices and addresses issues relating to health care for Asian, African, Spanish, European, and Native Americans. Challenges readers to become aware of their own beliefs about health and illness.

Tripp-Reimer T: Cross-cultural perspectives on patient teaching, *Nurs Clin North Am* 24(3):613, 1989.

Focuses on the importance of cultural understanding between the nurse and the client in facilitating patient teaching. Emphasizes that cultural diversity requires that nurses conduct thorough cultural assessments and use cultural negotiation to improve health teaching.

Chapter 5
Admission, Discharge, and Home Health Care

PREREQUISITE READING

Chapter 5, pp. 120 to 140

OBJECTIVES

Mastery of content in this chapter will enable the student to:

- Define selected terms related to the continuum of care.
- Describe the nurse's role in maintaining continuity of care from admission to an acute-care facility to transfer and discharge.
- Identify purposes of health care referrals.
- Identify clients in need of comprehensive discharge planning.
- Identify types of home health care agencies and reimbursement mechanisms.
- Identify forces that have influenced the development of home health nursing.
- Describe roles and responsibilities of nurses in home health care.
- Describe how regulatory standards and quality assurance guidelines affect the clinical practice of home health nursing.
- Identify at least two areas of specialized nursing care in the home.
- Identify future trends in home health care and the way they affect clinical practice.

REVIEW OF KEY CONCEPTS

1. Hospital admission and discharge processes are regulated by government and accrediting agencies. (True or false?)
2. State the importance of the Omnibus Budget Reconciliation Act (OBRA) of 1990 as it relates to client hospital admission.
3. Identify the four levels of outcomes to be included in a client's discharge plan.

   a.

   b.

   c.

   d.

4. List at least six risk factors creating client inability to meet health care needs after discharge.

   a.

   b.

   c.

   d.

   e.

   f.

5. To ensure successful client care after hospital discharge, planning participants should include:
   a. the doctor.
   b. the nurse.
   c. the client.
   d. every person caring for the client.
6. An effective professional nurse rarely needs to make referrals to professionals in other health disciplines. (True or false?)
7. Define an AMA discharge.
8. Define home health care.
9. Identify the primary focus of home health care.
10. Briefly describe each of the following types of home health care services in terms of assistance offered and mechanisms for reimbursement.
    a. Home health agencies
    b. Private duty agencies
    c. Durable medical equipment companies
11. Identify at least four conditions creating an increased demand for home health care.

    a.

    b.

    c.

    d.

12. The nurse may evaluate the client's need for home health care services without a medical order. (True or false?)

13. Identify the three factors that must be examined to determine client eligibility for home health services.

    a.

    b.

    c.

14. Identify at least five areas that must be assessed before planning home health care.

    a.

    b.

    c.

    d.

    e.

15. It is important for the nurse to maintain control over the home environment to provide optimal home health care. (True or false?)
16. Governmental and private insurers will pay for home visits only until the client or family has had time to learn procedures. (True or false?)
17. The government agency responsible for monitoring compliance with home care regulations and distributing funds for claims is:
    a. Community Health Accreditation Program (CHAP)
    b. Joint Commission on Accreditation of Healthcare Organizations (JCAHO)
    c. Health Care Financing Administration (HCFA)
    d. National Institutes of Health (NIH)
18. The most important action to ensure accreditation and reimbursement for home health care services is to:
    a. provide highly technical, innovative nursing care.
    b. carefully document nursing assessments, plans, actions, and client response.
    c. identify all professional and non-professional services that the client requests or requires.
    d. document the agency need for specialty nursing teams and implement continuing-education programs for staff.
19. Briefly describe at least three home health care trends for the 1990s.

    a.

    b.

    c.

CRITICAL THINKING AND EXPERIENTIAL EXERCISES

1. Admission and discharge standards
   Review the JCAHO Standards for Admission and Discharge (text, p. 122).
   a. Compare these to the standards of your institution.
   b. Identify the ways your institution meets the standards.
   c. Describe how your institution exceeds the standards.
2. Hospital admission process
   Follow a client through the entire admission process.
   a. Compare and contrast the hospital admission to the nursing division admission. What was the same? What was different?
   b. Describe the role and responsibilities of the professional nurse in this process. Which actions would you consider the most essential to the client's hospitalization? Why?
   c. Describe the role and responsibilities of the client in the admission process.
   d. Interview the client and a family member one to two days after hospital admission. What did they consider the most important information provided? What was least important or inaccurate? Was there anything else they wish they had been told?
   e. If you had the authority to modify the admissions procedure in your institution, what would you change? Why do you believe the change is appropriate? How would you go about implementing the change?
3. Institutional discharge planning
   a. Identify the individuals responsible for discharge planning or coordination of home health care services at your institution.
   b. Determine whether your institution has any formal protocols for planning clients' discharge and home care.
   c. Talk to staff nurses to determine their role and responsibilities concerning discharge planning.
4. Home health care needs
   After providing nursing care (or completing a nursing assessment) for a hospitalized client:
   a. Identify the client's risk for needing comprehensive discharge planning.
   b. Identify the current professional, paraprofessional, and health care equipment services being utilized by the client.
   c. Determine the services that the client will require at the time of discharge.
   d. Consult your instructor or your institution's home health coordinator or discharge planner to determine the client's eligibility for home health care.
5. Home health care agencies
   a. Survey a designated geographical area in your community to identify home health care agencies.
   b. Contact local home health care agencies to determine the nature of services offered and their primary sources of reimbursement for services.
   c. Interview a nurse employed by a home health care agency. Determine the nurse's level of academic preparation, area of clinical specializa-

tion or primary interest, experiences before employment by the agency, and job responsibilities.

ADDITIONAL READINGS

American Nurses Association: *Standards of nursing care for home health care practice*, Kansas City, Mo, 1986, The Association.

    Outlines the expectations for professional nursing care delivered in the home.

Bedrosian C: *Home health nursing: nursing diagnoses and care plans*, Norwalk, Conn, 1989, Appleton & Lange.

    Provides practical and concise guides to home care. Focuses on older adult clients. Useful reference for nurses in hospital and home care.

Shamansky S, editor: Home health care, *Nurs Clin North Am* 23(2), 1988.

    A series of articles written by experts from home care practice, administration, education, and research. Provides an overview of major issues and trends in a complex and rapidly changing industry.

Walsh H, Perrsons CB, Wieck L: *Manual of home health care nursing*, Philadelphia, 1987, Lippincott.

    Adapts acute care nursing techniques to the home setting. Each technique is presented using a nursing process framework with emphasis on family teaching.

Chapter 6
Assessment

PREREQUISITE READING

Chapter 6, pp. 144 to 165

OBJECTIVES

Mastery of content in this chapter will enable the student to:
- Define selected terms related to assessment.
- State the five components of the nursing process.
- Describe the three components of nursing assessment.
- Discuss the purposes of nursing assessment.
- Differentiate between objective and subjective data.
- State the sources of data for a nursing assessment.
- Describe the four interviewing techniques.
- State the purpose of a nursing history.
- State the purpose of a physical examination.
- Demonstrate the four skills of physical assessment.
- Conduct and record a nursing assessment.

REVIEW OF KEY CONCEPTS

1. Define nursing process.
2. List the five components of the nursing process in their appropriate sequence.

    a.

    b.

    c.

    d.

    e.

3. Fill in the component of the nursing process that most accurately matches the purpose described.
    a. To identify client's goals, determine priorities, design nursing strategies, and determine outcome criteria _____
    b. To gather, verify, and communicate data about the client to establish a data base _____
    c. To determine the extent to which goals of care have been achieved _____
    d. To complete nursing actions necessary for accomplishing the care plan _____.
    e. To identify the health care needs of the client _____

4. Define objective data.

5. Define subjective data.
6. Which of the following assessment data is subjective?
    a. Temperature of 39° C (102.2° F)
    b. Heart rate of 96 beats per minute
    c. Weight loss of 10 kg (22 pounds)
    d. Sharp leg pain lasting 2 hours
7. Identify five sources of data for nursing assessment.

    a.

    b.

    c.

    d.

    e.

8. In most circumstances, the best source of information for nursing assessment of the adult client is the:
    a. client.
    b. physician.
    c. nursing literature.
    d. medical record.
9. Identify four methods of data collection the nurse uses to establish a data base.

    a.

    b.

    c.

    d.

10. The interviewing technique most effective in strengthening the nurse-client relationship by demonstrating the nurse's willingness to hear the client's thoughts is:
    a. open-ended question.
    b. direct question.
    c. problem solving.
    d. problem seeking.
11. While obtaining a health history, the nurse asks Mr. Jones if he has noted any change in his activity tolerance. This is an example of which interview technique?
    a. Problem seeking
    b. Problem solving
    c. Direct question
    d. Open-ended question

12. Mr. Davis tells the nurse that he has been experiencing more frequent episodes of indigestion. The nurse asks whether the indigestion is associated with meals or a reclining position and what relieves the indigestion. This is an example of which interview technique?
    a. Problem seeking
    b. Problem solving
    c. Direct question
    d. Open-ended question
13. Identify and briefly describe the three phases of the interview.

    a.

    b.

    c.
14. Match the communication strategy with the most accurate description or definition.

Strategy

    a. Silence _____

    b. Attentive listening _____

    c. Conveying acceptance _____

    d. Planning related questions _____

    e. Paraphrasing _____

    f. Clarifying _____

    g. Focusing _____

    h. Stating observations _____

    i. Offering information _____

    j. Summarizing _____

Description
    1. Demonstrates willingness to listen to the client without being judgmental
    2. Condenses data into an organized review and validates data
    3. Asking the client to restate the information or provide an example
    4. Provides time to the nurse to make observations and for the client to organize thoughts
    5. Provides client with feedback about how nurse sees personal behavior or actions
    6. Activity facilitated by maintaining eye contact, remaining relaxed, and using appropriate touch techniques
    7. Allows nurse to clarify health-related issues, initiate teaching, and identify and correct misconceptions
    8. Formulation of client's statement by nurse, in more specific words, without changing meaning
    9. Use of words and word patterns in client's normal sociocultural context
    10. Limits area of discussion and helps nurse to direct attention to pertinent aspects of the client's message

15. Identify the four purposes (objectives) for obtaining a nursing health history.

    a.

    b.

    c.

    d.
16. The reason that the client is seeking health care consistently corresponds to the medical diagnosis. (True or false?)
17. A client is admitted with pain in the right shoulder. What specific information should the nurse obtain concerning this symptom?
18. During the development of the nursing history, the client is asked, "What outcomes do you expect from this hospitalization?" What purpose does this question serve?
19. During an admission interview a client reports an allergy to aspirin. What additional information should the nurse elicit?
20. Why is it important to explore lifestyle patterns and habits such as the use of alcohol, nonprescription or prescription drugs, caffeine, or tobacco?
21. Why is it important to assess the client's patterns of sleep, exercise, and nutrition?
22. The information obtained in a review of systems (ROS) is:
    a. objective.
    b. subjective.
    c. based on physical examination findings.
    d. based on the nurse's perspective.
23. What is the purpose of a physical examination?
24. Fill in the technique of physical examination with the description provided.
    a. The process of listening to sounds produced by the body. _____
    b. Use of the hands and sense of touch to gather data. _____
    c. Observation of responses, behaviors, and physical appearance. _____
    d. Tapping the body's surface to produce vibration and sound. _____
25. Identify at least two contributions that laboratory data make to the nursing assessment.

    a.

    b.
26. Comparing assessed data with another source to establish accuracy is the process of _____ .
27. Grouping related data to form a picture of the client's health needs is the process of _____ .
28. List three ways to validate information obtained during a nursing history.

    a.

    b.

    c.

29. All pertinent client data, normal or abnormal, obtained during assessment should be recorded. (True or false?)

CRITICAL THINKING AND EXPERIENTIAL EXERCISES

1. Nursing process
   a. Observe a nurse in any practice setting.
   b. Identify components of the nursing process that you observe and describe how these components are incorporated in the practice setting.
   c. Discuss your findings with your peers and instructor.
2. Nursing health history
   a. Review a completed nursing health history form found in a client's medical record or in your text.
   b. Analyze the client's health history using these guidelines.
      (1) Is each of the basic components for a nursing health history included in the health history form or tool?
      (2) What other data, if any, are present that are not identified in the basic components described in your text? Is this additional information important? Why or why not?
      (3) What sources were consulted while obtaining the needed data?
      (4) Identify data present in the health history as objective or subjective.
   c. Design your own health history form using available examples.
3. Nursing interview
   a. Observe a peer, nurse, or faculty member conducting a nursing interview (or view a videotaped interview).
   b. Analyze the interview using these guidelines.
      (1) Were the objectives of the nursing interview met?
      (2) Did you observe the three phrases of the interview? Describe their effectiveness.
      (3) What types of interview techniques were used?
      (4) What communication strategies were employed.
   c. Formulate alternative interview techniques and communication strategies to improve the nursing interview.
4. Laboratory data
   a. Review the medical record of a client.
   b. From the list presented in your text (p. 162), search for common laboratory and diagnostic tests that appear in the record.
   c. Identify the institutional norms for the data. Determine whether the client has any abnormal laboratory or diagnostic test results.
5. Clinical situation: client assessment
   Mary Anne Robinson, 29 years old, is admitted to the hospital with severe abdominal pain. She is alert, oriented, and able to describe her signs and symptoms. Mrs. Robinson's husband and mother have accompanied her to the hospital.
   a. List five sources of data collection about Mrs. Robinson.
   b. Formulate one or two sentences you might use while obtaining the nursing health history that reflect the nature of each of the three phases of an interview (orientation, working, and termination).
   c. Formulate at least four questions you would ask Mrs. Robinson about her abdominal pain.
   d. Is the information obtained from Mrs. Robinson considered objective or subjective data? Why?

SKILL AND TECHNIQUE ACTIVITIES

1. Interviewing technique
   a. Interview an individual (peer, family member, or client) about a topic of your choice.
   b. With the individual's permission, record the interview on videotape or audiotape. (If recording is not possible, write out the conversation as you recall it.)
   c. Analyze the interview, including type of technique, phases of the interview, and communication strategies.
   d. Formulate alternative techniques or strategies that you might have used in the interview.
   e. Submit your analysis to your instructor for feedback.
2. Nursing health history
   a. Obtain a nursing health history form (the one provided in your text or one currently being used in your institution).
   b. Elicit a nursing health history from a peer, friend, or family member.
   c. If feasible, record the interview on audiotape or videotape. (If recording is not possible, ask another peer to observe the interview and critique your performance.)
   d. Record the data obtained in the interview on the health history form.
   e. Analyze your technique and skills, including phases of the interview and communication strategies.
   f. Submit the health history form and interview analysis to your instructor for feedback.

ADDITIONAL READINGS

Bermost LS: Interviewing: a key to therapeutic communication in nursing practice, *Nurs Clin North Am* 1:205, 1966.
   Discusses principles of interviewing clients. Includes examples to clarify major points. Briefly analyzes examples of nurse-client interaction, enabling the learner to gain further insight into techniques.
Guzzetta C et al: *Clinical assessment tools for use with nursing diagnosis systems,* St Louis, 1989, Mosby–Year Book.
   A collection of focused assessment tools addressing specific age groups, body systems dysfunction, disease states, and rehabilitation.
Hickey PW: *Nursing process handbook,* St Louis, 1990, Mosby–Year Book.

Explains the nursing process in a clear, concise manner. Information is presented from the NANDA perspective. Appendices feature systems and head-to-toe assessment guides. A glossary of terms and index make this a particularly useful resource for students.

Malasanos L et al: *Health assessment,* ed 4, St Louis, 1989, Mosby–Year Book.

A comprehensive reference addressing the theoretical concepts and techniques needed to elicit a health history and perform a physical examination. Liberally illustrated to assist the student in understanding techniques of physical assessment. Discusses normal findings and describes abnormal conditions. Includes adults and pediatric assessment.

Norris L: Coaching the questions, *Nurs 86* 16(5):100, 1986.

Outlines 10 simple steps for assisting clients in obtaining information from health care providers about their health status and care plan.

Chapter 7
Nursing Diagnosis

PREREQUISITE READING
Chapter 7, pp. 168 to 185

OBJECTIVES
Mastery of content in this chapter will enable the student to:
- Define selected terms related to nursing diagnoses.
- Describe how defining characteristics and the etiological process individualize a nursing diagnosis.
- List and discuss the steps of the nursing diagnostic process.
- Demonstrate the nursing diagnostic process.
- Differentiate between a nursing diagnosis and a medical diagnosis.
- Explain what makes a nursing diagnosis correct.
- Discuss the advantages of nursing diagnoses for the client and the nursing profession.
- Discuss the limitations of nursing diagnoses.
- Formulate nursing diagnoses from a nursing assessment.

REVIEW OF KEY CONCEPTS
1. What is a nursing diagnosis?
2. Identify and briefly describe the two components of a nursing diagnosis.
3. Which component of the nursing diagnostic statement assists in individualization of the diagnosis and gives direction for planning client care?
4. Compare characteristics of medical and nursing diagnoses in each of the following areas:

	Medical Diagnosis	Nursing Diagnosis
Nature of diagnosis		
Goal		
Objective		

5. List the three steps of the nursing diagnostic process in the appropriate sequence.

   a.

   b.

   c.

6. Define defining characteristics.

7. The presence of one sign or symptom is adequate support for a nursing diagnostic label. (True or false?)
8. It is acceptable to use the medical diagnosis as the etiology of the nursing diagnosis. (True or false?)
9. List three advantages of nursing diagnoses.

   a.

   b.

   c.

10. List two limitations of nursing diagnoses.

   a.

   b.

11. Mrs. French is a 45-year-old mother of two who is 50 pounds overweight. She has a smoking history of two packs per day for 20 years. She is to have a hysterectomy tomorrow. Which nursing diagnosis should appear on Mrs. French's nursing care plan?
   a. Social isolation
   b. Potential uterine cancer
   c. Risk for ineffective airway clearance related to obesity and smoking
   d. Altered urinary elimination related to incisional pain
12. Mr. Margauz, a 52-year-old business executive, is admitted to the coronary care unit. During his admission interview he denies chest pain or shortness of breath. His pulse and blood pressure are normal. He appears tense and does not want the nurse to leave the bedside. When questioned, he states that he is very nervous. At this moment, which nursing diagnosis is most appropriate?
   a. Alteration in comfort, chest pain
   b. Alteration in bowel elimination related to restricted mobility
   c. High risk for altered cardiac output related to heart attack
   d. Anxiety related to intensive care unit admission
13. If a nurse were to record a client's nursing diagnosis as *high risk for malnutrition*, it would be incorrect because it is:
   a. stated as a medical diagnosis.
   b. stated as a nursing intervention.

c. an error of omission.

d. an error of commission.

14. If a nurse were to record a client's nursing diagnosis as *encourage client to verbalize fear,* it would be incorrect because it is:

a. stated as a medical diagnosis.

b. stated as a nursing intervention.

c. an error of omission.

d. an error of commission.

CRITICAL THINKING AND EXPERIENTIAL EXERCISES

1. Efficacy of nursing diagnoses in client care
   a. Divide a small group of peers into two groups (pro and con) to debate the use of nursing diagnoses in providing client care and advancing the profession.

2. NANDA classification system
   a. Visit your nursing library and find a text that addresses the topic of nursing diagnoses utilizing the NANDA classification system. Select one nursing diagnosis.
   b. Find the defining characteristics for that diagnosis.
   c. Find common etiologies for the diagnosis.
   d. Discuss how nursing care might be different for individuals with the same diagnosis but with different etiologies.
   e. Share your conclusions with your instructor.

3. Nursing diagnoses versus medical diagnosis: defining characteristics
   a. Review the medical record of a client in your institution. Identify the nursing diagnoses for your client.
   b. Identify the medical diagnoses for your client.
   c. Discuss the differences between these diagnoses.
   d. Select one of the nursing diagnoses.
      (1) List all the data present in the medical record supporting this diagnosis.
      (2) Identify the etiology of the nursing diagnosis.
      (3) Compare the data with the defining characteristics and etiologies as outlined in the NANDA classification system.

4. Formulating nursing diagnoses
   a. Obtain a nursing health history from a peer or a client (or review a completed nursing health history provided by your instructor).
   b. Validate the data utilizing other pertinent sources.
   c. Cluster the data.
   d. Identify general health care needs.
   e. Formulate nursing diagnoses.
   f. Submit your work to your instructor for feedback.

5. Clinical situation: Nursing diagnoses
   a. Working independently or in a small peer group, implement the steps of the diagnostic process (analysis and interpretation, identification of problems, and formulation of nursing diagnosis) with the case studies provided. Present infor-

mation in each section to your instructor for feedback.

Situation A: Jennifer Shampeon is a 16-year-old high school student who has experienced intermittent nausea and vomiting over the past 2 weeks. She has been admitted for diagnostic studies to determine the source of her physical problem.

During the nursing interview, Jennifer states that she hasn't had an appetite for the last 2 weeks and has eaten only toast or crackers with jelly, soda, gelatin, and tea. She tells the nurse that she is worried about what is wrong, feels "tense" and"jittery" most of the time, and has difficulty getting to sleep at night.

Jennifer's mother tells the nurse that her daughter "is just bored and sleeps only 3 to 4 hours each night because she doesn't do anything all day long." Jennifer responds that she is bored and misses her friends, classes, and social activities. She says the only thing to do at home and in the hospital is to "watch the soaps."

During the initial part of the physical examination, the following information is obtained:

Height: 5 feet, 2 inches
Current weight: 86 pounds
Normal weight: 92 pounds
Vital signs
  Temperature: 37°C (98.6° F)
  Pulse 80 beats per minute
  Respirations: 16 breaths per minute
  Blood pressure: 100/60 mm Hg
Pale skin color
Restless, frequently changing position in bed
Hands tremble when picking up water glass or peforming other self-care activities
Vomited 200 ml of greenish-colored emesis during the admission interview

Situation B: Mrs. Anderson, a 32-year-old single parent of two preschoolers, has been admitted to the hospital after a motor vehicle accident.

Mrs. Anderson sustained a fractured right arm, multiple cuts and bruises to her face, and a whiplash injury to her neck. Surgery was required to repair the right arm fracture. She returned from the operating room with a cast on her injured arm from above her elbow to her fingertips. She must also wear a cervical collar around her neck to help reduce muscle spasm.

Mrs. Anderson is right-handed. She is employed as a secretary. She states, "I don't know how I'm going to look after my children with this cast on my arm and my neck hurting so much. Right now my friend is looking after them, but she and her husband are leaving for Hawaii in 2 days. Also, I'm not sure what will happen with my job. I won't be able to type for at least 2 months. What if my boss lays me off! Look, I can't even cut the meat on my plate, so how can I help my kids?"

ADDITIONAL READINGS

Carpenito LJ: *Nursing diagnoses: application to clinical practice,* ed 4, Philadelphia, 1992, Lippincott.
   A comprehensive text for students and experienced practitioners. Overviews the development of nursing diagnosis

and its role in the nursing process. Includes an analysis of each currently accepted diagnostic category in terms of definition, defining characteristics, contributing and risk factors, assessment criteria, principles and rationale for nursing care interventions, and outcome criteria. Includes NANDA and other useful clinical diagnoses. Introduces a manual for collaborative problems. Excellent appendixes including age-specific assessment guides, pain-relief and stress-management techniques, crisis intervention, and play therapy.

Edel MK: Noncompliance: an appropriate nursing diagnosis? *Nurs Outlook* 33:183, 1985.

Discusses the concept of compliance and factors influencing compliant behavior. Proposes elimination of *noncompliance* as a nursing diagnosis and direct interventions toward the cause of the behavior, thus more appropriately meeting the client's real need. Upholds the client's need for independent decision making, informed choice, and responsibility for personal behaviors.

Gebbie KM, Lavin MA: Classifying nursing diagnoses, *Am J Nurs* 74:250, 1974.

Describes the original work of Gebbie and Lavin associated with the First National Conference on Classification of Nursing Diagnoses. Briefly discusses the proceedings and the development of the current classification system.

Iyer PW, Taptich BJ, Bernocchi-Losey D: *Nursing process and nursing diagnoses*, Philadelphia, 1986, Saunders.

Comprehensive text emphasizing the diagnostic phase of the nursing process. Straight forward approach to the care planning process. Includes multiple examples, self-test, and sample case studies to enhance understanding of concepts presented.

Leininger M: Issues, questions, and concerns related to the nursing diagnosis cultural movement from a transcultural nursing perspective, *J Transcultural Nurs* 2(1):23, 1990.

Discussion of the NANDA taxonomy from a transcultural perspective. Suggests that NANDA's wide application of diagnoses creates problems, ethical concerns, and critical questions regarding care of subcultures and minorities. Proposes that the taxonomy falls short of the ultimate goal of transcultural nursing: provision of culturally congruent, meaningful care.

Martens K: Let's diagnose strengths, not just problems, *Am J Nurs* 86:192, 1986.

Proposes that nurses direct care toward maintaining health through reinforcement of wellness behaviors. Supports use of diagnostic statements of strengths to provide the nurse with a more accurate picture of the client and enhance the quality and continuity of care. Includes methodology for formulation of diagnostic statements of client strengths.

Nettle C et al: Community nursing diagnosis, *J Community Health* 6(3):135, 1989.

Presents a tool developed for student use in community settings. Adapts Gordon's Health Problems (universal assessment structure) to the community as client.

Chapter 8
Planning

PREREQUISITE READING
Chapter 8, pp. 186 to 203

OBJECTIVES
Mastery of content in this chapter will enable the student to:
- Define selected terms related to the planning phase of the nursing process.
- Discuss the process of priority setting.
- Describe goal setting.
- List the seven guidelines for a written outcome statement.
- Discuss the difference between a goal and an expected outcome.
- Discuss the process of selecting nursing interventions.
- Define the three types of interventions.
- Discuss the differences among dependent, independent, and interdependent interventions.
- List the purposes of the nursing care plan.
- Describe the differences between care plans used in hospitals and those used in community health settings.
- Develop a care plan from a nursing assessment.
- List the six steps involved in consultation.
- Discuss the consultation process.

REVIEW OF KEY CONCEPTS
1. List the four activities involved in the planning process.

   a.

   b.

   c.

   d.

2. Mrs. Marks is a 50-year-old homemaker who had a cholecystectomy (removal of the gallbladder) 2 days ago. She complains of severe incision pain that interferes with her ability to ambulate, cough, and breathe deeply. She is extremely fearful and says that her best friend died after gallbladder surgery. Her nursing history reveals a 30 year history of smoking, chronic obstructive pulmonary disease (COPD), and obesity. She is the primary care giver for her 15-year-old mentally retarded son. Her husband, a businessman, travels frequently. According to Mrs. Marks, her husband has very little time for their son. Based on the information provided, prioritize Mrs. Marks' formulated nursing diagnoses as high (1), intermediate (2), or low (3).

   a. Altered nutrition: more than body requirements related to intake greater than metabolic need

   _____

   b. Pain (acute) related to abdominal incision

   _____

   c. High risk for infection related to invasive procedures (surgery or intravenous therapy), smoking, and COPD _____

   d. Ineffective family coping: compromised, related to adolescent mentally retarded son

   _____

   e. Fear related to perceived threat of death associated with surgical procedure _____

   f. Ineffective airway clearance related to pain, history of smoking, COPD, and obesity

   _____

3. Define goals of nursing care.
4. Identify the two purposes of writing client-centered goals.

   a.

   b.

5. Under what circumstance would the nurse or nursing team independently develop client-centered goals?
   a. when directed to do so by the physician
   b. when the hospital uses standardized care plans
   c. if the client is unable to participate in goal setting
   d. if the client is unable to read or write
6. Well-formulated, client-centered goals should:
   a. meet immediate client needs.
   b. include preventive health care.
   c. include rehabilitative needs.
   d. all of the above.
7. Describe the difference between short-term and long-term goals.
8. Define expected outcomes.

9. List three purposes for formulating expected outcomes.

a.

b.

c.

10. Describe the seven guidelines for writing goals and expected outcomes.

a.

b.

c.

d.

e.

f.

g.

11. The following statement appears on the nursing care plan for an immunosuppressed client: the client will remain free from infection throughout hospitalization. This statement is an example of a (an):
a. nursing diagnosis.
b. short-term goal.
c. long-term goal.
d. expected outcome.

12. The following statements appear on a nursing care plan for a client after a mastectomy: incision site approximated, absence of drainage or prolonged erythema at incision site, and client remains afebrile. These statements are examples of:
a. nursing interventions.
b. short-term goals.
c. long-term goals.
d. expected outcomes.

13. The following statement appears on a nursing care plan for a client who experienced a stroke with complete left-sided paralysis: client performs self-care activities independently. This statement is an example of a (an):
a. nursing diagnosis.
b. short-term goal.
c. long-term goal.
d. expected outcome.

14. An example of an independent nursing intervention is:
a. administering a prescribed pain medication.
b. administering a laxative according to a protocol.
c. turning a client every 2 hours to prevent skin breakdown.
d. ambulating a client according to a therapist's recommendation.

15. An example of a dependent nursing intervention is:
a. administering oral hygiene to a disabled client.
b. contacting a psychiatric nurse specialist about a depressed client.
c. teaching a client about relaxation techniques.
d. giving an enema to a client before x-ray studies.

16. An example of an interdependent nursing intervention is:
a. following admission protocol during an initial client interview.
b. assessing a client for side effects of medications.
c. administering a prescribed laxative.
d. providing counseling to a client having difficulty adjusting to an unplanned pregnancy.

17. Dependent interventions should automatically be implemented as prescribed. (True or false?)

18. Describe the three steps for selecting nursing interventions.

a.

b.

c.

19. List four purposes of a nursing care plan.

a.

b.

c.

d.

20. Briefly describe the differences among the following types of care plans:
a. Institutional
b. Standardized
c. Student

21. A scientific rationale is:
a. a projected outcome for client care derived from supporting literature.
b. the reason, based on supporting literature, a specific nursing action should be taken.
c. the reason a nursing diagnosis poses a risk to the client.
d. a scientific reason nursing care is required by the client.

22. What four questions evaluate whether nursing interventions are stated appropriately?

a.

b.

c.

d.

23. Which nursing intervention is correctly stated?
a. Ambulate client once each shift.
b. Nurse will provide oral hygiene 30 minutes before meals.
c. Nurse will observe client cough and deep breathe every 2 hours (even hours).
d. Client will request pain medication before daily physical therapy session.

24. Under what two circumstances would a nurse initiate a consultation?

a.

b.

25. List the six responsibilities of the nurse when seeking consultation.

a.

b.

c.

d.

e.

f.

CRITICAL THINKING AND EXPERIENTIAL EXERCISES

1. Review of nursing care plans
   a. Review the nursing care plan for a selected client in any health care setting. Is the plan an institutional, standardized, or student care plan?
   b. What components of the nursing process are included in the care plan?
   c. Are the goals, expected outcomes, and nursing interventions correctly stated?
   d. Are the goals, expected outcomes, and nursing interventions appropriate to the identified nursing diagnosis?
   e. How are the care plans used in the health care setting?
   f. If other care plans are available, compare characteristics of the plans used for clients in different health care settings: hospitals, clinics, and home health.
   g. If other care plans are available, compare characteristics of care plans used for a client during hospitalization and in preparation for discharge.

2. Designing a nursing care plan
   a. Develop a nursing care plan, based on a nursing history for an assigned (or simulated) client. Unless directed otherwise, include in your care plan two nursing diagnoses, one goal for each diagnosis, at least two expected outcomes for each goal, and at least two interventions (with rationales) for each goal. (Keep in mind that this is a practice exercise. In any care planning situation, the number of diagnoses, goals, expected outcomes, and interventions will be specific to the client's needs.)
   b. Discuss your care plan with a peer to determine whether your plan is clearly stated and replicable without additional information. Make any necessary revisions.
   c. Submit the care plan to your instructor for feedback.

3. Nurse practice acts and independent functions
   a. Review the nurse practice act for your state or province.
   b. Identify nursing activities described as independent interventions.
   c. Describe how the practice act shapes your client care.

4. Consultation
   a. Identify nursing specialists and other health team members in your health care setting who are available for consultation in client care.
   b. Determine the appropriate method for obtaining consultation.
   c. Explore the role of the primary nurse (student nurse) in the consultation process.
   d. Care for, or review the nursing assessment of, a client. Identify the areas in which consultation could benefit client care. List individuals available for consultation. With your instructor's assistance, initiate the consultation process.

5. Clinical situation: consultation
   Mr. Laine is a 29-year-old single parent. His only son, Jimmy, 9 years old, was diagnosed with insulin-dependent diabetes mellitus 8 months ago. The medical treatment for Jimmy includes a diabetic diet and insulin injections. During the last 6 months, Jimmy has been hospitalized three times because his diabetes was out of control. Jimmy refuses to adhere to his diet because he can't eat what his friends eat. Mr. Laine states that "Jimmy's diet isn't *that* important" and wants the physician to increase Jimmy's insulin dose to control his disease.
   a. Identify two problems that may require Jimmy's primary nurse to seek consultation.
   b. Assuming that the following consultants are available, select those most appropriate for Jimmy's needs.
      (1) Medical-surgical clinical nurse specialist
      (2) Psychiatric clinical nurse specialist
      (3) Social worker
      (4) Diabetes educator
      (5) Pediatric nurse practitioner
      (6) Nutritionist (dietitian)
   c. List three pieces of pertinent information the nurse should provide to the consultant.

ADDITIONAL READINGS

Please refer to readings cited in Chapters 6 and 7 that include sources for the care planning process. References previously cited are not included here.

Carpenito LJ: *Nursing care plans and documentation*, Philadephia, 1991, Lippincott.
   Overviews documentation of care, care planning systems, responses of the hospitalized adult, and the surgical experience. Details care plans for specific medical disorders, surgical interventions, and diagnostic and therapeutic procedures. Includes plans for collaborative problems and problems unique to nursing practice.

Ulrich SP, Canale SW, Wendell AS: *Nursing care planning guides: a nursing diagnosis approach*, ed 2, Philadelphia, 1990, Saunders.
   A comprehensive guide for the development of nursing care plans. Provides standardized care plans for medical-surgical conditions. Includes guidelines for individualizing plans for each client.

Chapter 9
Implementation

PREREQUISITE READING
Chapter 9, pp. 204 to 217

OBJECTIVES
Mastery of content in this chapter will enable the student to:
- Define selected terms related to the implementation phase of the nursing process.
- Discuss the differences between protocols and standing orders.
- Describe the information-processing model for selecting nursing interventions.
- List and discuss the five steps of the implementation process.
- Describe five different implementation methods.
- Select appropriate implementation methods for an assigned client.

REVIEW OF KEY CONCEPTS
1. Implementation is a continuous activity performed throughout the nursing process. (True or false?)
2. Written documents containing rules, procedures, and orders for client care in a specific clinical setting are

   _____ .

3. A written plan specifying procedures to be followed during the assessment or treatment of a client is

   called a _____ .
4. A nurse performing a dependent intervention ordered by the physician is not responsible for any complications that might occur. (True or false?)
5. Identify the sequence of activities when using the information-processing model for determining nursing interventions.

   a.

   b.

   c.

   d.
6. List and briefly describe the five steps of the nursing implementation process.

   a.

   b.

   c.

   d.

   e.
7. List three areas from which the nurse can seek assistance when implementing the nursing care plan.

   a.

   b.

   c.
8. Describe five different methods for implementing nursing interventions.

   a.

   b.

   c.

   d.

   e.
9. When delegating a client's care to another staff member, the nurse is responsible for ensuring that the interventions were completed correctly. (True or false?)

CRITICAL THINKING AND EXPERIENTIAL EXERCISES
1. Nursing interventions
   a. Review or design a nursing care plan for a selected client or observe a nurse caring for a client in any health care setting.
   b. Identify and describe at least three nursing actions for each type of nursing intervention: dependent, independent, and interdependent.
   c. Compare your findings to those of your peers.
   d. Discuss your findings with your instructor.
2. Methods of implementation
   a. Review or design a nursing care plan for a selected client or observe a nurse caring for a client in any health care setting.
   b. Identify and describe at least one example of each of the five methods for implementing nursing care.
   c. Compare your findings to those of your peers.
   d. Discuss your findings with your instructor.
3. Implementation process
   a. Design a nursing care plan for a selected client.

b. Perform the five steps of the implementation phase of the nursing process.

c. Describe and evaluate your activities for each of the five implementation steps; for example, what actions did you take, what worked well, what didn't work well, and how would you modify your activities in the future?

d. Discuss your activities and self-evaluation with your instructor.

4. Communication of nursing implementation

a. Review your institution's protocol for communicating nursing implementation in the nursing care plan and medical record.

b. Observe ways in which nurses communicate information about client care.

c. Based on an actual (or simulated) client situation, practice verbal and written communication about nursing implementation in a small peer group.

d. Provide an opportunity for critique of your written and verbal communication by your instructor.

5. Protocols and standing orders

a. Examine your institution's policies on protocols and standing orders.

b. Obtain a copy of a protocol and standing order for a specific client care setting. Compare these two documents. What do they describe? How are they similar? How are they different? What responsibility or authority is given to the nurse? Discuss your conclusions with your instructor.

c. Discuss protocols and standing orders with a staff nurse in a specific client care setting. What common protocols and standing orders are used? What are the advantages and disadvantages of protocols and standing orders in this nurse's practice? Share your findings with your peers and instructor.

d. Discuss with your instructor or nursing manager the specific responsibilities of nursing students in relation to institutional protocols and standing orders.

ADDITIONAL READINGS

Please refer to readings cited in Chapters 6, 7, and 8 that include sources for the care planning process. References previously cited are not included here.

Bulechek G, McCloskey J, editors: Nursing interventions, *Nurs Clin North Am* 27:2, 1992.

Describes work in the classification of nursing interventions intended to parallel the NANDA taxonomy of nursing diagnoses. Includes labels, definitions, and practice activities associated with interventions for specific categories of clients.

Marriner A: *The nursing process: a scientific approach to nursing care,* ed 4, St Louis, 1987, Mosby–Year Book.

A thorough discussion of the nursing process. Presents various concepts related to the components of the nursing process. Includes practical examples to enhance application of the nursing process.

Chapter 10
Evaluation

PREREQUISITE READING

Chapter 10, pp. 218 to 231

OBJECTIVES

Mastery of content in this chapter will enable the student to:

- Define key terms related to the evaluation phase of the nursing process.
- Explain the relationship between expected outcomes and goals of care.
- Describe the interaction of the components of the nursing process.
- Give examples of evaluation measures used to determine progress toward outcomes.
- Evaluate nursing actions selected for a client.
- Explain the differences and similarities between quality assurance and quality improvement.
- Give examples of the 10 steps to quality improvement.

REVIEW OF KEY CONCEPTS

1. Describe evaluation in the context of the nursing process.
2. The evaluation component of the nursing process is oriented toward the client receiving care and the providers of that care. (True or false?)
3. The criteria for determining the effectiveness of nursing action are based on:
   a. nursing diagnosis.
   b. expected outcomes.
   c. client satisfaction.
   d. nursing interventions.
4. Describe the steps for the objective evaluation of client goal achievement.

   a.

   b.

   c.

   d.
5. The primary source of data for evaluation is the:
   a. physician.
   b. client.
   c. nurse.
   d. medical record.

6. Explain the difference between expected outcomes and goals of care.
7. When a client-centered goal has not been met in the projected time frame, the most appropriate action by the nurse would be to:
   a. repeat the entire sequence of the nursing process to discover needed changes.
   b. conclude that the goal was in appropriate or unrealistic and eliminate it from the plan.
   c. continue with the same plan until the goal is met.
   d. rewrite the plan using different interventions.
8. Define quality assurance.
9. Quality improvement:
   a. focuses on the process of care.
   b. focuses on problems.
   c. separates analysis of effectiveness and efficacy.
   d. focuses on outcomes of care and continuous development.
10. Match each of the examples with the most representative component of the quality improvement program.

Examples

a. Nurses establish that 95% of their clients should be able to accurately take their own pulse. _____

b. Nurses compare the percentage of clients who can accurately take their own pulse to the established threshold of 95%. _____

c. Nurses working on a specific division make decisions about practice and monitor the quality of care administered. _____

d. The staff meet to share the outcomes of their quality-improvement process, identifying interventions that improved clients' abilities to take their own pulses. _____

e. A nursing unit admits adults with cardiac diseases. _____

f. Because only 85% of the clients assessed could accurately take their own pulse and all the successful clients were under the age of 60, nurses meet to identify alternative teaching approaches for older adults. _____

g. Nurses determine that effective education includes the clients' abilities to accurately take their own pulses. _____

h. Nurses remonitor the quality indicators. _____

i. Nurses identify three major activities that are central to nursing care for cardiac clients: client education, cardiac monitoring, and cardiac rehabilitation. _____

j. Nurses assess clients using the designated structure, process, or outcome indicators. _____

Compenent

1. Responsibility for the QI program
2. Scope of service
3. Key aspects of service
4. Developing quality indicators
5. Establishing thresholds for evaluation
6. Data collection and analysis
7. Evaluation of care
8. Resolution of problems
9. Evaluation of improvement
10. Communication of results

CRITICAL THINKING AND EXPERIENTIAL EXERCISES

1. Quality improvement
   a. Meet with a nursing manager to discuss the health care facility's quality improvement program. What are the components of the quality improvement program and how do they compare with the JCAHO's 10 steps for quality improvement?
   b. Interview a nurse providing direct client care. What quality improvement program is being implemented in the client care area? How do the nurses participate in the program? In what way(s) has the program influenced the delivery of care and client outcomes?
2. Evaluating client care
   a. Design and implement a nursing care plan for an assigned client.
   b. Compare the client's response to the expected outcomes.
   c. Analyze the reasons for the client's ability to meet or not meet the desired outcomes and goals. (For example: Was the assessment accurate and inclusive? Was the nursing diagnosis accurate? Were the goals realistic? Were the outcomes appropriate? Were the interventions performed correctly? Were the interventions appropriate and inclusive enough to assist the client in goal achievement?)

   d. Modify the care plan, providing rationale for your changes.
   e. Submit your work to your instructor for feedback.
3. Clinical situation: expected outcomes
   a. Using the following case study, develop nursing diagnoses, goals, and evaluation criteria (expected outcomes) you would use to measure Mr. Reynolds' response to nursing care and his progress toward achieving his health care goals. Submit your written work to your instructor for feedback.

Mr. Reynolds, a 48-year-old business executive, was admitted with a medical diagnosis of a myocardial infarction (heart attack). He is 6 feet (182.8 cm) tall and weighs 230 pounds (104.33 kg). His lifestyle is sedentary. He is recently divorced.

Mr. Reynolds smokes two packs of cigarettes per day and has one or two cocktails every night, usually more on weekends. He has been in the intensive care unit for five days and has just been transferred to a cardiac rehabilitation unit in preparation for discharge. He has no complaints of pain after being transferred but tells the nurse, "I'm dying for a cigarette." His physician has ordered a low-calorie, low-salt, reducing diet; smoking cessation; and a progressive aerobic exercise program. Mr. Reynolds angrily demands a telephone in his room because he is behind at work and has deadlines to meet. He also wants to talk to his teenage son about his recent decision to drop out of high school.

ADDITIONAL READINGS

Anderson PA, Davis SE: Nursing peer review: a developmental process, *Nurs Management* 18(1):46,1987.
> Describes a process-focused peer review model developed and implemented as part of a quality assurance program at a Midwest Veterans Administration hospital.

Beyers M, editor: Quality assurance, *Nurs Clin North Am* 23(3):617, 1988.
> A collection of articles addressing quality assurance in provision of nursing care. Includes discussion of JCAHO focus on nursing quality, institutional standards, program design, individual nursing performance, and monitoring methods.

Davis-Martin S: Outcome and accountability: getting into the consumer dimension, *Nurs Management* 17(10):25, 1986.
> Describes the increasing need for consumer satisfaction with health care delivery systems. Emphasizes that sensitivity to client's satisfaction is important to professional development. Presents a consumer tool used for nursing student evaluation and proposes similar tool development for utilization by staff nurses and nurse managers.

Mitty EL, editor: *Quality imperatives in long term care: the elusive agenda*, New York, 1992, National League for Nursing Press.
> Proceedings of the eighth National League for Nursing Invitational Long-Term Care Conference. Includes articles by experts from education, service, and provider organizations addressing quality in long-term care.

Chapter 11
Research

PREREQUISITE READING
Chapter 11, pp. 234 to 253

OBJECTIVES
Mastery of content in this chapter will enable the student to:
- Define selected terms related to nursing research.
- Compare the various ways to acquire knowledge.
- List the characteristics of scientific investigation.
- Compare methods for developing new nursing knowledge.
- Define scientific and nursing research.
- Compare the research process with the nursing process.
- List ANA's priorities for nursing research.
- Explain the rights of human research subjects.
- Explain the rights of other persons who assist in human research studies.
- Describe a typical research report.
- Discuss methods of locating research reports in nursing and related areas.
- Explain how to organize information from a research report.
- List the characteristics of a clinical nursing problem that can be researched.
- List the criteria for using research findings in nursing practice.

REVIEW OF KEY CONCEPTS
1. Match the examples provided with the method of knowledge acquisition.

Examples

a. For the last 3 years the nurse has used povidone-iodine (Betadine) to clean intravenous dressing sites. This technique seems to control infection. _____

b. The nursing staff is uncertain about the type of surface most effective in preventing bedsores in postoperative clients. They call a nurse specialist for advice. _____

c. Mrs. Theros has worked in critical care for 5 years. She believes her suctioning technique is most effective. _____

d. A nursing manager is concerned about controlling discomfort associated with long-term nasogastric tube placement. The manager and a clinical specialist plan to study the effects of applying cold compresses to the necks of clients with tubes inserted for more than 24 hours. _____

e. The nurse is frustrated while caring for Mr. Wilm's bedsore. It does not seem to be healing. One day, the physician orders heat lamp treatments. Two days later the nurses use povidone-iodine (Betadine) to clean the bedsore. Of all the treatments, thorough cleansing and keeping the client off the sore seem to work best. _____

Method
1. Trial and error
2. Tradition
3. Experience
4. Scientific method
5. Consulting experts

2. List the five characteristics of scientific investigation.

a.

b.

c.

d.

e.

3. Define scientific research.

4. Define nursing research.

5. Biomedical research focuses on:
   a. how clients and families cope with health problems.
   b. the psychological implications of health and illness.
   c. the study of health promotion behaviors.
   d. the causes and treatments of disease.

6. Match the type of research with the most accurate description.

Type of research

a. Historical _____

b. Exploratory _____

c. Evaluation _____

d. Descriptive _____

e. Experimental _____

f. Quasi-experimental _____

g. Correlational _____

Description

1. Researcher controls independent variables, but subjects cannot be randomly assigned to treatment conditions.
2. Tests how well a program, practice, or policy is working.
3. Explores interrelationships among variables of interest without any active intervention by the researcher.
4. Systematic collection and critical evaluation of data relating to past events.
5. Investigator controls independent variable and randomly assigns subjects to different conditions.
6. Purpose is to identify characteristics of persons, situations, or groups and the frequency with which certain events or characteristics occur.
7. Study designed to develop or refine research questions or to test and refine data collection methods.

7. In an experimental study:
   a. subjects are randomly assigned to the experimental and control groups.
   b. the control group receives the therapy being studied.
   c. conditions affecting the subjects are left uncontrolled to allow generalization of findings.
   d. clients most likely to perform the best are assigned to the experimental group.
8. Explain the difference between qualitative and quantitative research.
9. Match the component of the nursing process with the correlative activity of nursing research.

Component

a. Assessment _____

b. Diagnosis _____

c. Planning _____

d. Implementation _____

e. Evaluation _____

Activity

1. Nurse publishes results of a research study for use by other nurses.
2. Nurse uses a new treatment method on an experimental group and records the results.
3. Nurse identifies the anticipated response of clients to the experimental treatment.
4. Nurse identifies the factors to be measured in determining effects of new treatment.

5. Nurse determines the type of statistical tests that will be used to measure results of study.

10. The purpose of the ANA's priorities for nursing research is:
    a. to review nurse researchers' ethical standards.
    b. to identify areas of nursing practice needing further knowledge to improve client care.
    c. to assess the quality of nursing research proposals.
    d. to identify the educational preparation required of nurse researchers.

11. List at least 5 of the 11 ANA priorities for nursing research.

    a.

    b.

    c.

    d.

    e.

12. The researcher's refusal to disclose the name of subjects is:
    a. confidentiality.
    b. anonymity.
    c. informed consent.
    d. protection of clients.

13. Any nurse has the right to refuse to carry out any research procedure about which the nurse has ethical concerns. (True or false?)

14. The purpose of an institutional review board is to:
    a. ensure that federal funds are equitably appropriated.
    b. conduct research benefiting the public.
    c. determine the risk status of clients in research projects.
    d. ensure that ethical principles are observed in human-subject research.

15. Research studies can most easily be identified by:
    a. looking for the word "research" in the title of the report.
    b. looking for the study only in research journals.
    c. examining the contents of the report.
    d. reading the abstract and conclusion of the report.

16. Which statement concerning research reports is accurate?
    a. Nursing textbooks are primary sources of information.
    b. Primary sources are those written by one of the researchers in the study.
    c. The fact that a report is a primary source guarantees its accuracy.
    d. Secondary sources are the best source of information about the research study.

17. To find articles on a particular subject, the nurse first checks:
    a. the citation list at the end of the article.
    b. through pages of other, related journals.
    c. other articles written by the same authors.
    d. the subject headings in a cumulative index.

18. A computerized search for research articles is obtained through:
   a. MEDLINE.
   b. *Cumulative Index to Nursing*.
   c. *Index Medicus*.
   d. *Annual Review of Nursing Research*.

19. A research report includes all of the following except:
   a. a summary of literature used to identify the research problem.
   b. the researcher's interpretation of the study results.
   c. a summary of other research studies with the same results.
   d. a description of methods used to conduct the study.

20. List at least three characteristics of a clinical nursing problem with the potential to be researched.

   a.

   b.

   c.

21. List four criteria used to determine whether research findings should be applied to nursing practice.

   a.

   b.

   c.

   d.

22. Explain the meaning of the following statement and its relevance to nursing practice: "Some people estimate that the half-life of knowledge in the health care field is 5 years."

CRITICAL THINKING AND EXPERIENTIAL EXERCISES

1. Clinical nursing problems
   a. Working independently or with a small peer group, formulate a list of clinical nursing problems you would be interested in studying.
   b. Develop relevant research questions about each problem.
   c. Share this information with your instructor.

2. Organizing information from a research study
   a. Select a topic of interest related to clinical nursing practice.
   b. Using the *Cumulative Index to Nursing and Allied Health Literature (CINAHL)* or another appropriate cumulative index, select a research article (primary source article) from the nursing journal of your choice.
   c. Locate the article in your nursing library.
   d. Read the article.
   e. Write an index card for the article using the sample on p. 245 of your textbook.

3. Application of research findings
   a. Review a primary source research article addressing a clinical nursing problem.

   b. Identify whether the research report includes all the pertinent sections and components of a typical research report (based on information presented in your text).
   c. Analyze the applicability of the research findings to clinical practice based on the criteria described in Question 21.

4. Nurse researchers
   a. Interview a nurse who is researching a clinical problem to discuss the activities, rewards, and frustrations encountered in the research process.

5. Clinical situation: rights of human subjects
   Robert Maury, a nursing student, finds the physician explaining an experimental drug study to a client. The client appears anxious, and his questions suggest that he is confused about the study. When the physician leaves the room, the client says: "I don't know what to do, but I'm afraid my doctor will be upset if I don't agree to take the drug."
   a. Review the clinical situation with a peer group.
   b. Answer the following questions:
      (1) What are the client's rights in this situation?
      (2) What are the physician's responsibilities?
      (3) What must the physician explain about the drug?
      (4) What are the nursing student's roles and responsibilities to the client?
      (5) Assuming that the student is qualified to administer medications, what rights does the student have in this situation?
   c. Share your answers with your instructor.

6. Clinical situation: nursing research process
   Kalleen O'Malley is a professional nurse interested in studying the effects of environmental factors on the visitors in an intensive care unit (ICU). Throughout her 6 years of coronary care unit experience, Kalleen has seen visitors become anxious when they enter the unit. Whenever a client is surrounded by equipment or hospital staff, family members seem hesitant to touch their loved one.
   a. Review the clinical situation independently or in a small peer group.
   b. Answer the following questions:
      (1) Which method for acquiring knowledge has influenced Kalleen's impressions about the effects of the ICU on family members?
      (2) What methods could be used to study the problems faced by ICU visitors? Which of these methods would be considered the most reliable?
      (3) Kalleen is not aware of studies previously conducted involving family members of ICU clients. What steps should she take before planning a formal study? (Kalleen decides to study 75 family members by giving them a questionnaire measuring feelings and perceptions about ICU events. Three different ICUs will be used.)

(4) How will Kalleen maintain confidentiality of the subjects?

(5) What specific actions must be taken to ensure that ethical principles of informed consent are followed?

(6) Kalleen must formulate a hypothesis before conducting the study. What should her hypothesis describe?

(7) Why is it important for Kalleen to include a description of the setting when reporting study findings?

c. Share your answers with a peer. Discuss the rationale for your responses.

d. Discuss your answers with your instructor.

ADDITIONAL READINGS

Brown JJ, Fanner CA, Padrick KP: Nursing's search for scientific knowledge, *Nurs Res* 33:26, 1984.
  Analysis of characteristics of current nursing research through examination of trends and changes throughout the past 30 years. Makes recommendations for future research based on the analysis presented.

Castles MR: *Primer of nursing research*, Philadelphia, 1987, Saunders.
  Presents the language and process of nursing research in simple terms to help students understand research and apply findings to clinical practice.

LoBiondo-Wood G, Haber J: *Nursing research: methods, clinical appraisal, and utilization*, ed 2, St Louis, 1990, Mosby–Year Book.
  Clear overview of research methodology for consumers of nursing research, as well as the nurse researcher. Includes separate chapters detailing various experimental designs and methods of data analysis.

Sarter B, editor: *Paths to knowledge: innovative research methods for nursing*, New York, 1988, National League for Nursing.
  Introduces methodologies rarely used in nursing research and provides insights into the trends of current research methodology.

Tanner C, Lindeman C, editors: *Using nursing research*, New York, 1989, National League for Nursing.
  Text directed toward nursing faculty and students for use at an undergraduate level. Introduces basic concepts of nursing research. Includes analysis of research articles by nursing students, recent graduates, and faculty.

Chapter 12
Values

PREREQUISITE READING
Chapter 12, pp. 256 to 271

OBJECTIVES
Mastery of content in this chapter will enable the student to:
- Define selected terms associated with personal and professional values.
- Describe the ways in which values influence behavior and attitudes.
- Discuss the ways in which values are learned.
- Contrast and compare modes of value transmission.
- Compare how values are formed at different stages of development.
- Discuss the influence of caring on professional nursing practice.
- Identify the seven values defined by the American Association of Colleges of Nursing as essential for professional nursing.
- Explain the relationship between the nurse's values and clinical decision making.
- Discuss how the pressures within the health care system can threaten a nurse's ability to exercise caring values.
- Describe the process of values clarification.
- Discuss the advantages of values clarification in nursing.
- Use a values clarification strategy to examine personal values.
- Discuss techniques used to help clients clarify values.
- Analyze personal values as a nursing student.

REVIEW OF KEY CONCEPTS
1. Define a value.
2. Define an attitude.
3. The type of care administered to clients is influenced by the nurse's personal and professional values. (True or false?)
4. Which statement about values is correct?
   a. Most individuals possess many personal values.
   b. A person's values about health will determine decisions about health promotion activities.
   c. Extrinsic values are associated with the maintenance of life.

   d. Personal values rarely influence an individual's perception of others.
5. Describe the five traditional modes of value transmission.

   a.

   b.

   c.

   d.

   e.
6. The mode of value transmission viewed as promoting greater understanding of an individual's personal

   values is _____ .
7. A nursing instructor is comforting a grieving parent. By actions, the instructor may be transmitting a value of caring through which mode?
   a. modeling
   b. moralizing
   c. laissez-faire
   d. responsible behavior
8. Children's developmental stage, during which parents may actively begin directing their child toward valued behaviors, is:
   a. adolescence.
   b. school age.
   c. preschool age.
   d. infancy.
9. An adult's established values may be threatened by advancing age. (True or false?)
10. List the four criteria that define caring as a value and ethical standard for nursing practice.

    a.

    b.

    c.

    d.

11. List and define the seven essential nursing values and behaviors recognized by the American Association of Colleges of Nursing.

a.

b.

c.

d.

e.

f.

g.

12. A process to improve insight into an individual's personal values is called _____

13. List the three major phases of values clarification.

a.

b.

c.

14. Values clarification is an effective guide for solving ethical dilemmas. (True of false?)

15. Identify and briefly describe at least one strategy for assisting a client in clarifying values.

16. List three characteristics of a clarifying response.

a.

b.

c.

17. In the first step of the values clarification process, which of the following behaviors would reflect appropriate client support?

a. Encouraging the client to state personal values

b. Assisting the client in examining alternative values

c. Helping the client plan ways to translate values into behaviors

d. Offering a set of values from which the client may choose those preferred

CRITICAL THINKING AND EXPERIENTIAL EXERCISES

1. Personal values and professional practice

a. Identify three of your own personal values.

b. Determine factors you believe contributed to your acquiring these values.

c. Describe how each value may influence your professional practice.

d. Share your information with other nursing students in a small group discussion.

2. Essential values and behaviors

a. Compare and contrast the traditional modes of value transmission in the table. Note ways parents use each mode and cite examples of potential desirable and undesirable outcomes of each mode.

Modes of value transmission	Parent's behavior	Desirable effect	Undesirable effect
Modeling			
Moralizing			
Laissez-faire			
Responsible choice			

3. Essential values and behaviors

a. Provide care to a client or observe a nurse providing care in any setting.

b. Identify how each of the seven essential values (according to the American Association of Colleges of Nursing) was evident in professional behaviors you performed or observed.

4. Developmental value formation

Give an example of how values are formed in each developmental stage.

a. Infancy

b. Toddler age

c. Preschool age

d. School age

e. Adolescence

f. Adulthood

(1) Young adult

(2) Middle-age adult

(3) Older adult

5. Personal values clarification

a. Independently, or in a small group, complete the health values scale (p. 266 in your text). Identify factors contributing to your acquisition of these values. Discuss your ranking of the values with other group members.

b. In a small group, independently complete the rank ordering tool (p. 266 in your text). If possible, include an experienced nursing student, staff nurse, head nurse, or instructor in your group. Identify factors contributing to acquisition of these values. Discuss your ranking of the values with other group members.

c. File the values clarification exercises that you have just completed. Review your value ranking when you have completed the first year of your nursing program to determine whether professional growth has altered your values system. (If possible, review these exercises when you complete the nursing program.)

6. Values clarification with clients

a. After a client-care experience, identify a client (or nurse) who may be a candidate for values clarification.

b. Describe the client's (nurse's) behaviors that indicate the potential need for values clarification.

c. Discuss how values clarification might benefit the client (nurse).

d. Describe the strategies that you might use to assist the client (nurse) in the values clarification process.

7. Clinical situation: values clarification

Mr. Barnes, 26 years old, is hospitalized after a gunshot wound to the spinal cord. The injury has left him with complete paralysis of his legs and partial paralysis of his arms. You learn that Mr. Barnes was shot during a police raid on his home, during which a large supply of illegal drugs was confiscated. Mr. Barnes requests narcotic pain medication frequently.

   a. Discuss how strategies for values clarification might assist you in caring for this client.
   b. Identify resources in your nursing program and health care setting to assist you in the values clarification process.

8. Clinical situation: clarifying responses

Mr. Watkins is admitted to the hospital with severe cardiac failure. The physician informs Mr. Watkins that his condition will not improve with medication and he will be severely limited in his ability to carry out activities of daily living (ADLs) for the remainder of his life.

   The physician tells Mr. Watkins that the only other treatment option is surgery, which *may* improve his condition, but the risk of death associated with the procedure is extremely high. Mr. Watkins tells the nursing student, "I just don't know what to do. I want to do what's right. What do you think?"

   a. What behaviors indicate that values clarification may be helpful in this situation?
   b. In a small group, use role-playing to enact this situation, with one student as Mr. Watkins and another as the nursing student. Be sure to structure your responses according to the five char-

acteristics described in your text. Attempt to work through the situation using the seven steps of the values clarification process.

   c. Evaluate the role-playing situation. Identify what strategies that were most successful and those that were least successful. Determine how your own values influenced role playing as the nursing student and as Mr. Watkins. Discuss your conclusions with your peers and instructor.

ADDITIONAL READINGS

Bernal EW: Values clarification: a critique, *J Nurs Educ* 24: 174, 1985.

   Describes the concept of values clarification. Points out the limitations of values clarification in resolving ethical dilemmas. Emphasizes the need for nurses to become skillful in ethical reasoning.

Coletta SS: Values clarification in nursing: why? *Am J Nurs* 78:1057, 1978.

   Briefly reviews the seven steps of the values clarification process. Explains the importance of values clarification in nursing practice.

Fry ST: Toward a theory of nursing ethics, *ANS* 11(4):9, 1989.

   Proposes that nursing ethics should not parallel development of biomedical ethics. Explores the foundations of nursing ethics, derived from the nature of the nurse-patient relationship.

Omery A: Values, moral reasoning, and ethics. *Nurs Clin North Am* 24(2):499, 1989.

   Explores complex concepts becoming central to nursing practice in the 21st century.

Uustal DB: Values clarification in nursing: application to practice, *Am J Nurs* 78:2058, 1978.

   Discusses the theoretical concepts guiding values clarification. Presents 10 strategies to be used in personal or professional values clarification exercises.

Chapter 13
Ethics

PREREQUISITE READING
Chapter 13, pp. 272 to 289

OBJECTIVES
Mastery of content in this chapter will enable the student to:
- Define terms associated with ethics in nursing practice.
- Discuss the influence of ethics on nursing practice.
- Discuss the influence of personal and professional values on ethical decisions.
- Compare responsibility and accountability in nursing practice.
- Identify the purposes of a professional code of ethics.
- Identify and apply the primary and secondary principles of ethics to clinical situations.
- Discuss the types of ethical conflicts confronted by nurses.
- Discuss and apply to a clinical situation the process used to resolve ethical problems.
- Identify and analyze the ethical dilemma of any clinical situation for presentation to an ethics committee.

REVIEW OF KEY CONCEPTS
1. Define ethics.
2. Define ethical dilemma.
3. A healthcare issue often becomes an ethical dilemma because:
   a. a client's legal rights coexist with a health professional's obligations.
   b. decisions must be made quickly, often under stressful conditions.
   c. decisions must be made based on value systems.
   d. the choices involved do not appear to be clearly right or wrong.
4. The personal conviction that something is absolutely right or wrong in all situations is a (an):
   a. legal obligation.
   b. personal value.
   c. moral belief.
   d. ethical issue.
5. Define each principle underlying ethical codes for professional nurses.
   a. Autonomy
   b. Beneficence
   c. Nonmaleficence
   d. Justice
   e. Veracity
   f. Fidelity
   g. Confidentiality
6. Compare responsibility and accountability in professional nursing practice.
7. A basic structure against which competent care is objectively measured is a:
   a. law.
   b. principle.
   c. standard.
   d. code.
8. Discuss the intent and implications of the Patient Self-Determination Act (Advanced Directives Act) of 1990.
9. A document that lists the medical treatment a person chooses to refuse if unable to make decisions is the:
   a. durable power of attorney.
   b. informed consent.
   c. medical record.
   d. living will.
10. List and briefly describe the six steps in the model for ethical decision making.

    a.

    b.

    c.

    d.

    e.

    f.
11. Which statement about an institutional ethics committee is correct?
    a. The ethics committee is an additional resource for clients and health care professionals.
    b. The ethics committee relieves health care professionals from dealing with ethical issues.
    c. The ethics committee would be the first option in addressing an ethical dilemma.
    d. The ethics committee replaces decision making by the client and health care providers.

CRITICAL THINKING AND EXPERIENTIAL EXERCISES

1. Codes of ethics
   a. Discuss the American Nurses Association (ANA), International Council of Nurses (ICN), or Canadian Nurses Association (CNA) Code of Ethics as it relates to each of the following:
      (1) Standards of nursing care
      (2) Responsibility to the clients
      (3) Responsibility to the profession
      (4) Role in society
   b. Compare and contrast the ANA, ICN, or CNA Code of Ethics to the nurse practice act of your state or province in each of the following areas:
      (1) Professional responsibility
      (2) Professional accountability
      (3) Client advocacy
      (4) Legal obligations
2. Professional accountability
   Describe at least two ways that nursing students are able to maintain professional accountability to each of the following individuals or groups.
   a. Personal (self)
   b. Client
   c. Profession
   d. Educational institution or health care institution
   e. Society
3. Ethical dilemmas in nursing
   a. Independently or in a small group, contact nurses practicing in different areas of your institution or community. Ask them to identify at least three ethical issues they have encountered in their particular practice setting. Ask them to describe the ways in which the ethical issue was addressed and the resources available to assist them in the process.
   b. After an observational experience or after providing client care in any health care setting, identify ethical issues that would be considered unique to the practice setting or your particular client situation. Support your identification of the issue as an ethical problem. How would you present this situation to a hospital ethics committee?
   c. Invite an experienced staff nurse to discuss an ethical dilemma encountered in clinical practice. Compare the method used by the nurse to resolve the dilemma with the process outlined in your text.
4. Clinical situation: resolution of ethical dilemmas
   Independently, or in a small group, apply the process for resolving ethical problems to the following hypothetical situations. For each step, identify the information you would gather and describe the actions you would take to resolve the dilemma.
   a. *Situation A:* You are performing an assessment on an assigned client. You think that you hear crackles during auscultation of the lungs, but the co-assigned staff nurse records that the client's lungs are clear. The client tells you that you are the only person who has listened to her chest that morning.
   b. *Situation B:* You are working in the campus clinic when Jean, an undergraduate, comes in for treatment of a severe headache. You take some classes with Jean and have seen her take a friend's narcotic pain medication regularly. Jean tells the clinic physician that she only takes aspirin and acetaminophen for headaches and that it provides little relief. She is requesting something stronger for pain.

ADDITIONAL READINGS

American Nurses Association: Code for nurses, *Am J Nurs* 50:196, 392, 1950.
   Original publication of principles guiding professional nursing practice. Developed by the ANA Committee on Ethics.

Aroskar MA: Nurses as decision makers: ethical dimensions, *Imprint* 39:29, 1985.
   Detailed discussion of ethical problems, principles, and the ethical decision-making process.

Chinn P, editor: *Ethical issues in nursing,* Rockville, Md, 1986, Aspen.
   Selected articles from two nursing journals (*Advances in Nursing Science* and *Topics in Clinical Nursing*) addressing ethical issues associated with nursing practice.

Chinn P, editor: Ethical issues, *ANS* 11(3), 1989.
   A series of articles addressing ethical issues in nursing practice.

Scott RS: When it isn't life or death, *Am J Nurs* 85:19, 1985.
   Examines a common ethical dilemma encountered by middle-age children and their chronically ill parents. Presents a four-step framework for ethical decision making as it applies to this ethical problem.

Weeks LC et al: How can a hospital ethics committee help? *Am J Nurs* 90:651, 1989.
   Explores the valuable resources available through a hospital ethics committee. Especially useful for nurses new to professional practice.

Chapter 14
Legal Issues

PREREQUISITE READING
Chapter 14, pp. 290 to 307

OBJECTIVES
Mastery of content in this chapter will enable the student to:
- Define selected legal terms associated with nursing practice.
- Explain legal concepts that apply to nurses.
- Describe the legal responsibilities and obligations of nurses.
- List sources for standards of care for nurses.
- Define legal aspects of nurse-client, nurse-physician, nurse-nurse, and nurse-employer relationships.
- Give examples of legal issues that arise in nursing practice.

REVIEW OF KEY CONCEPTS

1. Identify three sources for standards of nursing care.

   a.

   b.

   c.

2. Nurses in an intensive care unit or operating room are held to the same standards of care and skill as general duty nurses. (True or false?)
3. The state or provincial board of nursing has the authority to suspend or revoke a nurse's license. (True or false?)
4. Which statement about the nursing student's legal liability is correct?
   a. A student who has safely administered oral medications may perform this task when employed as a nurse's aide.
   b. Students are expected to perform at the level of professional nurses.
   c. A student's instructor may share liability when a student's action or inaction injures a client.
   d. A student cannot be held liable for performing tasks that are being learned.
5. Match the most accurate description with the sources and categories of contemporary law.

Description
   a. Law created by elected legislative bodies

   _____

   b. Law created by judicial decision _____
   c. Law concerned with protection of a person's rights _____
   d. Law concerned with acts threatening society _____

Category
   1. Civil law
   2. Criminal law
   3. Statutory law
   4. Common law
6. A civil wrong committed against a person or property is a _____ .
7. Define negligence.
8. List the four criteria that must be established in a malpractice law suit against a nurse.

   a.

   b.

   c.

   d.

9. Discuss ways that the nurse may avoid being named in a lawsuit.
10. An institution's liability insurance usually offers adequate protection for professional nurses. (True or false?)
11. The nurse accidentally leaves a crib side down. The child falls out of bed and suffers a skull fracture. The nurse could be charged with:
    a. assault.
    b. battery.
    c. intentional tort.
    d. malpractice.
12. The physician orders an injectable tranquilizer for an uncooperative client in the emergency room. The nurse asks the student to hold the client's arm so the nurse can safely give the injection. The student could be accused of:
    a. assault.
    b. battery.
    c. negligence.
    d. malpractice.

13. Mr. Neilson, a nursing student, tells his peers that he is caring for Sam Jones, a local politician suffering from acquired immunodeficiency syndrome (AIDS). Mr. Neilson could be charged with:
   a. invasion of privacy.
   b. defamation of character.
   c. libel
   d. negligence.
14. The Patient's Bill of Rights (American Hospital Association, 1972):
   a. is a formal legal document.
   b. provides a guideline for interaction with clients.
   c. provides a written standard of care for clients.
   d. is only applicable to hospitalized clients.
15. List the four conditions that must be present for informed consent to be valid.

   a.

   b.

   c.

   d.
16. A signed consent form is required for:
   a. routine treatment.
   b. surgical procedures.
   c. invasive diagnostic procedures.
   d. all of the above.
17. It is the nurse's responsibility to obtain client consent for medical or surgical procedures. (True or false?)
18. Mr. Treat is scheduled for a cholecystectomy and has already signed the consent form. As the nurse enters the room to administer the preoperative injection, Mr. Treat says he isn't sure if he wants to have the surgery. Which nursing action would be appropriate?
   a. Give Mr. Treat his preoperative injection because it will help him to relax.
   b. Remind Mr. Treat that he consented to the surgery the evening before and the operating team is waiting for him.
   c. Withhold the injection and notify the surgeon that Mr. Treat is having second thoughts about the surgery.
   d. Encourage Mr. Treat to have the surgery because it will ultimately make him feel better.
19. What is the most important factor in legally determining death?
20. Nurses are legally obligated to treat a corpse with dignity and care. (True or false?)
21. A nurse following an inaccurate physician's order is legally responsible for any harm suffered by the client. (True or false?)
22. Ms. Watson, an experienced pediatric nurse, has been assigned charge nurse responsibilities on the evening shift. Because of a staffing shortage and a high pediatric census, she is told that she must be in charge and provide primary care for six children. Which action by Ms. Watson would place her at greatest risk of legal liability?

   a. Informing the supervisor that she is not qualified for the assignment
   b. Refusing the assignment
   c. Informing the supervisor that she is leaving the hospital
   d. Submitting a written protest to nursing administration
23. What is the purpose of an incident report?
24. What is the purpose of a Good Samaritan law?
25. An oral contract with a client is as legally binding as a written contract. (True or false?)
26. Mrs. Taylor, a registered nurse (RN), is offered a job in the operating rooms. In this institution, three or four therapeutic abortions are done each working day. Mrs. Taylor is strongly opposed to abortion but likes all other aspects of the job. Mrs. Taylor should:
   a. ask if the employer has a "conscience clause" that would allow her to refuse to assist with abortions.
   b. assist with abortions, remembering that her personal values should not influence her professional actions.
   c. contact the local pro-life group to discuss her rights in assisting with the abortions.
   d. reject the job offer and seek employment elsewhere.

CRITICAL THINKING AND EXPERIENTIAL EXERCISES

1. Risk management
   Interview a health care agency attorney or risk management consultant. Include some of the following questions in your discussion.
   a. What are the agency's policies and procedures regarding incident reports?
   b. What recommendations does the attorney or consultant have about liability insurance for professional nurses and nursing students?
   c. How does the institution meet the legal regulations regarding the Patient Determination Act and the Uniform Anatomical Gift Acts?
   d. How does the institution execute its ethical responsibilities in the Patient Determination Act and the Uniform Anatomical Gift Acts?
2. Contracts
   a. Review the contract that your educational institution has with your assigned clinical agency. Identify the areas of responsibility for students, instructors, and nursing staff.
3. Licensure
   Review the nursing licensure statute for your state or province.
   a. Identify the licensure requirements.
   b. What circumstances are cited as grounds for license suspension or revocation?
   c. What activities are defined as nursing practice?
4. Legal issues in practice
   a. Independently, or in a small group, survey nurses practicing in a variety of clinical areas or settings.

b. Ask each nurse to identify legal issues most often encountered in clinical practice.

c. What actions does the nurse take to limit legal liabilities?

d. Which legal issues are common among all nurses surveyed?

e. Which legal issues are unique to specialty areas?

5. Patient's Bill of Rights

After a client care or observational experience, review the Patient's Bill of Rights (AHA, 1972, on p. 295 of your text).

a. Which of the client's rights were actively preserved? What actions did you observe that preserved these rights?

b. Were any of the rights violated or not met? What measures might be taken in future situations to ensure that these rights are preserved?

6. Clinical situation: incident reports and malpractice

Mr. Thompson, RN, has been caring for Mrs. Adams for the past week. Mr. Thompson enters Mrs. Adams' room to administer her 10 AM medications. This is the third time he has given medications to Mrs. Adams on this shift, so he does not check her identification band before administering the medications. Just before administering medications to his second client, Mrs. Peters, he realizes he has mixed up the drugs and given the wrong ones to Mrs. Adams.

a. What is the nature of Mr. Thompson's legal liability in this situation?

b. What actions should Mr. Thompson take at this time?

c. What documentation should be made about this incident? (If possible, obtain a sample of your institution's incident report and complete it as part of the exercise.)

d. How could Mr. Thompson approach Mrs. Adams about what has just occurred? What should he say? What should he do?

e. What actions should be taken to avoid this situation in the future?

7. Clinical situation: informed consent

a. Mr. Bolden is scheduled for a bone marrow biopsy. The physician explained the procedure and obtained informed consent yesterday. Mrs. Bolden was present during the physician's explanation, and the consent was witnessed by the assistant head nurse. You are assigned to care for Mr. Bolden and will remain with him during the biopsy. The physician enters the room and begins the procedure. Mr. Bolden is extremely anxious and cries out in pain. He states, "Please stop, I'm not sure if I want to go through with this." The physician tells Mr. Bolden he will be giving him some medication to relax, and the biopsy will be over soon. Describe the actions you would take and provide the rationale for them.

8. Clinical situation: client rights

Mr. James is admitted with acute gastrointestinal bleeding and hypotension. The physician has ordered packed red blood cells to be transfused immediately. The admitting nurse is aware that Mr. James' religious beliefs prohibit any form of blood or blood product transfusion. The nurse is also aware that Mr. James' condition is rapidly deteriorating and that the transfusion may prevent him from going into shock.

a. What are the patient's rights in this situation?

b. What are the nurse's responsibilities to the client?

c. Who should be involved or consulted in this situation?

d. What documentation must be made about this situation?

ADDITIONAL READINGS

Creighton H: *Law every nurse should know*, ed 5, Philadelphia, 1986, Saunders.

Comprehensive presentation of legal facts associated with nursing practice. Information presented in clear, nontechnical manner; applicable to student nurses and experienced nurse practitioners.

Fiesta J: *The law and legal liability: a guide for nurses*, ed 2, New York, 1988, Wiley.

Provides introduction to legal issues encountered in professional practice. Uses case study method to illustrate major legal principles.

Feutz SA: Professional liability insurance. In Northrop CA, Kelly ME: *Legal issues in nursing*, St Louis, 1987, Mosby–Year Book.

Discussion of issues associated with liability insurance for the professional nurse.

Northrop C: Student nurses and legal accountability, *Imprint* 32:16,1985.

Summarizes nursing students' legal accountability for actions during clinical practice.

Northrop CE, Kelly ME: *Legal issues in nursing*, St Louis, 1987, Mosby–Year Book.

Comprehensive resource addressing legal issues influencing nursing practice. Written in a clear, nontechnical manner; applicable to student nurses or experienced nurse practitioners.

Chapter 15
Communication

PREREQUISITE READING

Chapter 15, pp. 308 to 345

OBJECTIVES

Mastery of content in this chapter will enable the student to:

- Define selected terms associated with communication in nursing practice.
- Describe differences among the three levels of communication.
- Identify characteristics of verbal and nonverbal communication.
- Discuss the functions of communication in the nurse-client relationship.
- Explain the role of communication in the nursing process.
- Describe each element of the communication process.
- Identify factors that promote and inhibit communication.
- Give examples of techniques that promote therapeutic communication.
- List and discuss the phases of a therapeutic helping relationship.
- Explain the dimensions of a helping relationship.
- Discuss nursing care measures for clients with communication alterations.

REVIEW OF KEY CONCEPTS

1. Define communication.
2. List and briefly describe the three levels of communication.

    a.

    b.

    c.

3. The nurse enters Mr. Ford's room and notes the client's facial expression of discomfort. The nurse considers the factors that may be causing Mr. Ford's pain. This level of communication is best described as:
    a. public.
    b. private.
    c. interpersonal.
    d. intrapersonal.
4. Fill in the element of the communication process with the description provided.

    a. The person to whom the message is sent

    _____

    b. The receiver returns a message to the sender

    _____

    c. The information that is sent _____

    d. Methods for conveying information

    _____

    e. The person who initiates the interpersonal communication _____

    f. The factor that motivates a person to communicate _____

5. In demonstrating the method for deep breathing exercises, the nurse places the hands on the client's abdomen to explain diaphragmatic movement. This technique involves the use of which communication element?
    a. Feedback
    b. Tactile channel
    c. Referent
    d. Message
6. Match the verbal communication technique with the appropriate description or example.

Description

    a. Describing the client's illness without using medical terminology _____

    b. Waiting until a client's pain is relieved before discussing the importance of exercise _____

    c. Avoiding prolonged pauses or rapid shifts to other subjects _____

    d. Providing examples and repeating important parts of a message _____

Technique

    1. Pacing
    2. Timing
    3. Clarity
    4. Vocabulary

7. Compare the major characteristics of verbal and nonverbal communication.

8. Which statement about nonverbal communication is correct?
   a. It is easy for a nurse to judge the meaning of a client's facial expressions.
   b. The nurse's verbal messages should be reinforced by nonverbal cues.
   c. The physical appearance of the nurse rarely influences nurse-client interaction.
   d. Words convey meanings that are usually more significant than nonverbal communication.
9. The term referring to the sender's attitude toward the self, the message, and the listener is:
   a. nonverbal communication.
   b. meta communication.
   c. connotative meaning.
   d. denotative meaning.
10. List at least five means of nonverbal communication.
   a.
   b.
   c.
   d.
   e.
11. List and define five factors that influence interpersonal communication.
   a.
   b.
   c.
   d.
   e.
12. To establish a therapeutic relationship, it is important for the nurse to discuss personal emotions with the client. (True or false?)
13. Communication is more effective when the participants remain aware of their roles in a relationship. (True or false?)
14. A client's personal space:
   a. is clearly visible to others.
   b. is the same as the client's territoriality.
   c. can be separated from the client.
   d. is highly mobile.
15. List the three dimensions of an individual's personal space, including the actual distance characteristic of each dimension.
   a.
   b.
   c.
16. Interpersonal communication is least threatening at a:
   a. social distance.
   b. personal distance.
   c. intimate distance.
   d. territorial distance.

17. Social interaction with a client is inappropriate when attempting to establish a therapeutic relationship. (True or false?)
18. List and describe four skills facilitating attentive listening.
   a.
   b.
   c.
   d.
19. List two actions that convey the nurse's acceptance of what the client is saying.
   a.
   b.
20. When a nurse conveys acceptance of a client, it means that the nurse agrees with the client. (True or false?)
21. Which communication technique would be most effective in eliciting detailed information from a client?
   a. Maintaining silence
   b. Open-ended questions
   c. Stating observations
   d. Summarizing
22. Identify the communication technique illustrated in each of the sample interactions.

Interaction

a. _____ *Client:* The medication always seems to upset my stomach.
   Nurse: That may be because you aren't taking it with meals. The drug can cause stomach irritation.
b. _____ *Client:* This test tomorrow—the doctor says it's painless, but I've heard differently from my friends. I'm not sure if I want it.
   Nurse: It sounds as if you're frightened about the test.
c. _____ *Client:* Well, when I seem to move wrong, the pain gets worse.
   Nurse: Tell me what you mean by "move wrong."
d. _____ *Nurse:* Tell me what medications you are taking.
   Client: I take Inderal and occasionally Valium.
   Nurse: How long have you taken each drug?
   Client: About 2 years for each.
   Nurse: What dose do you take of each drug?

Technique
   1. Paraphrasing
   2. Asking related questions
   3. Focusing
   4. Offering information

23. List four nontherapeutic communication techniques and briefly describe the reason that each inhibits communication.

    a.

    b.

    c.

    d.

24. Which of the following statements by the nurse could be considered false reassurance to the client?
    a. "I understand your concern about the surgery, but at your age there's nothing to worry about."
    b. "I know that it must be frightening to be in the hospital, but you'll receive the care you need."
    c. "It's a difficult time for you, but be assured that I'm willing to listen to anything you have to say."
    d. "No, I've never lost a close relative to cancer, but I can understand how difficult it must be for you."

25. List at least four general conditions in which verbal reassurance may be offered to the client.

    a.

    b.

    c.

    d.

26. Define therapeutic relationship.
27. List and briefly describe the five characteristics of any helping relationship.

    a.

    b.

    c.

    d.

    e.

28. Describe the difference between empathy and sympathy.
29. Match the phase of a helping relationship with the characteristic behaviors or goals described.

Behavior or goal

    a. The nurse chooses the location and setting for the interaction. _____
    b. The nurse helps the client adjust to changes of illness. _____
    c. The nurse's initial goal is to direct the conversation to help the client feel at ease. _____
    d. The client tests the nurse's genuineness in wanting to help. _____
    e. The nurse and client evaluate goals and their outcomes. _____

f. The nurse uses communication skills while performing routine care measures. _____
g. The nurse and client identify mutual goals. ___

Phase
1. Preinteraction
2. Orientation
3. Working phase
4. Termination

30. The client should be informed about the termination of a relationship during which phase of the working relationship?
    a. Preinteraction
    b. Orientation
    c. Working phase
    d. Termination
31. List and briefly describe two communication skills that promote client self-understanding.

    a.

    b.

32. The following interaction occurs between Ms. Russ, a 70-year-old client with heart disease, and her nurse:
    Ms. Russ: I'm afraid I won't be able to do the things I enjoy any more.
    Nurse: I'd like to understand your concern. Tell me more, and perhaps I can explain how your condition might affect you.
    Ms. Russ: It's important to me to be able to visit my friends.
    Nurse: I believe we can find ways that will allow you to continue your visits.
    This interaction is an example of:
    a. clarifying roles.
    b. separation.
    c. testing.
    d. building trust.
33. Mr. Towns has a rare blood disorder and is in the hospital for tests to adjust his medications. The nurse enters the room:
    Nurse: Mr. Towns, I'm Ms. Long. I'll be caring for you today.
    Mr. Towns: You're a different nurse than the one I had yesterday.
    Nurse: Yes, but I'm aware of the test you had yesterday and thought you might want to talk about what's planned for today.
    Mr. Towns: Are you sure you can explain what I need to know?
    This interaction is an example of:
    a. asking related questions.
    b. testing.
    c. contract formation.
    d. identifying problems.
34. Communication skills are of importance only in low-visibility tasks associated with the psychological,

spiritual, and socioeconomic needs of the client. (True or false?)

35. Client communication may be impaired by:
 a. physical changes associated with disease states or therapies.
 b. psychological alterations associated with coping or social interaction.
 c. environmental conditions.
 d. all of the above.

36. List five alternate methods for communicating with clients who have physical conditions creating barriers to interaction.

 a.

 b.

 c.

 d.

 e.

37. List three methods of environmental control to facilitate interpersonal communication.

 a.

 b.

 c.

38. All of the following are important factors when communicating with clients. Which is the most important in establishing effective communication with a child?
 a. Meeting the child at eye level
 b. Providing a quiet, comfortable environment
 c. Informing the child about any discomfort associated with a procedure.
 d. Understanding the influence of development on language and thought processes.

39. List three interactions to facilitate communication with a client who is hearing impaired.

 a.

 b.

 c.

40. The nurse maximizes communication with the aphasic client by:
 a. speaking very loudly.
 b. avoiding the use of visual cues.
 c. asking "yes" and "no" questions.
 d. interrupting to provide appropriate words.

41. Nurses do not need to be concerned about communication and interaction when caring for an unconscious client. (True or false?)

CRITICAL THINKING AND EXPERIENTIAL EXERCISES

1. Elements of the communication process
 a. Conduct a 5-minute observation of two people interacting (nurse-client, student-instructor, student-student, or two family members).

 b. List and give examples of the modes of communication you observed.
  (1) Verbal
  (2) Nonverbal
 c. List and give examples of the elements of the communication process you observed.
  (1) Referent
  (2) Sender
  (3) Message
  (4) Channels
  (5) Receiver
  (6) Intrapersonal variables

2. Communication and the nursing process
 After an observation or after providing care for an assigned client, identify the communication skills that were used in each step of the nursing process.
 a. Assessment
 b. Diagnosis
 c. Planning
 d. Implementation
 e. Evaluation

3. Clinical situation: therapeutic communication
 Read the hypothetical interaction between a nurse and client.
 Client: You see, Ms. Williams, I am 68 years old and now my doctor has told me that I have cancer. I've always felt I could live forever. I guess that was foolish.
 Nurse: I want to understand how you feel. Please go on.
 Client: How can you understand? You are so young.
 Nurse: Oh, that's silly. I'm not that young.
 Client: Well, of course you are. Anyway, it seems as though I will either have to take chemotherapy or choose surgery.
 Nurse: Maybe you should get another opinion.
 Client: Oh? I've always liked Dr. Rose. He has taken care of most of my family and has always done a good job when we needed him.
 Nurse: You're saying that you trust him?
 Client: Yes, I do. He's suggested I try chemotherapy.
 Nurse: By the way, have you taken any pain medications recently?
 Client: What? Oh yes, but only before I go to bed so I can sleep.
 a. List therapeutic communication techniques.
 b. List techniques that inhibit communication and explain why communication is inhibited.
 c. Formulate an alternative approach to the nontherapeutic techniques listed.

SKILL AND TECHNIQUE ACTIVITIES

1. Therapeutic communication techniques
 a. During interactions with peers or family members, practice using each of the 11 therapeutic communication skills described in your text.

(Many students find it helpful to focus on one skill at a time.)
  (1) Identify the skills that are most comfortable for you.
  (2) Identify and continue to practice the skills you find awkward or uncomfortable.

b. Record on an audiotape or videotape a role-playing situation or interaction with a peer. Attempt to use the therapeutic techniques described in your text. Play back the tape and critique your performance in each of the following areas:
  (1) Factors that influenced the communication
  (2) Effective therapeutic communication techniques
  (3) Nontherapeutic or ineffective therapeutic communication techniques
  (4) Alternative approaches to communication

c. Transcribe a segment of an interaction with an assigned client. (Although this will not be an exact recording, try to recall the points discussed and the techniques used.) Analyze your interaction, including:
  (1) factors that influenced communication.
  (2) nonverbal communication that you observed in the client or transmitted yourself.
  (3) therapeutic communication skills used.
  (4) barriers to communication and techniques that might have been used to minimize them.
  (5) nontherapeutic communication skills that you used and alternative responses that are more therapeutic.

ADDITIONAL READINGS

Bradley J, Edenberg MA: *Communication in the nursing context,* ed 3, Norwalk, Conn, 1990, Appleton & Lange.
  Presents theories and techniques of communication. Focuses on communication skills as they apply to clinical practice. Highlights discussion with practice exercise.

Dreher BB: *Communication skills for working with elders,* New York, 1987, Springer.
  Details approaches for successful interaction with older adult clients.

Knowles RD: Building rapport through neuro-linguistic programming, *Am J Nurs* 83:1011, 1983.
  Examines the effect of visual, auditory, and kinesthetic messages on the communication process. Proposes that most individuals' communications reflect a preference for one of three transmission methods. Recommends techniques that may enhance interactions when implementing these neurolinguistic modes.

Murray RB: Therapeutic communication for emotional care. In Murray RB, Huelskoetter MM: *Psychiatric–mental health nursing: giving emotional care,* Englewood Cliffs, NJ, 1987, Prentice-Hall.
  Clearly presents principles of communication and techniques to facilitate the interviewing process. Addresses techniques appropriate for specific client behaviors frequently encountered by the nurse. Also describes techniques appropriate for each developmental level.

Purtilo R: *Health professionals–patient interaction,* ed 4, Philadelphia, 1990, Saunders.
  Discusses the basis for achieving effective client interations. Describes methods fostering therapeutic relationships.

Chapter 16
Teaching-Learning Process

PREREQUISITE READING
Chapter 16, pp. 346 to 381

OBJECTIVES
Mastery of content in this chapter will enable the student to:
- Define selected terms associated with teaching and learning.
- Describe the similarities and differences between teaching and learning.
- Identify the purposes of client education.
- Describe how to incorporate communication principles into the teaching-learning process.
- Describe the domains of learning.
- Differentiate factors that determine the motivation to learn from those that determine the ability to learn.
- Compare the nursing process with the teaching process.
- Write learning objectives for a teaching plan.
- Describe characteristics of a good learning environment.
- Identify different teaching approaches to use for clients with specific learning needs.
- Describe the instructional method best suited for a client with a specific learning need.
- Describe ways to incorporate teaching into routine nursing care.
- Identify methods for evaluating learning.

REVIEW OF KEY CONCEPTS
1. List the three major purposes of client education.

   a.

   b.

   c.
2. Define teaching.
3. Define learning.
4. Accrediting agencies require that health care institutions provide clients with health care education. (True or false?)
5. Match the element of the communication process with the corresponding activity in the teaching-learning process.

Element
   a. Referent _____

   b. Sender _____

   c. Intrapersonal variables of the sender _____

   d. Message _____

   e. Channels _____

   f. Receiver _____

   g. Intrapersonal variables of the receiver _____

   h. Feedback _____

Activity
   1. Content or information taught
   2. Perceived need to provide information
   3. Teacher's knowledge, approach, values, and emotions
   4. Determining achievement of learning objectives
   5. Learner
   6. Teacher
   7. Teaching methods
   8. Willingness and ability to learn
6. Learning is most effective when a single sensory channel is used. (True or false?)
7. Fill in the name of each learning domain described below.
   a. Learning that deals with expression of feelings and acceptance of attitudes, opinions, or values _____
   b. Learning that involves acquisition of skills requiring integration of mental and muscular activity _____
   c. Learning that involves development of intellectual behaviors _____
8. List and briefly describe the three conditions necessary for learning.

   a.

   b.

   c.
9. Learning readiness is influenced by all of the following except:
   a. the ability to concentrate on information to be learned.
   b. internal impulses that cause a person to take action.

c. the individual's level of development.

d. the individual's psychosocial adaptation to illness.

10. Which level of anxiety is most likely to motivate an individual to learn?
   a. Absence of anxiety
   b. Mild level of anxiety
   c. Moderate level of anxiety
   d. High level of anxiety

11. Define compliance.

12. List four health beliefs necessary for initiation of a health action.

   a.

   b.

   c.

   d.

13. Mr. Miller was involved in an automobile accident resulting in the loss of his right leg. Which comment by Mr. Miller indicates that he is ready for teaching related to self-care on discharge?
   a. "If those ambulance people would have done their jobs right, this would have never happened."
   b. "You know, they said my leg is gone, but I still feel it. I'll be ready to get up and walk in a few days."
   c. "Nothing in my life needs to change, so long as I do everything you and the doctor tell me."
   d. Without my leg, I'm not sure how I'll be able to work. I feel helpless."

14. A plan for client teaching is best introduced during which stage of the grieving process.
   a. Acceptance
   b. Bargaining
   c. Denial
   d. Anger

15. Identify the three major factors influencing an individual's ability to learn.

   a.

   b.

   c.

16. The use of role playing would be an effective teaching methods for which developmental level?
   a. Toddler
   b. Preschooler
   c. Adolescent
   d. Older adult

17. Mr. Dennis, a newly diagnosed diabetic, must learn self-injection of insulin. Which physical attribute would not relate to his ability to perform this psychomotor task?
   a. Size
   b. Strength
   c. Coordination
   d. Sensory acuity

18. List at least five factors to consider when selecting the learning setting.

   a.

   b.

   c.

   d.

   e.

19. Match the teaching activity with the corresponding step of the nursing process.

Activity

   a. Writing learning objectives _____
   b. Determining available teaching resources _____
   c. Organizing group discussions _____
   d. Identifying learning needs _____
   e. Determining the client's ability to perform a new skill independently _____

Step

   1. Assessment
   2. Nursing diagnosis
   3. Planning
   4. Implementation
   5. Evaluation

20. List the five major areas requiring assessment in the teaching process.

   a.

   b.

   c.

   d.

   e.

21. Ms. Derring, a 21-year-old college student, has come to the campus clinic for a routine health check. During the physical examination, the nurse determines that Ms. Derring does not know that regular breast self-examination is important. Which nursing diagnosis would be most appropriate for this client situation?
   a. Noncompliance with cancer prevention activities
   b. Knowledge deficit (affective) related to anxiety about cancer
   c. Knowledge deficit (psychomotor) related to inability to perform breast self-examination
   d. Altered health maintenance related to lack of information about breast self-examination

22. List and briefly describe the three components of a learning objective.

   a.

   b.

   c.

23. Which behavioral objective is the most accurately stated?
    a. Client will describe how to change the abdominal dressing.
    b. Client will demonstrate abdominal dressing change.
    c. Client will change abdominal dressing using clean technique before hospital discharge.
    d. Client will know the correct technique for abdominal dressing change before hospital discharge.
24. Which verb should the nurse avoid when writing a behavioral learning objective?
    a. Explain
    b. Understand
    c. Identify
    d. State
25. Why is it important to develop a written teaching plan for clients?
26. How is the approach to teaching different from teaching methodology?
27. Describe at least seven principles to apply in any teaching plan.

    a.

    b.

    c.

    d.

    e.

    f.

    g.
28. Mr. Browner needs to learn to perform back-strengthening exercises. The best teaching method for his need is:
    a. group discussion.
    b. demonstration.
    c. formal lecture.
    d. watching a slide program.
29. Which teaching method would be most appropriate in stimulating affective learning?
    a. Discussion
    b. Lecture
    c. Teaching booklets
    d. Demonstration
30. Identify at least six teaching strategies especially important for older adult clients.

    a.

    b.

    c.

    d.

    e.

    f.

31. The most important factor to consider when developing a teaching plan for a child is:
    a. the information to be taught.
    b. the amount of time available to teach.
    c. the developmental level of the child.
    d. the chronological age of the child.
32. Which statement about teaching methodology is accurate?
    a. More difficult, complex content should be presented first.
    b. Repetition should be avoided to prevent client boredom.
    c. The most essential information should be presented last.
    d. Frequent sessions of 20 to 30 minutes are most beneficial.
33. The most effective way to evaluate effectiveness of client teaching is to:
    a. ask the client whether he or she understands what was taught.
    b. measure performance of the expected behavior.
    c. ask the client questions about the information taught.
    d. request that the client repeat exactly what he or she has learned.
34. List the three areas to be included when documenting client teaching.

    a.

    b.

    c.

CRITICAL THINKING AND EXPERIENTIAL EXERCISES

1. Teaching process during routine client care
    a. Review a clinical experience in which you observed or provided client care. Identify the opportunities and potential topics for client education during routine morning care.
2. Learning environment
   After an observational experience in any health care setting:
    a. Identify factors in the environment conducive to client education.
    b. Identify factors in the environment that could create barriers to client education.
    c. Describe nursing actions that could overcome or control the environmental factors inhibiting client learning.
3. Learning objectives
   Formulate a behavioral learning objective for each of the following situations:
    a. Your client needs to know how to take a pulse before going home from the hospital.
    b. A client at home is unfamiliar with the side effects of new medications.
    c. Your client needs to develop a daily menu for a weight reduction program recently joined.

d. Your client is expected to report any signs of visual loss to the physician.

4. Developmentally appropriate teaching strategies
For each developmental level listed, describe the teaching method or methods and the approach you would use to teach the client about oral hygiene.
a. Infant
b. Toddler
c. Preschooler
d. School-age child
e. Adolescent
f. Young or middle-age adult
g. Older adult

5. Clinical situation: communication and the teaching-learning process
a. Using the information provided in the following situation and the figure below, fill in the data appropriate to the teaching process as they correlate with the elements of communication.

Ms. Loomis has rheumatoid arthritis and is unaware of the types of exercises to perform to maintain joint motion. Ms. Loomis lives with her sister and is anxious to remain as independent as possible. Her vision is reduced, but she can read the large print in newspapers and magazines. Mr. Rosen, her nurse, plans to teach Ms. Loomis exercises by explaining their purpose and directing Ms. Loomis through each exercise. Mr. Rosen often works with clients with arthritis and can readily adjust exercises to the client's abilities. After the teaching session, Ms. Loomis will demonstrate each exercise.

6. Clinical situation: domains of learning
Mr. Gasen is 48 years old and recovering from a heart attack. His physician has prescribed new medication, an exercise program, and a low-cholesterol diet. Mrs. Gasen is concerned about her husband's return home because she is unfamiliar with his treatment plan and discharge restrictions. Identify at least two examples of knowledge or skills that Mr. Gasen and his wife will need to acquire in each of the learning domains:
a. Cognitive
b. Affective
c. Psychomotor

7. Clinical situation: teaching-learning process
Ms. Jeffries has had arthritis for several years. She lives in a six-room home with her husband, who is semi-retired and works 3 days each week. Ms. Jeffries has considerable joint pain and takes an analgesic every 6 hours. She is limited in her ability to perform any activity for an extended time because of discomfort and fatigue. Ms. Jeffries tells the nurse, "I wish I knew why this arthritis affects me like it does." A home health nurse who previously worked with Ms. Jeffries began to teach her alternative pain control methods, but Ms. Jeffries was admitted to the hospital for a week before the teaching plan had been completed. Now you are responsible for Ms. Jeffries' home care. Develop a teaching plan for Ms. Jeffries, including:
a. three factors you would assess to determine her ability to learn.

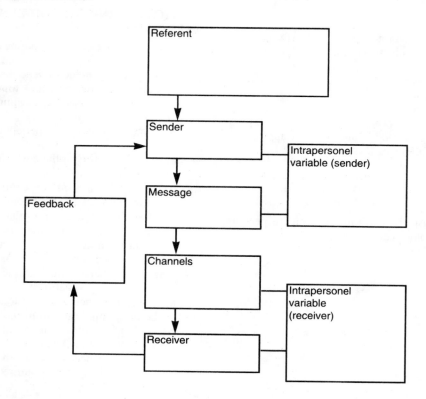

b. three factors you would assess to determine her readiness to learn.
c. two diagnoses of learning needs.
d. three learning objectives.
e. specific teaching methods.
f. potential methods of reinforcement
g. a description of evaluation techniques to measure client learning.

SKILL AND TECHNIQUE ACTIVITIES

1. Teaching methodologies
   a. Identify a specific target audience.
   b. Select a health maintenance topic such as breast self-examination, testicular self-examination, cancer warning signs, cancer prevention, or prudent living for a healthy heart.
   c. Organize a 10-minute teaching session that could be used for client education. Attempt to use more than one teaching technique.
   d. Record the teaching session on audiotape or videotape or present it to a peer group.
   e. Review the tape for self-evaluation and/or elicit peer and instructor feedback on your approach and methods.
2. Assessment of learning needs
   a. Conduct an assessment of an assigned client (or role play with a peer) to determine learning needs, motivation, ability to learn, teaching environment, and resources for learning.
   b. Formulate a prioritized list of diagnoses related to learning needs.
   c. Submit your assessment to your instructor for feedback.
3. Development of a teaching plan.
   a. After client assessment and diagnosis of a knowledge deficit, formulate learning objectives, outcome criteria, and specific teaching interventions. Submit your plan to your instructor for feedback before implementation.
   b. Evaluate your teaching session based on the stated outcome criteria and learning objectives.

Were the outcome criteria met? What contributed to a successful or unsuccessful outcome?
c. Describe modifications and revisions that would strengthen the teaching-learning experience.

ADDITIONAL READINGS

Barron S: Documentation of patient education, *Patient Educ Counsel* 9:81, 1987.
   Identifies major trends that require improved documentation of client education. Describes three specific standards to be incorporated into all documentation of client teaching. Discusses the processs of chart audit and development of a form for documentation of client education.
Fox V: Patient teaching: understanding the needs of the adult learner, *AORN J* 44:234, 1986.
   Contrasts pedagogical (teacher-directed) and androgogical (self-directed) teaching-learning styles. Briefly explores androgogical teaching strategies for the adult learner.
Leff EW: Ethics and patient teaching, *MCN* 11:375,1986.
   Examines ethical and legal dimensions of the nurse's teaching role and the dilemma that occurs when benefits perceived by the nurse conflict with the client's desire to know. Emphasizes the nurse's responsibilities to respect the client's autonomy in structuring a teaching program.
McHugh NG, Christman NJ, Honson JE: Prepatory information: what helps and why, *Am J Nurs* 82:780, 1982.
   Discusses study that revealed that sensory information was most useful in preparing clients for health care procedures. Presents guidelines for structuring preparatory information.
Moss RC: Overcoming fear: a review of research on patient, family instruction, *AORN J* 43:1107, 1986.
   Well-referenced discussion of current research addressing client preoperative instruction.
Redman BK: *The process of patient education*, ed 6, St Louis, 1988, Mosby–Year Book.
   A comprehensive text addressing theoretical and practical issues associated with client education. A valuable resource for students and experienced nurses.
Ward DB: Why patient teaching fails, *RN* 49:45, 1986.
   Identifies and describes six obstacles preventing clients from learning. Discusses nursing approaches to remove barriers and facilitate learning.

Chapter 17
Leadership and Management

PREREQUISITE READING
Chapter 17, pp. 382 to 393

OBJECTIVES
Mastery of content in this chapter will enable the student to:
- Define selected terms associated with leadership and management.
- Differentiate between leadership and management.
- Compare and contrast management theories in respect to their perspectives for improving productivity.
- Describe and give examples of the four classic leadership styles: authoritarian, democratic, laissez-faire, and situational.
- List and give examples of the four primary types of leadership skills that student nurses can begin to develop.
- Describe three phases of a change process.

REVIEW OF KEY CONCEPTS
1. Identify the major difference between leadership and management.
2. Match the leadership theory with the description provided.

Theory
   a. Trait development theory _____

   b. Scientific management theory _____

   c. Human relations movement _____

   d. Management process theory _____

   e. Theory X and theory Y _____

   f. Theory Z _____

Description
1. Proposes that managers' functions are the same regardless of setting and include planning, organizing, directing, and controlling
2. Proposes that power within an organization is derived from the interpersonal relationships within the work environment; emphasizes feelings and attitudes of employees
3. Proposes that leaders are born with certain qualities that determine their ability to lead
4. Proposes that employees have a predisposition to one of two specific attitudes and behaviors and the manager must address the specific traits to be effective in the leadership role
5. Emphasizes that job commitment and higher productivity are linked to employee participation in management or management decisions
6. Emphasizes technology as the basis for increasing productivity; uses time and motion studies to analyze tasks and improve efficiency

3. Describe the four styles of leadership behavior in situational management:
   a. Directing
   b. Coaching
   c. Supporting
   d. Delegating

4. Mr. Massie is the team leader on a busy surgical floor. The team members are upset with the evening client assignments. Mr. Massie tells the team members to work things out for themselves and that whatever they decide will be satisfactory. Mr. Massie's leadership style could best be described as:
   a. authoritarian.
   b. democratic.
   c. laissez-faire.
   d. situational.

5. The effective nurse manager is able to use different styles and leadership skills depending on the specific situation and the maturity of the employees. This is an example of which leadership style?
   a. Authoritarian
   b. Democratic
   c. Laissez-faire
   d. Situational

6. The authoritarian leader:
   a. promotes individual initiative and creativity.
   b. is concerned primarily about tasks and goals.
   c. establishes a two-way group communication pattern.
   d. distributes authority and responsibility to others.

7. During a cardiac arrest, which leadership style would be most effective?
   a. Authoritarian
   b. Democratic
   c. Laissez-faire
   d. Situational
8. List and describe the three stages of the change process.

   a.

   b.

   c.
9. Successful change is most likely when:
   a. the change is introduced quickly.
   b. the plan for change is loosely structured.
   c. the change is introduced by a specified leader.
   d. a need for the change is established.
10. List the four primary leadership skills for nurses and describe at least two behaviors characteristic of each skill.

    a.

    b.

    c.

    d.

CRITICAL THINKING AND EXPERIENTIAL EXERCISES

1. Leadership styles
   a. Identify a leader with whom you have worked. Describe the leadership style used by the leader. Provide examples of the leader's behaviors reflecting that style.
   b. Identify the leadership style or styles you believe create the best environment for your work productivity and personal development.
   c. Identify the leadership style with which you are most uncomfortable in the work or educational setting. How can you effectively work with a colleague who uses this leadership style?
   d. Examine the primary leadership skills for nurses that appear on p. 390 of your text. Complete a self-assessment, indicating which skills you believe you already possess and those you need to develop. For those needing development, identify at least one strategy for your personal development plan. Share the plan with your instructor.

2. Clinical situation: leadership styles
   Ms. White, a recent nursing graduate, has been assigned to provide care for five clients. She is having difficulty organizing her nursing activities to meet the demands of each client and those imposed by the established routine of the nursing unit. The head nurse is aware of Ms. White's problem. Provide an example illustrating the possible approach each of the following head nurses might use when addressing Ms. White's problem using the situational leadership mode.
   a. The head nurse who uses directing
   b. The head nurse who uses coaching
   c. The head nurse who uses supporting
   d. The head nurse who uses delegating
      If you were the new nurse in this situation, which leadership approach would you prefer? Why?

ADDITIONAL READINGS

Berhard L, Walsh M: *Leadership: the key to professionalization of nursing,* ed 2, St Louis, 1990, Mosby–Year Book.
   Approaches the development of leadership in nursing from a conceptual base. Explores various functions of the nurse leader in detail.
Douglas LM: *The effective nurse: leader and manager,* ed 4, St Louis, 1992, Mosby–Year Book.
   Comprehensively addresses a variety of topics related to leadership and management in nursing practice. Correlates management strategies with patterns of nursing care delivery and the nursing process. Devotes special sections to discussion of communication skills, conflict resolution, control, and legal and ethical issues. Is well referenced for additional direction in reading.
Hein E, Nicholson M: *Contemporary leadership behavior: selected readings,* ed 2, Boston, 1986, Little, Brown.
   Presents a variety of leadership behaviors that may be incorporated into progressive nursing practice. Organizes the collection of articles into areas, including the culture of nursing, modern leadership theories, contemporary leadership behaviors, evolving health organization settings, and the future of nursing practice. Is well referenced for additional reading.
McGovern W, Rogers J: Change theory, Am J Nurs 86:556, 1986.
   Discusses client care situations in which change theory was applied. Clearly links theory to practice.
Welch LB, editor: The nurse as change agent, *Nurs Clin North Am* 14(2), 1979.
   A collection of articles about change theory and strategies for the nurse to implement in the role of change agent. Presents the nurse as change agent in nursing service and education.

Chapter 18
Infection Control

PREREQUISITE READING
Chapter 18, pp. 396 to 453

OBJECTIVES
Mastery of content in this chapter will enable the student to:
- Define selected terms related to immunological function and infection control.
- Explain how each element of the infection-control chain contributes to infection.
- Identify the body's normal defenses against infection.
- Discuss the events in the inflammatory response.
- Explain the difference between cell-mediated and humoral immunity.
- Describe the nature of signs of a localized and systemic infection.
- Identify clients most at risk for acquiring infection.
- Explain conditions that promote the onset of nosocomial infections.
- Explain the difference between medical and surgical asepsis.
- Give an example for preventing infection for each element of the infection chain.
- Compare body substance isolation with universal blood and body fluid precautions.
- Identify principles of surgical asepsis.
- Correctly perform protective isolation techniques.
- Perform proper procedures for handwashing.
- Explain how infection-control measures may differ in the home versus the hospital.
- Properly apply a surgical mask, sterile gown, and sterile gloves.

REVIEW OF KEY CONCEPTS
1. Define infection.
2. List the six elements (in the chain) required to produce an infection.

   a.

   b.

   c.

   d.

   e.

   f.

3. Match the term associated with the chain of infection with the correct definition or description.

Chain of Infection
   a. Resident pathogen _____

   b. Carriers _____

   c. Aerobic bacteria _____

   d. Transient pathogens _____

   e. Anaerobic bacteria _____

   f. Virulence _____

   g. Susceptibility _____

Definition
1. Pathogenicity or strength of a disease-producing microorganism
2. Microorganisms usually picked up by the hands during activities of daily living (ADLs)
3. Degree of resistance to pathogens
4. Microorganisms normally present on the skin, not easily removed by washing
5. Persons or animals without symptoms of illness who are reservoirs of pathogens
6. Bacteria requiring free oxygen for survival
7. Bacteria that thrive in environments with little or no oxygen

4. The same microorganisms can be transmitted by more than one route. (True or false?)
5. List the four major routes through which microorganisms are transmitted from the reservoir to the host.

   a.

   b.

   c.

   d.

6. The severity of a client's illness will depend on all of the following except:
   a. extent of infection.
   b. pathogenicity of the microorganism.
   c. susceptibility of the host.
   d. incubation period.

7. Match the stages of the course of infection with the correct description.

Stage

   a. Prodromal period _____

   b. Convalescence _____

   c. Illness _____

   d. Incubation _____

Description

   1. Recovery period
   2. Interval between entrance of pathogen and symptom appearance
   3. Appearance of nonspecific symptoms
   4. Appearance of infection-specific symptoms

8. List the body's normal defenses against infection.

   a.

   b.

   c.

   d.

9. Norma flora:
   a. cause disease.
   b. maintain health.
   c. produce cellular injury.
   d. induce antibody production.

10. For each body system or organ, identify at least one defense mechanism and the primary action to prevent infection.

System/Organ	Defense mechanism	Action
Skin		
Mouth		
Respiratory tract		
Urinary tract		
Gastrointestinal tract		

11. Define inflammation.
12. Signs of local inflammation are also signs of local infection. (True or false?)
13. Identify five signs and symptoms of local inflammation.

   a.

   b.

   c.

   d.

   e.

14. Describe the three major events in the inflammatory response.

   a.

   b.

   c.

15. List seven signs and symptoms of systemic inflammation.

   a.

   b.

   c.

   d.

   e.

   f.

   g.

16. Match the term describing a component of immunity with the correct definition.

Component of immunity

   a. Immune response _____

   b. Cell-mediated response _____

   c. Humoral immune response _____

   d. Antibodies _____

   e. Foreign materials in the body _____

   f. Complement _____

   g. Interferon _____

Definition

   1. Antigens
   2. Synthesis of antibodies that destroy antigens
   3. Body response to foreign materials
   4. Proliferation of lymphocytes in response to a specific antigen.
   5. Immunoglobulins
   6. Substance that interferes with the ability of a virus to produce disease
   7. Enzyme activated when an antigen and antibody bind, causing cytolysis

17. Indicate the sequence of events in the immune response.

   a. Cell-mediated release of lymphocytes _____

   b. Antibodies circulating throughout the body _____

   c. Antigen entering the blood and lymphatic system _____

   d. Synthesis of antibodies _____

   e. Antibodies destroying the foreign antigen _____

18. Immunization against diseases is based on the immunological response of:
   a. antigen formation.
   b. cell-mediated reponse
   c. antibody formation.
   d. lymphocyte production.
19. Fill in the term that best completes each sentence.
   a. Infections resulting from health care delivery within a health care facility are _____ infections.
   b. Infections resulting from diagnostic or therapeutic procedures are _____ infections.
   c. Nosocomial infections caused by microorganisms that do not exist as normal flora are _____ infections.
   d. Nosocomial infections caused by an alteration and over growth in the client's body flora are _____ infections.
20. Describe at least three factors increasing a hospitalized client's risk of acquiring a nosocomial infection.

   a.

   b.

   c.
21. Which of the following clients would be at risk for infection related to inadequate primary defenses?
   a. Chronic smoker
   b. Client with anemia
   c. Client with leukopenia
   d. Client taking steroids
22. List six factors that influence an individual's susceptibility to infection.

   a.

   b.

   c.

   d.

   e.

   f.
23. An individual is most susceptible to infection during which segments of the life span?
   a. Infancy and childhood years
   b. Infancy and older adult years
   c. Adolescence and young adult years
   d. Middle and older adult years
24. A negative nitrogen balance will result in:
   a. increased resistance to infection.
   b. decreased resistance to infection.
   c. enhanced wound healing.
   d. increased protein breakdown.
25. Match each of the terms related to asepsis with the correct definition.

Term
   a. Asepsis _____
   b. Medical asepsis _____
   c. Surgical asepsis _____
   d. Sterile _____
   e. Contamination _____
   f. Disinfection _____
   g. Bacteriostatic _____
   h. Bacteriocidal _____

Definition
   1. Process by which an object becomes unsterile or unclean
   2. Term that describes an object free of microorganisms
   3. Absence of germs or pathogens
   4. Substance that kills bacteria but not spores
   5. Procedure used to eliminate microorganisms
   6. Process of destroying all pathogens except spores
   7. Procedure used to reduce the number of microorganisms and prevent their spread
   8. Substance that prevents bacterial growth
26. The most important and most basic technique in preventing and controlling the transmission of pathogens is _____
27. Identify six situations in which it is recommended that nurses wash their hands.

   a.

   b.

   c.

   d.

   e.

   f.
28. Match the nursing action with the element of the infection chain that is being controlled. (Answers may be used more than once.)

Nursing action
   a. Providing a client with a balanced diet _____
   b. Properly disposing of contaminated needles _____
   c. Changing wet or soiled dressings _____
   d. Washing hands _____
   e. Cleaning soiled equipment _____
   f. Wearing gloves when handling body fluids or exudates _____

g. Keeping the urinary drainage bag below the level of the client's bladder _____

h. Wearing a mask when working with a mild cold _____

i. Providing clients with personal sets of care items (e.g., bedpan, bath basin, thermometer) _____

Element of infection chain

1. Control or eliminate infection agents
2. Control or eliminate reservoirs
3. Control portals of exit
4. Control transmission
5. Control portals of entry
6. Protect susceptible host

29. List three goals for the client with an actual or potential risk for infection.

a.

b.

c.

30. List the two major nursing responsibilities in controlling infection.

a.

b.

31. When cleaning equipment is soiled by organic matter, the nurse should use:

a.

b.

c.

d.

32. The least expensive and most practical method for sterilizing items in the home is:
a. soaking in isopropyl alcohol for 60 minutes.
b. baking at 350 degrees for 30 minutes.
c. boiling in water for 15 minutes.
d. steaming in a pressure cooker for 10 minutes.

33. The technique used to control transmission of pathogens through barrier methods is:
a. surgical asepsis.
b. medical asepsis.
c. isolation.
d. sterilization.

34. List and describe the two systems used in implementing isolation.

a.

b.

35. Describe the purpose of each category-specific isolation technique.
a. Strict
b. Contact
c. Respiratory

d. Enteric precautions
e. Tuberculosis isolation
f. Drainage and secretion precautions
g. Universal blood and body fluid precautions
h. Care of the severely compromised client

36. Place an X under the barriers required to maintain protective asepsis for each category-specific isolation technique in the following table.

Type of isolation	Room	Gown	Gloves	Mask
Strict				
Contact				
Respiratory				
Enteric precautions				
Tuberculosis isolation				
Drainage and secretion precautions				
Universal blood and body fluid precautions				
Care of the severely compromised client				

37. Body substance isolation and universal blood and body fluid precautions include the same procedures. (True or false?)

38. Respond to option a or b.
a. List the 11 guidelines for universal precautions according to the Centers for Disease Control.
b. List the nine guidelines for body-substance isolation (BSI).

39. Describe the four basic principles of any isolation system.

a.

b.

c.

d.

40. List two major nursing actions reducing the negative psychological effects of isolation.

a.

b.

41. Individuals visiting an isolated client should wash their hands:
a. before entering and immediately after leaving the isolation room.
b. after entering and before leaving the isolation room.
c. every time they touch the client.
d. after leaving the isolation room.

42. The primary reason for gowning during protective asepsis is to:
   a. keep warm because the isolation room is usually cool.
   b. ensure that the client is not exposed to the organisms on the nurse's uniform.
   c. maintain a sterile environment when providing client care.
   d. prevent soiling of clothing during contact with the client.

43. When gloves are used during protective asepsis, they should be changed after coming in contact with any infected material, even if the client's care has not been completed. (True or false?)

44. When a client on respiratory isolation must be transported to another part of the hospital, the nurse:
   a. places a mask on the client before leaving the room.
   b. obtains a physician's order to prohibit the client from being transported.
   c. advises other health team members to wear masks and gowns when coming in contact with the client.
   d. instructs the client to cover the mouth and nose with a tissue when coughing or sneezing.

45. To ensure maximal effectiveness of masks worn in an isolation room, the nurse should do all of the following *except:*
   a. discard the mask if it becomes moist.
   b. reuse the mask if it has not been contaminated.
   c. change the mask every hour.
   d. fit the mask snugly over the mouth and nose.

46. A single, impervious, sturdy bag is adequate for discarding or wrapping items being removed from an isolated environment. (True or false?)

47. Indicate the proper sequence that the nurse follows when removing protective clothing that has been worn in an isolation room.
   a. Remove mask. _____
   b. Wash hands. _____
   c. Remove gloves. _____
   d. Leave room. _____
   e. Remove gown. _____

48. List five responsibilities of the infection-control nurse.
   a.
   b.
   c.
   d.
   e.

49. Surgical aseptic techniques are only practiced in specialized areas such as the operating room or the labor and delivery area. (True or false?)

50. List three teaching points to to reduce the risk of client-associated contamination during sterile procedures or treatments.
   a.
   b.
   c.

51. Based on principles of sterile technique, analyze each situation and determine whether sterile items would remain sterile (S) or would be rendered contaminated (C).
   a. A sterile tray is set up on a client's over-bed tray below the level of the nurse's waist. _____
   b. A nurse's ungloved hand positions a sterile drape by grasping the outer 1-inch border. _____
   c. A sterile tray is covered with a clean towel. _____
   d. A client's sterile dressing is being applied while the roommate's bed is being made. _____
   e. The nurse holds the tips of forceps, previously stored in disinfectant, with the tips down. _____
   f. A sealed, sterile dressing package is placed on a wet table surface. _____

52. A staff nurse is performing a sterile dressing change assisted by the head nurse. The staff nurse thinks that the sterile glove may have been contaminated by a brush against the client's arm. The nurse should:
   a. ask the head nurse whether he or she observed sterile technique being broken.
   b. ask the client whether he or she felt the nurse touch the arm.
   c. continue with the dressing change.
   d. stop and ask the head nurse to get another set of sterile gloves.

53. Indicate the sequence that should be followed to maintain sterile asepsis in the operating room.
   a. Wash hands. _____
   b. Put on sterile gloves. _____
   c. Put on mask and cap. _____
   d. Put on sterile gown. _____

54. When a surgical mask becomes moist, the nurse in the delivery room should:
   a. leave the delivery room and change masks.
   b. reposition the mask so that the area over the mouth and nose will be dry.
   c. apply a second mask over the first.
   d. remain in the room and change masks.

55. Describe the method for surgical handwashing using the following criteria:
   a. Disposition of jewelry
   b. Care of the nails
   c. Areas to be washed

d. Duration of scrub
e. Equipment required
f. Position of hands and arms
g. Method for drying

56. When the color of a chemical tape on a sterile item remains unchanged, the item is considered sterile. (True or false?)
57. When opening commercially packaged sterile items, the nurse tears the wrapper away from the body. (True or false?)
58. When adding sterile supplies to a sterile field, it is acceptable to flip or toss objects onto the field to minimize contamination. (True or false?)
59. To maintain sterility of solutions, it is important for the nurse to:
    a. place the lid sterile side down on a clean surface.
    b. pour a small amount of solution to cleanse the lip of the bottle.
    c. hold the bottle high over the sterile field to avoid splashing.
    d. pour the solution quickly to avoid contaminating the bottle.
60. What part of a sterile gown is considered sterile?
    a. Back
    b. Anterior surface—below the collar to the waist
    c. Anterior and posterior surface of the arms
    d. All of the above
61. Describe the seven steps for application of a sterile drape with ungloved hands.

    a.

    b.

    c.

    d.

    e.

    f.

    g.

62. In most home situations, it is aceptable for clients to use clean rather than sterile techniques. (True or false?)
63. List seven topics that may be incorporated into a client teaching session addressing infection prevention and control.

    a.

    b.

    c.

    d.

    e.

    f.

    g.

CRITICAL THINKING AND EXPERIENTAL EXERCISES

1. Microorganism transmission
   a. After an observation or client care experience, identify how microorganism spread may be facilitated in a health care setting. For each of the four major routes of transmission, cite at least one method for organism transmission and at least one action that the nurse can take to break this link in the infection chain.

Route	Transmission method	Nursing action
Contact		
Air		
Vehicle		
Vectors		

2. Nosocomial infection
   a. After an observational or client care experience in an institutional setting, list at least two causes or sources of nosocomial infection for each of the sites listed.
   b. For each of the causes or sources of infection listed, describe nursing actions you observed or enacted that helped to reduce the risk of nosocomial infection.

Site	Source or Cause of Infection	Preventive Measures
Urinary tract		
Surgical wounds		
Respiratory tract		
Bloodstream		

3. Isolation
   Care for, interview, or review the medical record of a client requiring isolation. Answer the following questions and include specific examples to illustrate these concepts.
   a. For what organism has the client been isolated?
   b. What is the means of transmission for the organism?
   c. What barrier methods must be used to protect individuals coming in contact with the client?
   d. What instructions should be given to the client's visitors about using isolation precautions?
   e. Develop three nursing diagnoses addressing the psychological implications of isolation. For each diagnosis, identify one goal and describe at least two pertinent nursing interventions.
4. Client education: infection control
   a. Terry Summers, 37 years old, is a single parent of two school-age children. Two weeks before, Ms. Summers was in an automobile accident.

The traumatic injury she sustained became infected. Although she has recovered sufficiently to return home, she continues to have a draining leg wound infected with *Staphyloccoccus* organisms. A home health care nurse will be visiting to perform needed dressing changes. Devise a teaching plan for Ms. Summers to promote compliance with infection-control and infection-prevention practices.

5. Clinical situation: susceptibility to infection
James Miller, 83 years old, is admitted to the hospital for abdominal surgery. Although he previously has been able to care for himself, Mr. Miller's appearance indicates that he has been unable to bathe or perform oral hygiene. Because of his physical condition, Mr. Miller has also been unable to prepare or eat solid foods for several days and reports that his diet has been composed primarily of ginger ale and soup. He has a 50-year history of cigarette smoking. He currently has intravenous (IV) fluids infusing in his right hand.
   a. Which of Mr. Miller's normal body system defense mechanisms have been altered, increasing the risk of infection.
   b. What other factors increase Mr. Miller's susceptibility to infection. For each factor, describe the associated physiological changes reducing resistance to infection.
   c. The presence of an IV line predisposes Mr. Miller to local infection (phlebitis).
      (1) What observations would indicate that this complication has occurred?
      (2) Describe the physiological mechanisms that produce these signs and symptoms.
   d. After surgery, Mr. Miller requires oral and nasotracheal suctioning. Explain why oral suctioning requires medical aseptic technique and nasotracheal suctioning requires sterile technique.

SKILL AND TECHNIQUE ACTIVITIES

1. Hand-washing technique
   a. Practice the proper procedure for handwashing while a peer observes and critiques your performance.
   b. Elicit an instructor's evaluation of your handwashing technique during a clinical laboratory experience.
2. Isolation techniques
   a. Examine your institution's infection control policies. Determine whether your institution uses body-substance isolation, universal precautions, category-specific guidelines or disease-specific isolation guidelines.
   b. Examine isolation equipment/materials for client care in your institution.
   c. Practice masking, gowning, and gloving techniques for isolation while a peer observes and critiques your performance.
   d. Elicit an instructor's evaluation of your masking, gowning, and gloving techniques for isolation.
   e. Identify a client hospitalized with a communicable disease. Using your institution's infection control protocol, determine the barrier methods that must be applied.
   f. Observe other hospital staff members as they implement protective isolation techniques. Discuss your observations with your instructor.
3. Surgical aseptic technique
   a. Examine your institution's policies about surgical handwashing techniques.
   b. Practice surgical handwashing techniques while a peer observes and critiques your performance.
   c. Elicit an instructor's evaluation of your surgical handwashing technique.
   d. Practice the series of steps to maintain surgical aseptic technique (mask, cap, surgical handwashing, sterile gown and gloves) while a peer observes and critiques your performance.
   e. Elicit an instructor's evaluation of your surgical aseptic technique.
   f. Practice handwashing and open-gloving techniques (used in general care areas) while a peer observes and critiques your performance.
   g. Elicit an instructor's evaluation of your handwashing and open-gloving technique.
   h. Observe other hospital staff members as they use sterile technique. Discuss your observations with your instructor.
   i. Practice setting up a sterile field with items provided by your instructor. Have a peer observe and critique your performance.
   j. Elicit and instructor's evaluation as you set up a sterile field.

ADDITIONAL READINGS

Bennett J: Nurses talk about the challenge of AIDS, *Am J Nurs* 87:1150, 1987.
   Presents eight clinicians discussing their concerns and opinions about care of the client with acquired immunodeficiency syndrome (AIDS).
Bjerke NB, editor: Infection control in critical care units, *Crit Care Nurs Q* 11(4), 1989.
   Addresses infection in the intensive care unit in a series of articles. Presents techniques applicable to any acute care setting. Covers asepsis in client care, wound care, nosocomial infections, and antimicrobial toxicity.
Burtis R, Evangelisti J: Will universal precautions protect me? A look at the staff nurse's attitudes, *Nurs Outlook* 40(3):133, 1992.
   Reports the results of a survey of nurses' attitudes in caring for clients with AIDS and hepatitis B. Expresses concern that nurses are uninformed about modes of disease transmission.

Grady C, editor: AIDS, *Nurs Clin North Am* 23:4, 1988.
    Addresess, in a series, the epidemiology, pathophysiology, and treatment of AIDS. Examines complex nursing care needs of adults and children infected with the human immunodeficiency virus (HIV). Discusses ethical and other practice-related issues associated with the care of clients with HIV.

Larson EL: Handwashing: it's essential even when you use gloves, *Am J Nurs* 89:934, 1989.
    Reports on research regarding handwashing and glove-wearing techniques. Describes the level of protection offered by gloves. Reemphasizes the importance of handwashing techniques.

Chapter 19
Vital Signs

PREREQUISITE READING
Chapter 19, pp. 454 to 505

OBJECTIVES
Mastery of content in this chapter will enable the student to:
- Define selected terms associated with vital sign measurement.
- Identify when vital signs should be taken.
- Explain the principles and mechanisms of thermoregulation.
- Discuss the rationale for a care plan for a client with a fever.
- Identify steps used to assess oral, rectal, axillary, and tympanic membrane temperature.
- Explain the physiology for the regulation of temperature, pulse, respirations, and blood pressure.
- Describe the types of factors normally causing variations in body temperature, pulse, respirations, and blood pressure.
- Identify steps used to assess pulse, respirations, and blood pressure.
- Identify normal vital signs for an adult and an infant.
- Explain variations in technique used to assess an infant's and a child's vital signs.
- Describe the benefits and precautions involving self-measurement of blood pressure.
- Accurately record and report vital sign measurements.

REVIEW OF KEY CONCEPTS
1. List at least five situations in which it is necessary to take a client's vital signs.
   a.
   b.
   c.
   d.
   e.
2. A person's normal body temperature may vary above or below 37° C (98.6° F). (True or false?)
3. The part of the brain responsible for controlling body temperature is the _____ .
4. The skin plays a role in temperature regulation by:
   a. insulating the body.
   b. constricting blood vessels.
   c. sensing external temperature variations.
   d. all of the above.
5. List four sources or mechanisms for heat production.
   a.

   b.

   c.

   d.
6. Match the mechanisms for body heat loss with the example provided.

Mechanism
   a. Conduction _____
   b. Convection _____
   c. Radiation _____
   d. Evaporation _____

Example
   1. Bathing the client in tepid water
   2. Placing a cooling blanket over a febrile client
   3. Release of sweat in response to temperature elevation
   4. Wearing lightweight, light-colored clothing
7. List three groups of clients who may experience difficulty in maintaining body temperature and briefly explain why this may occur.
   a.
   b.
   c.
8. In the absence of fever, the nurse expects a client's body temperature to peak between:
   a. 1 and 4 AM.
   b. 6 and 10 AM.
   c. 10 AM and 2 PM.
   d. 4 and 7 PM.
9. Define fever.
10. Which statement about fever is incorrect?
   a. Chilling occurs as the body's attempt to increase heat loss.
   b. Fever results from an alteration in the hypothalamic set point.

c. Metabolism and oxygen consumption increase during fever.

d. Fever may be caused by conditions other than infection.

11. Health care providers generally agree that all fever should be treated. (True or false?)

12. In children under age 5, rapidly elevated temperature may cause _____ .

13. List at least five assessment areas for the febrile client.

a.

b.

c.

d.

e.

14. Describe how antipyretic medications act to reduce fever.

15. Mr. Silverman is experiencing a fever of 39° C (102.2° F). Which nursing measure would be appropriate during the course of the fever?

a. Bathe the client in cold water.

b. Raise the room temperature to avoid chills.

c. Encourage activity to maintain energy levels.

d. Provide at least 3000 ml of fluid per day.

16. Identify at least three goals for care of a client with fever.

a.

b.

c.

17. A thermal disorder characterized by hot, dry skin; elevated temperature; tachycardia; and hypotension is:

a. hypothermia.

b. heat exhaustion.

c. heat stroke.

d. fever.

18. The assessment site most closely reflecting core body temperature is:

a. oral.

b. rectal.

c. axillary.

d. tympanic.

19. In the examples given, indicate the acceptable method(s) for measuring the client's temperature: O, oral; R, rectal; R, axillary; T, tympanic. (Tympanic is not available in all settings.)

a. An infant who is restless, irritable, and crying _____

b. An adult after surgical repair of a fractured mandible _____

c. An adult receiving continuous oxygen therapy through nasal cannula _____

d. An adolescent who is confused and has traction applied to the left leg _____

e. An adult who is alert and ambulatory _____

20. Disposable gloves should be worn when taking an oral or rectal temperature. (True or false?)

21. Compare and contrast the three methods for assessing temperature of adults and children by completing the table below.

Site	Type of glass thermometer	Time left in place	Client's position	Special precautions
Oral				
Rectal				
Axillary				

22. Convert the following temperature readings:

a. 100.4° F to C

b. 38.3° C to F

c. 98° F to C

d. 39.4° C to F

23. Which of the following statements about pulse regulation is inaccurate?

a. The medulla regulates heart rate through sympathetic and parasympathetic stimulation.

b. The heart maintains a relatively constant blood flow despite heart rate variations.

c. Mechanical, neural, and chemical factors influence heart contractions.

d. The pulse rate provides a direct measurement of cardiac output.

24. With each ventricular contraction the heart pumps 80 ml of blood. Assessment of the heart rate for 15 seconds reveals a value of 18.

a. What is the pulse rate?

b. What is the cardiac output?

c. Is the cardiac output normal?

25. When a client's condition suddenly deteriorates, where is the best pulse assessment site?

a. Radial

b. Apical

c. Carotid

d. Femoral

26. List three situations in which it is preferable to assess the apical pulse.

a.

b.

c.

27. The best site for assessing an infant's or young child's pulse is:

a. carotid.

b. brachial.

c. femoral.

d. apical.

28. List four characteristics to identify during peripheral pulse assessment. By using an asterisk, specify the

two characteristics evaluated when assessing an apical pulse.

a.

b.

c.

d.

29. To accurately assess pulse rate, the nurse should:
   a. know that the pulse typically increases with age.
   b. know that postural changes will not alter the pulse.
   c. recognize that anxiety lowers the heart rate.
   d. measure the pulse when the client is at rest.
30. Match the term with the most accurate description or definition.

Term

a. Tachycardia _____

b. Bradycardia _____

c. Dysrhythmia _____

d. Pulse deficit _____

e. Doppler _____

f. Diaphragm _____

g. Telemetry _____

h. Bell _____

Description

1. Electronic stethoscope that magnifies sounds
2. Abnormal, irregular heart rhythm
3. Stethoscope chest piece that best amplifies heart and vascular sounds
4. Adult heart rate greater than 100 beats/min
5. Concurrent pulses: apical 110, radial 90
6. Adult heart rate less than 60 beats/min
7. Stethoscope chest piece that best amplifies bowel and lung sounds
8. Continuous monitoring transmitted to a stationary monitor screen

31. Compare and contrast the three methods for pulse assessment by completing the table.

Site	Equipment needed	Length of time	Indications	Special techniques or precautions
Radial				
Apical				
Apical-radial				

32. Match the terms associated with respiration with the definitions provided.

Term

a. External respiration _____

b. Internal respiration _____

c. Ventilation _____

d. Conduction _____

e. Diffusion _____

f. Perfusion _____

Definition

1. Distribution of blood through pulmonary capillaries
2. Mechanical movement of air to and from the lungs
3. Movement of air between the environment and lungs
4. Movement of oxygen and carbon dioxide between alveoli and red blood cells (RBCs)
5. Movement of oxygen between hemoglobin and single cells
6. Movement of air through lungs and other airways

33. The most important factor controlling ventilation in the typical adult is the arterial blood:
   a. oxygen.
   b. carbon dioxide.
   c. pH.
   d. hemoglobin.
34. a. What is the breathing stimulus for a client with chronic lung disease?
   b. Why does this occur?
35. Describe how each of the following conditions may affect ventilatory movements.
   a. Chest wall pain
   b. Anemia
   c. Pneumothorax
   d. Emphysema
36. List three objective measurements used in respiratory status assessment.

   a.

   b.

   c.

37. Respiratory rate may decrease with:
   a. fever.
   b. exercise.
   c. pain.
   d. narcotic analgesics.
38. Fill in the blank with the most appropraite term associated with respiratory assessment.

   a. Difficulty in breathing _____
   b. A harsh, crowing sound associated with airway obstruction _____
   c. Regular but abnormally rapid breathing

   _____

d. Temporary cessation of respirations _____

e. Inability to breathe comfortably while lying down _____

39. Label the two alterations in respirations by comparing each with the normal respiratory pattern included.

a. _____

b. _____

c. _____

40. Fill in each group's normal respiratory rates.

a. Infants _____

b. Children _____

c. Adults _____

41. List four areas to incorporate into the respiratory status assessment (other than rate, depth, and rhythm).

a.

b.

c.

d.

42. Define the following terms.

a. Blood pressure

b. Systolic

c. Diastolic

43. The client's blood pressure is 116/59.

a. What is the diastolic pressure?

b. What is the systolic pressure?

c. What is the pulse pressure?

44. Indicate the effect of each variable on blood pressure by writing ↑ BP (for increased blood pressure) or ↓ BP (for decreased blood pressure).

a. Diuretic medication _____

b. Decreased cardiac output _____

c. Acute pain _____

d. Increased blood volume _____

e. Increased blood viscosity _____

f. Anxiety _____

g. Hemorrhage _____

h. Advancing age _____

i. Increased peripheral vascular resistance _____

45. What are the criteria for diagnosis of hypertension in an adult?

46. When a nurse assesses a client's blood pressure for the first time it is especially important to:

a. compare blood pressures in both arms.

b. have the client lie down for the first reading.

c. have the client perform light exercise before measurement.

d. use the bell of the stethoscope for auscultation.

47. Which sphygmomanometer provides the most consistent, accurate blood pressure measurement?

a. Aneroid

b. Mercury

c. Portable home monitoring devices

d. Stationary automated machines

48. The nurse is auscultating Mrs. McKinnon's blood pressure. The nurse inflates the cuff to 180 mm Hg. At 156 mm Hg the nurse hears the onset of a tapping sound. At 130 mm Hg the sound changes to a murmur or swishing. At 100 mm Hg the sound momentarily becomes sharper, and at 92 mm Hg it becomes muffled. At 88 mm Hg the sound disappears.

a. What is Mrs. McKinnon's blood pressure?

b. Is it within normal limits?

49. Place the following steps for auscultating blood pressure in their proper sequence.

a. Palpate radial pulse and inflate cuff 30 mm Hg above point pulsation disappears. _____

b. Slowly release valve at 2 to 3 mm Hg per second. _____

c. Palpate brachial artery and place cuff 2.5 cm (1 inch) above pulsation site. _____

d. Place stethoscope's diaphragm over brachial artery. _____

e. Note point on manometer at which sound disappears. _____

f. Inflate cuff 30 mm Hg above client's normal systolic value. _____

g. Deflate cuff rapidly and wait 30 seconds. _____

h. Note point on manometer at which first sound is heard. _____

50. Which of the following statements about blood pressure assessment is accurate?

a. Systolic pressure in the legs is usually lower than in the brachial artery.

b. Blood pressure should be measured in the arm with the lower pressure.

c. Two minutes should elapse before repeating measurements in the same arm.

d. A difference of 12 mm Hg in readings between arms is considered normal.

51. Describe auscultatory gap.

52. List two methods the nurse may use to assess blood pressure when Korotkoff sounds are not audible with the standard stethoscope.

    a.

    b.

53. Clients should be advised that stationary automated blood pressure machines in public places are often unreliable. (True or false?)

CRITICAL THINKING AND EXPERIENTIAL EXERCISES

1. Client with fever
Care for, or review the medical record of, a client experiencing a fever.
    a. Assess the client and identify defining characteristics associated with fever.
    b. Trace the fever pattern manifested by the client. Determine whether the pattern is characteristic of those described in your text.
    c. Formulate nursing diagnoses that relate to the problems associated with the client's fever. For each diagnosis, identify at least one goal and describe at least two pertinent nursing interventions and their rationales.
    d. Compare the medical therapies prescribed for the client with those described in your text.

2. Clinical situation: vital sign assessment
Mr. West is admitted to the hospital complaining of chest pain and feeling dizzy for the last 24 hours.
    a. To assess Mr. West's vital signs accurately, the nurse needs to obtain what three categories of information from a previous medical record?
    b. The physician examines Mr. West and orders oxygen therapy. Blood samples are also ordered. A medication is ordered to improve cardiac function. Mr. West is scheduled to have a cardiac catheterization to diagnose the extent of any heart disease. In relation to this information, when should the nurse assess Mr. West's vital signs?
    c. At 0800 (8 AM) Mr. West's radial pulse is 88 and regular. At 1200 (noon) the nurse assesses the radial pulse to be 100 and irregular. What actions should the nurse take at this time?
    d. Mr. West is very anxious about the hospitalization. He has never received heart medications before. Even though he is feeling better, the chest pain occasionally recurs. The physician has discussed the plan of care with Mr. West and orders a fat-free, low-sodium diet. Which of the conditions just described could affect Mr. West's pulse rate? Why?
    e. Late one evening, the nurse enters Mr. West's room to find him in respiratory distress. He states, "I can't get my breath." His respiratory rate is approximately 32 breaths/min. Respirations are shallow with evidence of increased chest wall movement. The rhythm of respirations is regular.

        (1) How would these respirations be described?
        (2) What changes might you expect in Mr. West's other vital signs?
    f. During the episode of respiratory distress, Mr. West's nurse assesses a blood pressure of 90/70. A second nurse immediately checks the blood pressure again and gets a reading of 114/60. Assuming the second reading is accurate, what factors might have caused the first nurse to assess the pressure of 90/70?

3. Clinical situation: client education, heat stroke
    a. A group of Boy Scouts (ages 10 to 12) invites you to talk to the group about heat stroke in preparation for the group's annual summer hike. Devise a developmentally appropriate teaching program for the scouts, including prevention measures, symptoms, and treatment.

4. Clinical situation: client education, hypertension
Mr. Williams is a 50-year-old black man recently diagnosed with hypertension. His history indicates that he is 20% above his desired body weight, smokes about 10 cigarettes per day, and enjoys a glass of wine before dinner. He reports that his work is extremely stressful and often requires him to travel two or three times per month. His physician has prescribed antihypertensive drugs, home blood pressure monitoring, and lifestyle changes. Mr. Williams is concerned that his children (10 and 24 years old) are at risk. He repeatedly states that his blood pressure is "back to normal" and he feels fine. He tells you, the nurse, "You know, lots of people have high blood pressure; it's no big thing."
    a. How would you explain hypertension and its effects on the body to Mr. Williams?
    b. What are the risks for Mr. Williams' children? What factors may increase their risk for development of hypertension?
    c. Mr. Williams is uncomfortable with the idea of checking his own blood pressure with the mercury sphygmomanometer and asks about using the electronic digital readout devices or the automated machines he sees at airports and drug stores. How would you advise Mr. Williams about these different types of blood pressure monitoring equipment?
    d. Devise a teaching plan for Mr. Williams designed to promote compliance with his medical regimen and successful control of his blood pressure.

SKILL AND TECHNIQUE ACTIVITIES

1. Temperature assessment
    a. Examine your institution's policy and procedures for temperature assessment.
    b. Examine the variety of thermometers available within your institution. Practice handling the thermometer that you will be using in the clinical setting.

BARNES HOSPITAL
GRAPHIC SHEET B - 1

TEMPERATURE

STAMP ADDRESSOGRAPH PLATE HERE

Centigrade

O = Oral
R = Rectal
A = Axilliary

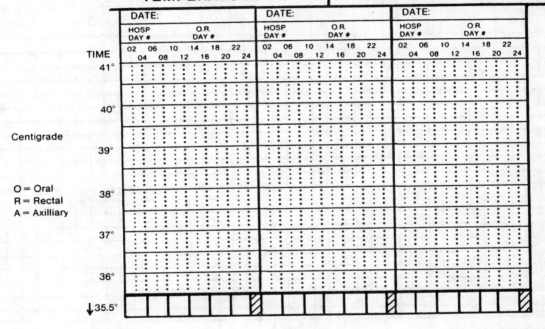

PULSE

X = Pulse
a = Apical

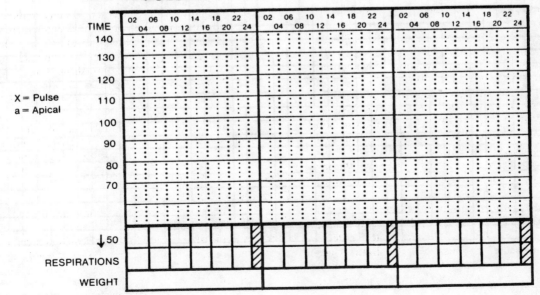

RESPIRATIONS

WEIGHT

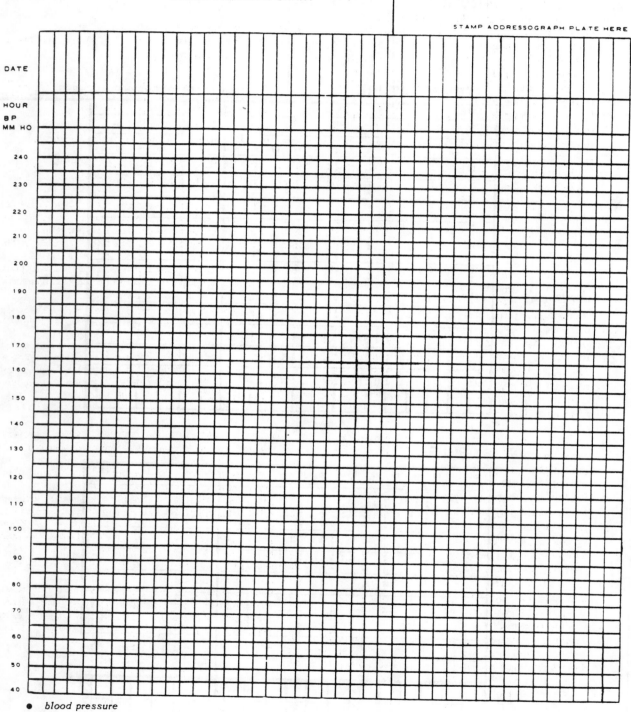

BARNES HOSPITAL
BLOOD PRESSURE CHART

c. Practice the proper procedure for taking an oral temperature while a peer observes and critiques your performance.

d. Using a mannequin in your nursing laboratory, practice the proper procedure for taking a rectal and an axillary temperature while a peer observes and critiques your performance.

e. Obtain several mercury-in-glass thermometers. In a small group, have each member assess and record his or her own temperature. Clean the thermometer with alcohol, but do not "shake down" the thermometer. Exchange thermometers and read the registered temperature. Compare results.

f. Elicit an instructor's evaluation of your temperature assessment technique, including validation of the temperature reading.

2. Pulse assessment
   a. With a partner, locate the following sites for pulse assessment: temporal, carotid, brachial, radial, femoral, popliteal, posterior tibial, dorsalis pedis, and apical.
   b. Practice the technique for obtaining radial and apical pulses. Ask a peer to critique your performance.
   c. In groups of three, practice obtaining a radial-apical pulse rate.
   d. Elicit an instructor's evaluation of your pulse assessment technique, including validation of the pulse rate.

3. Respiration assessment
   a. Practice the technique for measuring respirations. Ask a peer to critique your performance.
   b. Elicit an instructor's evaluation of your respiration assessment technique, including validation of the respiratory rate.

4. Blood pressure assessment
   a. Examine aneroid and mercury sphygmomanometers. Practice handling the pieces of each type with particular attention to reading the scale and opening and closing the bulb with one hand.
   b. Practice the technique for blood pressure assessment. Ask a peer to critique your performance.
   c. If a teaching stethoscope (one chest piece, two sets of ear pieces) is available, obtain one. Practice assessing blood pressure with an instructor or experienced student listening with you.
   d. Elicit an instructor's evaluation of your blood pressure assessment technique, including validation of the blood pressure reading.

5. Vital sign assessment
   a. Practice obtaining temperature, radial pulse, respirations, and blood pressure in an organized fashion. Ask a peer to critique your performance.

b. Set up a blood pressure screening session with other students at your school. Be sure to involve a nursing faculty member who can serve as a consultant.

c. As your confidence and skill increase, participate in a blood pressure screening program in your community.

6. Recording vital signs
   a. Obtain and examine vital sign graphic sheets or charts used at your institution.
   b. Obtain a set of vital signs on a partner (or create a set of vital signs) and record these on the forms supplied by your institution (or on the forms provided on pp. 69 and 70).
   c. Submit your vital sign charting to your instructor to confirm the accuracy of your recordings.

ADDITIONAL READINGS

Birdsall C: How accurate are your blood pressures? *Am J Nurs* 84(11):1414, 1984.

Summarizes four critical components of blood pressure measurement techniques. Places emphasis on ways to increase accuracy of blood pressure assessment.

Birdsall C: How do you interpret pulses? *Am J Nurs* 85(7):786, 1985.

Brief overview of characteristics to evaluate during pulse assessment. Includes descriptions of a variety of diagnostic pulses.

Erickson R, Yount S: Comparison of tympanic membrane and oral temperatures in surgical patients, *Nurs Res* 40(2):90, 1991.

Presents study of tympanic and oral temperature readings in preoperative clients. Demonstrates that tympanic temperature is more sensitive to effects of intervention than oral temperature. Indicates close correlation between tympanic and oral temperature readings.

McCarron K: Fever: the cardinal vital sign, *Crit Care Q* 9(1):15, 1986.

Brief overview of thermoregulation, fever mechanisms, and current research addressing fever management.

Norman E, Gadaleta D, Griffin CC: An evaluation of three blood pressure methods in a stabilized acute trauma population, *Nurs Res* 40(2):86, 1991.

Discusses indirect blood pressure measurement using the bell and diaphragm methods with the direct internal arterial measurement. Suggests that determination of Korotkoff sounds 1, 4, and 5 through direct and indirect methods is not significantly different in stable patients.

Reeves-Swift R: Rational management of a child's acute fever, *MCN* 15(2):82, 1990.

Overviews the physiological basis of fever. Emphasizes the therapeutic benefits of fever and provides guidelines for nursing management. Includes possible complications associated with fever and briefly addresses use of antipyretics.

Chapter 20
Physical Examination and Health Assessment

PREREQUISITE READING
Chapter 20, pp. 506 to 609

OBJECTIVES
Mastery of content in this chapter will enable the student to:
- Define selected terms related to physical examination and health assessment.
- Discuss the purposes of physical assessment.
- Describe the techniques used with each physical assessment skill.
- Describe the proper position for the client during each phase of the examination.
- List techniques used to promote the client's physical and psychological comfort during an examination.
- Make environmental preparations before an examination.
- Identify information to collect from the nursing history before an examination.
- Discuss normal physical findings for a young and middle-age adult compared with those for an older adult.
- Discuss ways to incorporate health teaching into the examination.
- Conduct physical assessments in an organized and proper fashion.
- Describe physical measurements made in the assessment of each body system.
- Identify self-screening examination commonly performed by clients.

REVIEW OF KEY CONCEPTS
1. List five nursing purposes for performing a physical assessment.

   a.

   b.

   c.

   d.

   e.
2. Baseline data refer to the normal values or findings expected during physical examination. (True or false?)

3. List four principles to facilitate accurate inspection of body parts.

   a.

   b.

   c.

   d.
4. Which statement describing the technique of palpation is accurate?
   a. Tender areas should be palpated first to reduce client apprehension.
   b. Light palpation requires that tissues be depressed approximately 2 cm (1 inch).
   c. Student nurses should only attempt deep palpation with an instructor's assistance.
   d. The client should be encouraged to hold the breath to minimize abdominal wall movement.
5. Identify the parts of the hand used to assess each of the following:
   a. Temperature
   b. Pulsations
   c. Vibrations
   d. Turgor
6. Describe the bimanual palpation technique.
7. What information is obtained through percussion?
8. To correctly perform indirect percussion, the nurse:
   a. keeps the wrist extended and tensed when striking the finger.
   b. places the middle finger of the dominant hand over the body's surface.
   c. delivers a sharp, quick stroke to the finger placed against the body.
   d. quickly strikes the body surface directly with one or two fingers.
9. Match the anatomical area with the percussion sound expected.

Sound
   a. Middle of the anterior surface of the thigh ____
   b. Left lower anterior aspect of the rib cage ____

c. Posterior aspect of the thorax _____

d. Right seventh intercostal space _____

Anatomical area

1. Tympany
2. Dullness
3. Resonance
4. Flatness

10. To auscultate body parts correctly, the nurse:
    a. stretches the tubing its full length before placing the chest piece.
    b. learns the normal characteristics for each type of sound auscultated.
    c. uses the bell for assessment of lung and bowel sounds.
    d. holds the bell firmly against the skin.

11. The sense of smell may help the nurse detect abnormalities that cannot be recognized by any other means. (True or false?)

12. List at least three environmental factors that the nurse should attempt to control before performing a physical examination.

    a.

    b.

    c.

13. The component that should receive the highest priority before a physical examination is:
    a. preparation of the environment.
    b. preparation of the equipment.
    c. physical preparation of the client.
    d. psychological preparation of the client.

14. Match the client position or positions with the body part to be examined. (There may be more than one correct position for selected body parts.)

Body part

a. Heart _____

b. Abdomen _____

c. Posterior aspect of the thorax _____

d. Female genitalia _____

e. Prostate _____

Position

1. Supine
2. Lithotomy
3. Dorsal recumbent
4. Sims'
5. Sitting

15. The purpose of having a third person who is of the client's gender in the room during the physical examination is to:
    a. observe the client's emotional responses and inform the examiner.
    b. assure the client that the examiner will behave in an ethical manner.

c. respond to the client's questions so that the examiner may work without interruption.

d. validate any abnormal findings that the examiner elicits.

16. Identify at least one variation in the nurse's interview style appropriate for an individual from each of the specified age groups.
    a. Infants and younger children
    b. Older children
    c. Adolescents
    d. Older adults

17. List three assessment components of the general survey.

    a.

    b.

    c.

18. List eight specific observations included in the assessment of the client's general appearance and behavior.

    a.

    b.

    c.

    d.

    e.

    f.

    g.

    h.

19. Before measuring a client's height and weight, the nurse should:
    a. ask the client his or her height and weight.
    b. ask if there has been a recent change in weight.
    c. calibrate the scale by setting the weight at zero.
    d. all of the above.

20. List three actions that should be taken to ensure accurate weight measurement of a hospitalized client.

    a.

    b.

    c.

21. Describe how a nurse would measure the height of a client unable to stand or bear weight.

22. For each skin color variation, identify the mechanism producing color change, common causes of the variation, and optimal sites for assessment.

Skin Color	Mechanisms	Causes	Assessment Sites
Cyanosis			
Pallor			
Jaundice			
Erythema			

23. Increased skin color in selected body areas is known as _____.

24. The skin assessment parameter essential in evaluating clients at risk for impaired peripheral circulation is:
    a. temperature.
    b. turgor.
    c. moisture.
    d. texture.

25. Define skin turgor and describe normal findings.

26. Tiny, pinpoint-size, red or purple spots on the skin caused by small hemorrhages into the skin layers are called _____.

27. List at least six criteria for lesion assessment.
    a.
    b.
    c.
    d.
    e.
    f.

28. Supply the correct term for each skin condition from the following list.

    Macule   Papule   Nodule   Atrophy
    Wheal   Vesicle   Pustule   Ulcer

    a. Deep loss of the skin's surface _____
    b. Thinning of the skin with loss of normal appearance _____
    c. Flat, nonpalpable change in skin color, such as a freckle _____
    d. Circumscribed elevation of skin filled with pus, such as acne _____
    e. Circumscribed elevation of skin filled with serous fluid, such as a blister _____
    f. Irregularly shaped, elevated area, such as a hive _____
    g. Palpable, circumscribed, solid skin elevation _____
    h. Elevated, solid mass, deeper and firmer than a papule, such as a wart _____

29. Answer the following:
    a. How does the nurse assess a client for pitting edema?
    b. Describe what is meant by the assessment finding "2+ pitting edema."

30. List at least two teaching points related to skin cancer prevention.
    a.
    b.

31. What type of abnormality is expected in a client with unusual distribution and growth of body hair?

32. An absence of hair growth over the lower extremities may indicate:
    a. a genetic abnormality.
    b. circulatory insufficiency.
    c. febrile illness.
    d. poor nutrition.

33. Define alopecia.

34. During inspection of the hair follicles on the scalp and pubic areas, the nurse is more likely to observe the eggs from lice than the lice themselves. (True or false?)

35. Nail clubbing is characterized by:
    a. red or brown linear streaks in the nail bed.
    b. transverse depressions in the nail bed.
    c. approximately a 160-degree angle between the nail plate and nail base.
    d. a softened nail bed, nail flattening, and enlarged fingertips.

36. A disorder caused by excessive growth hormone resulting in enlarged jaw and facial bones is _____.

37. Identify the components of the eye examination described:
    a. Reading the letters on the Snellen chart _____
    b. Asking the client to follow movement of the nurse's finger along the eight directions of gaze _____
    c. Instructing a client to state when the nurse's finger enters the field of vision _____
    d. Moving a penlight from the side of the client's face, shining the light on the pupil _____

38. Match the name of the common visual problem with the most accurate description.

Description
    a. Abnormal elevation of pressure within the eye _____
    b. Impaired near vision in middle-age and older adults _____
    c. Ability to see distant but not close objects _____
    d. Loss of transparency of the lens _____
    e. Lack of coordination of muscles controlling eye movement _____
    f. Ability to see close objects but not distant objects _____

Problem
    1. Hyperopia
    2. Myopia
    3. Presbyopia

4. Strabismus
5. Cataract
6. Glaucoma

39. What is the easiest way to assess a client's visual acuity?

40. What does the following assess men finding mean? "Vision 20/60 s̄c"

41. Warning signs of eye disease include all of the following except:
a. diplopia.
b. halos around lights.
c. floaters.
d. consensual constriction.

42. Supply the correct term for the description associated with examination of the eye from the list provided.

Arcus senilis   Conjunctivitis   Exophthalmos
Nystagmus   Photophobia   Ptosis
Red reflex

a. Fine, rhythmical ocillation of the eyes

_____

b. Bulging or protrusion of the eyes

_____

c. Abnormal drooping of the eyelid over the pupil _____

d. Inflammation of the membrane covering the surface of the eyeball and the lining of the eyelids _____

e. Thin, white ring along the margin of the iris _____

f. Bright orange glow in response to light on the pupil _____

g. Sensitivity to light _____

43. Define PERRLA.

44. The pupils normally dilate when focusing on a near object. (True or false?)

45. List three normal findings expected during an ophthalmoscopic examination.

a.

b.

c.

46. Annual eye examinations are recommended for all clients after age:
a. 15.
b. 30.
c. 40.
d. 65.

47. List at least three risk factors for hearing problems.

a.

b.

c.

48. Place the mechanisms for sound transmission in their appropriate sequence.
a. The cochlea receives the sound vibration.

_____

b. The sound waves reach the tympanic membrane, causing it to vibrate. _____

c. Sound waves in the air enter the external ear, passing through the outer ear canal. _____

d. Nerve impulses from the cochlea travel to the auditory nerve and the cerebral cortex. _____

e. Vibrations are transmitted through the middle ear by way of the bony ossicular chain to the oval window at the opening of the inner ear. _____

49. If no pain is elicited on palpation of the auricle and tragus, the nurse may rule out an ear infection. (True or false?)

50. Which otoscopic assessment finding is considered abnormal?
a. Presence of dark yellow or brown cerumen
b. Pearly gray or translucent eardrum
c. Shiny, reddened ear canal
d. Cone-shaped light reflection in ear canal

51. Describe the correct method for ear speculum insertion in:
a. infants and small children.
b. older children and adults.

52. List and briefly describe the three types of hearing loss.

a.

b.

c.

53. Sounds can normally be heard longer through air conduction than through bone conduction. (True or false?)

54. What is the meaning of a negative Rinne test?

55. A pale nasal mucosa with clear discharge is a sign of infection. (True or false?)

56. Describe the normal characteristics of the following mouth structures:
a. Soft palate
b. Tongue
c. Teeth
d. Gingiva

57. List three early warning signs of oral cancer.

a.

b.

c.

58. Which statement about lymph node assessment is accurate?
a. Small, mobile, nontender nodes are uncommon.
b. Normally nodes are easily palpable.

c. Malignant nodes are usually tender.

d. Infections can cause permanent node enlargement.

59. Which statement about thyroid gland assessment is accurate?

a. Masses or nodules may be signs of malignant disease.

b. Enlargement is a normal finding.

c. Normally the thyroid gland is easily visualized.

d. Normally the thyroid gland descends during swallowing.

60. Complete the table describing assessment finding of the thorax.

Assessment Findings	Assessment Skill Used	Explanation or Possible Cause
Bulging		
Reduced tactile fremitus		
Reduced excursion		
Resonance over posterior aspect of thorax		
Retraction		
Anteroposterior diameter 1:1		

61. Which statement describes normal breath sounds?

a. Bronchial sounds are audible over the posterior part of the thorax.

b. Inspiratory and expiratory phases of vesicular sounds are equal.

c. Vesicular sounds are audible over the peripheral area of the lung.

d. Bronchovesicular sounds are audible over the trachea.

62. Complete the table describing adventitious breath sounds.

Sound	Auscultation Site	Cause	Character
Pleural friction rub			Grating quality heard on inspiration does not clear with cough
Rhonchi	Primarily over trachea and bronchi; if loud, over most lung fields	Severely narrowed bronchus	
Crackles			

63. Answer the following:

a. What is the PMI?

b. Where is the PMI normally located in the infant and young child?

c. Where is the PMI normally located in the older child and adult?

d. What techniques may be used to locate the PMI in an adult?

64. From the list provided, label the diagram, describing each of the cardiac assessment areas and the sites at which each of the four sounds would be most clearly audible.

Aortic area	Pulmonic area	S_1	S_3
Mitral area	Tricuspid area	S_2	S_4

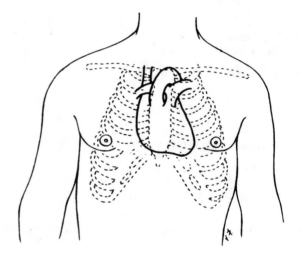

65. Which statement about extra heart sounds and murmurs is correct?

a. S_3 and S_4 are normal in children.

b. Abnormal heart sounds are best heard with the client in a right side-lying position.

c. Murmurs are best heard with the diaphragm of the stethoscope.

d. Abnormal heart sounds are best heard over the aortic area.

66. List the six factors to be assessed when a murmur is detected.

a.

b.

c.

d.

e.

f.

67. A continuous palpable sensation, like the purring of a cat, that may accompany a murmur is

a _____ .

68. The blowing or swishing sound that is created by blood flow through a narrowed vessel is

a _____ .

69. List and state the rationale for two precautions the nurse must take to avoid client injury when palpating the carotid artery.

a.

b.

70. A bruit is a normal assessment finding when auscultating the carotid arteries. (True or false?)

71. When the client is lying flat, bilaterial jugular vein distention is considered abnormal (True or false?)

72. The rating assigned to a peripheral pulse that is easy to palpate and not easy to obliterate is:
a. 0.
b. 1+.
c. 3+.
d. 4+.

73. Identify each assessment finding as a circulatory alteration associated with arterial insufficiency (A) or venous insufficiency (V).
a. Decreased or absent pulse _____
b. Cyanotic skin color _____
c. Dusky red color in dependent extremity _____
d. Normal skin temperature _____
e. Marked edema _____
f. Shiny skin with thickened nails _____

74. Describe the assessment techniques and expected findings for a client with phlebitis.

75. Breast examination is a necessary component of the physical assessment for a male client. (True or false?)

76. The proper technique for palpating breast tissue is:
a. using the palm of the hand to compress underlying tissue.
b. palpating each quadrant and the tail of the breast slowly and methodically.
c. palpating only the tail when lymph node enlargement is present.
d. palpating the breast with a mass before proceeding to the unaffected breast.

77. Write "N" for normal or "A" for abnormal to describe the assessment findings from the breast examinations described.
a. A 26-year-old pregnant woman with a yellowish fluid draining from her nipples _____
b. A 35-year-old woman with tissue retraction in the right breast when raising her arms above her head _____
c. A 20-year-old woman with breasts that are nontender and without masses, but the right breast is larger than the left with nipple asymmetry _____
d. A 30-year-old woman with palpable lymph nodes in the right axilla _____
e. A 24-year-old man with a small, hard, fixed, nontender mass in the lower outer quadrant _____
f. A 78-year-old woman with breast tissue that feels stringy and nodular _____

78. List five characteristics that should be included when describing an abnormal breast mass.

a.

b.

c.

d.

e.

79. Label the abdominal diagram, including quadrants, liver, stomach, transverse colon, small intestine, ascending colon, descending colon, and sigmoid colon.

80. The anatomic landmark for kidney assessment is the _____ .

81. Describe four techniques used to help the client relax during abdominal assessment.

a.

b.

c.

d.

82. What is the correct sequence for abdominal assessment?
a. Inspection, palpation, percussion, auscultation
b. Auscultation, inspection, palpation, percussion
c. Palpation, auscultation, percussion, inspection
d. Inspection, auscultation, percussion, palpation

83. Match the physical finding of abdominal assessment with the most appropriate description.

Description

a. Abdominal skin taut; flanks that do not bulge _____

b. Symmetrical abdomen appearing to sink into the muscular wall _____

c. Large, protruding abdomen with rolls of adipose tissue along the flanks _____

d. Abdominal skin taut; dependent protuberance in the side-lying position _____

Finding

1. Gaseous distention
2. Fluid distention
3. Obesity
4. Concave abdomen

84. Which abdominal assessment finding would be considered abnormal?
  a. Abdomen symmetrically flat or rounded
  b. Venous patterns prominent and distinct
  c. Umbilicus flat or concave
  d. Regular midline pulsations present only in thin clients

85. When assessing bowel sounds, the nurse knows that:
  a. normal sounds are loud and "growling."
  b. if no sounds are heard within 1 minute, the client has no gastric motility.
  c. bowel sounds are normally soft, gurgling, and irregular in frequency.
  d. inflamed bowel usually causes reduced motility.

86. What action would the nurse take to ensure accurate auscultation of bowel sounds in a client with a nasogastric tube connected to suction?

87. How long is it necessary to listen for bowel sounds before determining that they are absent?

88. Loud, "growling" bowel sounds indicating increased gastrointestinal motility are _____

89. Tenderness in response to percussion over the costovertebral angle indicates
  a. liver enlargement.
  b. bowel inflammation.
  c. kidney inflammation.
  d. spinal cord injury.

90. A voluntary tightening of underlying abdominal muscles in response to palpation of a sensitive area is _____

91. Answer the following:
  a. Describe the correct technique for assessing rebound tenderness.
  b. What does a positive rebound tenderness test indicate?

92. What would a smooth, dome-shaped elevation over the symphysis pubis indicate?

93. Identify three warning signs of colorectal cancer.
  a.
  b.
  c.

94. Complete the table, describing assessment findings of the female and male genitalia.

Assessment findings	Normal or abnormal	Assessment technique	Possible cause (if abnormal)
Bulging at inguinal ring			
Smooth, round, firm prostate			
Yellow drainage at cervical os			
Labia minora thin and darker in color than surrounding skin			
Left testicle lower than right			
Small, pea-sized lump on front of testicle			

95. The testicles shrink and soften in the older man. (True or false?)

96. A hernia is the protrusion of the spermatic cord through the inguinal canal. (True or false?)

97. Fill in the blank with the musculoskeletal condition described.
  a. Lateral spinal curvature _____
  b. Muscle that feels flabby; position determined by gravity _____
  c. "Hunchback," or an exaggeration of the thoracic spinal curvature _____
  d. Crackling sound associated with joint movement _____
  e. "Swayback," or an increased lumbar curvature _____
  f. Considerable resistance of a muscle to passive movement _____

98. The nurse might use a goniometer to measure:
  a. a client's muscle strength.
  b. joint range of motion before and after exercise.
  c. vibration sense.
  d. a client's balance.

99. Describe two maneuvers used to assess muscle strength and identify the muscle group being tested.

100. A client must be aroused to maximal alertness before level of consciousness can be assessed. (True or false?)

101. Describe the correct technique for application of painful stimuli during neurological assessment.

102. A client who understands written and verbal speech but who cannot write or speak appropriately has:
   a. sensory aphasia.
   b. receptive aphasia.
   c. motor aphasia.
   d. mental retardation.

103. Match the nurse's assessment questions with the mental or emotional area being tested.

Questions
   a. "Mr. Mays, tell me what the phrase 'A rolling stone gathers no moss' means." _____
   b. "Who visited you this morning, Mrs. Klein?" _____
   c. "Tell me what you know about the new medication you are taking." _____
   d. "What is the year? What is the name of this place?" _____

Area
   1. Knowledge
   2. Orientation
   3. Abstract thinking
   4. Memory

104. Match the assessment technique with the appropriate cranial nerve.

Technique
   a. Ask client to identify sour, salty, or sweet tastes. _____
   b. Ask client to shrug shoulders. _____
   c. Ask client to clench teeth. _____
   d. Ask client to read breakfast menu. _____
   e. Ask client to smile and to raise and lower eyebrows. _____
   f. Ask client to identify aroma of coffee. _____
   g. Elicit a gag reflex. _____
   h. Check pupil constriction in response to light. _____

Cranial nerve
   1. Olfactory (I)
   2. Optic (II)
   3. Oculomotor (III)
   4. Trochlear (IV)
   5. Trigeminal (V)
   6. Abducens (VI)
   7. Facial (VII)
   8. Auditory (VIII)
   9. Glossopharyngeal (IX)
   10. Vagus (X)
   11. Spinal accessory (XI)
   12. Hypoglossal(XII)

105. All sensory testing is performed with the client's eyes closed. (True or false?)

106. Coordination of muscle activity and maintenance of balance and equilibrium occur in the _____ .

107. Describe one maneuver to evaluate:
   a. coordination.
   b. balance.

108. To correctly assess reflexes the nurse:
   a. asks the client to flex the limb to be tested.
   b. holds the reflex hammer firmly and strikes it lightly against the tendon.
   c. asks the client to relax the limb to be tested and then applies a slight stretch to the muscle.
   d. compares the speed of all reflexes on one side of the body.

109. A deep tendon reflex described as 2+ is:
   a. diminished.
   b. normal.
   c. brisker than normal but not necessarily indicative of disease.
   d. hyperactive and often associated with spinal cord disorders.

CRITICAL THINKING AND EXPERIENTIAL EXERCISES

1. Physical assessment
   During any client care observation or experience:
   a. Observe an experienced nurse perform a physical assessment of a client.
   b. Note modifications used in techniques and determine the rationale for such modifications.
   c. Compare your observations with those of students who have observed in other settings or with those of other nurses. Share your impressions with your instructor.

2. Integration of physical assessment and nursing care
   Independently or in a small group, determine specific components of the physical examination that may be assessed during each of the following routine client care activities.
   a. Bathing a client
   b. Assisting a client with oral care
   c. Assisting a client with a meal
   d. Walking a client to the bathroom

3. Disease prevention education
   Working in a small group, have each member select an area for client education from the list provided (or independently develop a list of teaching points for each area listed). Present the major points to be included in a client teaching plan addressing the selected topic. Critique peer performance, or elicit instructor evaluation of a written or verbal presentation.
   a. Early warning signs of cancer
   b. Skin cancer prevention
   c. Lung disease prevention

    d. Heart disease prevention
    e. American Cancer Society guidelines for detection of breast cancer
    f. American Cancer Society guidelines for detection of testicular cancer
    g. Colon cancer prevention

4. Glasgow Coma Scale
Provide care for or observe a client with an altered level of consciousness.
    a. Assess the client using the Glasgow Coma Scale.
    b. Compare your assessment with that of an experienced staff nurse or your instructor.
    c. List factors contributing to the client's altered level of consciousness.
    d. Based on your findings, identify nursing diagnoses and related nursing care.
    e. Submit your written work to your instructor for feedback.

5. Clinical situation: preparation for physical examination
Mr. Clancy is a 69-year-old client with a long history of serious lung disease and a recent onset of chest pain. He is short of breath with a respiratory rate of 28 breaths/min and complains of a dull, aching sensation in the center of his chest. He is diaphoretic and appears anxious as he intently watches the nursing staff.
    a. What is the best position for examination of Mr. Clancy?
    b. What positions should be avoided during the examination?
    c. How might the nurse organize the assessment?
    d. What examination elements are essential and which may be deferred?
    e. What should be done to prepare Mr. Clancy psychologically for this examination?

SKILL AND TECHNIQUE ACTIVITIES

1. Physical examination techniques
    a. Check with your instructor or nursing library personnel to find audiovisual material that demonstrate techniques or illustrate common findings of physical assessment. Review these materials in preparation for laboratory practice sessions and client assessment. Contact your instructor to clarify any questions.
    b. Check with your instructor or nursing library personnel to find models or mannequins that may be used to practice assessment techniques and evaluate specific physical findings. Practice your skills using these models. Contact your instructor for additional guidance or direct assistance.
    c. Using a nursing assessment form as a guide, write a list of all of the equipment needed to conduct a physical assessment on a client. Find and prepare all of the necessary equipment on your assigned clinical area or in your nursing arts laboratory.
    d. With a partner, practice using the techniques of light palpation and direct and indirect percussion.
    e. With a partner, practice using your stethoscope to evaluate breath, heart, and bowel sounds.
    f. With a partner and the assistance of an instructor, practice using the otoscope, ophthalmoscope, percussion hammer, tuning fork, or other special pieces of equipment required to perform physical assessment.
    g. Audiotape a recording of the explanations you would give clients in preparation for the physical examination. Include as your clients a toddler, adolescent, and adult. Perform a self-evaluation, or submit your tape to a peer or instructor for feedback.
    h. Practice assisting a partner into the various positions for examination. Be sure to identify the name of the position and provide your simulated client with appropriate physical and psychological support while he or she assumes the selected position.
    i. Using a nursing assessment form or a self-developed assessment tool, perform a general survey of a partner. Record your findings on the form or tool. Formulate nursing diagnoses based on your findings. Submit your work to your instructor for feedback.
    j. Using a nursing assessment form or a self-developed assessment tool, perform a complete or partial head-to-toe or systems assessment of a partner. Record your findings on the form or tool. Formulate nursing diagnoses based on your findings. Submit your work to your instructor for feedback.
    k. Perform a complete or partial assessment of a partner. Elicit an instructor's feedback of your performance and validate your physical findings.

2. Testicular self-examination
    a. For male students, compare your testicular self-examination techniques with those presented in the text. Modify your personal technique to comply with the guidelines of the American Cancer Society. Clarify questions about the technique with an instructor or clinical specialist.
    b. For all students, audiotape a teaching session in which you provide instruction to a simulated client about the technique of testicular self-examination (or present the information to a peer for critique).

3. Breast self-examination
    a. For female students, compare your breast self-examination techniques with those presented in the text. Modify your personal technique to comply with the guidelines of the American Cancer Society. Clarify questions about the technique with an instructor or clinical specialist.

b. For all students, audiotape a teaching session in which you provide instruction to a simulated client about the technique of breast self-examination (or present the information to a peer for critique).

ADDITIONAL READINGS

Bates B: *A guide to physical examination,* ed 4, Philadephia, 1987, Lippincott.

Comprehensive, clearly written, extensively illustrated text describing techniques for obtaining a health history and performing a physical examination. Illustrates normal and abnormal findings; includes adult and pediatric assessment.

Champion VL: Effect of knowledge, teaching method, confidence and social influence on breast self-examination behavior, *Image J Nurs Sch* 21(2):76, 1989.

Identifies variables influencing breast self-examination behaviors. Findings provide insight into the development of teaching approach to provide optimal compliance.

Dennison R: Cardiopulmonary assessment, *Nurs 86* 16(4):34, 1986.

Presents 15 practical tips to improve the quality of cardiopulmonary assessment.

Fraser MC, McGuire DB: Skin cancer's early warning system, *Am J Nurs* 84:1232, 1984.

Colored photographs clearly illustrate malignant and premalignant conditions associated with malignant melanoma. Includes overveiw of melanoma, prevention guides, and client education. Heavily referenced to guide the learner to additional information.

Kain C, Reilly N, Schultz E: The older adult: a comparative assessment, *Nurs Clin North Am* 25(4):833, 1990.

Provides an overview of the physiological changes associated with the aging process. Differentiates between aging and pathological changes. Focuses on unique changes in men and women particularly as they relate to genitourinary and reproductive systems. Also describes normal changes in laboratory studies associated with aging.

Malasanos L et al: *Health assessment,* ed 4, St Louis, 1990, Mosby–Year Book.

Comprehensive reference presents concepts and techniques needed to elicit a health history and perform a physical examination. Liberally illustrated with photographs and drawings to assist in correctly performing physical assessment. Illustrates normal and abnormal findings. Includes adult and pediatric assessment.

Manning ML: Health assessment of the early adolescent: challenges and clinical issues, *Nurs Clin North Am* 25(4):823, 1990.

Emphasizes the importance of understanding developmental characteristics of young adolescents in providing health care services. Identifies behaviors potentially threatening the health of adolescents.

Whaley LF, Wong DL: *Nursing care of infants and children,* ed 4, St Louis, 1991, Mosby–Year Book.

A comprehensive pediatric nursing text. Includes a developmental approach to assessment. An excellent resource to assist in identification of normal and abnormal assessment findings based on disease states of infants and children.

Chapter 21
Administration of Medications

PREREQUISITE READING
Chapter 21, pp. 610 to 693

OBJECTIVES
Mastery of content in this chapter will enable the student to:
- Define selected terms related to medication administration.
- Discuss the nurse's legal responsibilities in drug prescription and administration.
- Describe the physiological mechanisms of drug action including absorption, distribution, metabolism, and excretion of medications.
- Differentiate among toxic, idiosyncratic, allergic, and side effects of drugs.
- Discuss developmental factors that influence drug pharmacokinetics.
- Discuss factors that influence drug actions.
- Discuss methods of educating a client about prescribed medications.
- Describe the roles of the pharmacist, physician, and nurse in drug administration.
- Describe factors to consider in choosing routes of administration.
- Correctly calculate a prescribed drug dosage.
- Discuss factors to include in assessing needs for and responses to drug therapy.
- List the "five rights" of drug administration.
- Correctly prepare and administer subcutaneous, intramuscular, and intradermal injections and intravenous (IV) medication; insulin injections; oral medications; topical skin preparations; eye, ear, and nose drops; vaginal installations; rectal suppositories; and inhalants.

REVIEW OF KEY CONCEPTS
1. Match the drug name with the correct description.

Description

   a. Name listed in the United States Pharmacopoeia (USP) _____

   b. Name the drug manufacturer uses to market the drug _____

   c. Name describing the drug's composition _____

   d. Name given by the first developer/manufacturer of the drug _____

Drug name
1. Brand name
2. Chemical name
3. Generic name
4. Official name

2. A drug classification indicates:
   a. the effect on a body system.
   b. the symptoms relieved.
   c. the desired effect.
   d. all of the above.

3. Fill in the form of medication with the description provided.

Caplet   Capsule   Elixir   Enteric-coated tablet
Lotion   Ointment   Paste   Pill
Solution   Suppository   Suspension   Syrup
Tablet   Tincture   Troche   Transdermal patch or disk

   a. Oral medication of finely divided particles dispersed in a liquid medium _____

   b. Flat, round dosage form dissolved in the mouth to released the drug _____

   c. Medication encased by a gelatin shell _____

   d. Semisolid, externally applied preparation, usually containing one or more drugs _____

   e. Medicine dissolved in a concentrated sugar solution _____

   f. Oral tablet coated with materials to prevent dissolving in the stomach _____

   g. Drug in liquid suspension, applied externally to protect the skin _____

h. Powdered medication compressed into hard disks _____

i. Semisolid preparation, thicker and stiffer than ointment and absorbed more slowly than ointment _____

j. Oral medication of clear fluid containing water and alcohol _____

k. Medication contained within a semipermiable membrane that allows slow skin absorption over an extended time _____

4. What actions may be taken against a nurse who fails to follow legal provisions when administering controlled substances?

5. Define pharmocokinetics.

6. Dispersal of a drug to body tissues, organs, and specific action sites is:
  a. absorption.
  b. metabolism.
  c. distribution.
  d. excretion.

7. Which statement correctly characterizes drug absorption?
  a. Most drugs must enter systemic circulation to have their therapeutic effect.
  b. Mucous membranes are relatively impermeable to chemicals, making absorption slow.
  c. Oral medications are absorbed more quickly when administered with meals.
  d. Drugs administered subcutaneously are absorbed more quickly than those injected intramuscularly.

8. Systemic distribution of a parenteral drug would be increased by:
  a. local vasoconstriction.
  b. low serum albumin levels.
  c. application of cold over the injection site.
  d. enhanced protein binding.

9. Most drug biotransformation occurs in the:
  a. kidneys.
  b. blood.
  c. intestines.
  d. liver.

10. Most drug excretion occurs through the:
  a. kidneys.
  b. intestines.
  c. liver.
  d. lungs.

11. Define therapeutic drug effect.

12. Match the unpredicted or unintended effect of a drug with the best definition or description.

Description

  a. Severe reaction characterized by wheezing, shortness of breath, and hypotension _____

  b. Reaction characterized by urticaria, eczema, pruritis, or rhinitis _____

  c. Response to excess amounts of a drug within the body _____

  d. Reaction to a drug that is different from the normal or expected response _____

  e. Unintended, secondary effects of a drug _____ _____

Effect

  1. Side effect
  2. Toxic effect
  3. Idiosyncratic reaction
  4. Allergic reaction
  5. Anaphylactic reaction

13. Describe synergistic drug interaction.

14. Drug interactions are typically undesirable and nontherapeutic. (True or false?)

15. Define serum half-life.

16. Fill in the drug action time interval described.
  a. Maintenance of blood serum concentration of a drug after repeated, fixed doses _____
  b. Time required for a drug to reach its highest effective concentration _____
  c. Time drug is present in concentrations sufficient to produce a response _____
  d. Time required for a drug to produce a response after administration _____

17. List three physiological variables that influence drug metabolism.
  a.
  b.
  c.

18. A client's response to a medication may be influenced by environmental conditions at the time the drug is administered. (True or false?)

19. The nurse's behavior when administering a medication can significantly affect the client's response to the drug. (True or false?)

20. Which nursing decision would be beyond the scope of nursing practice?
  a. Selecting the injection site for an intramuscular medication.
  b. Determining whether the client should receive an oral medication in liquid or tablet form.
  c. Increasing the frequency of pain medication administration.
  d. Holding a medication when the client presents with possible drug side effects.

21. Mrs. Carr will receive an antibiotic intramuscularly. Which factor might influence the nurse's method of administration?
  a. Client's level of alertness
  b. Presence of renal disease

c. Condition of muscle tissue

d. Permeability of skin surface

22. The route of choice for medicating clients with poor peripheral perfusion is:
    a. oral.
    b. rectal.
    c. subcutaneous.
    d. intravenous.

23. Local medications, such as those applied to the skin, may cause systemic effects. (True or false?)

24. Describe at least two instructions to give a client before administering sublingual or buccal medication.

    a.

    b.

25. List the four major types of parenteral medication injection.

    a.

    b.

    c.

    d.

26. Why is it necessary to maintain strict sterile technique when preparing medications for parenteral injection?

27. Identify the corresponding basic units of metric measurement and the abbreviation for each:
    a. Length
    b. Weight
    c. Volume

28. In which direction is the decimal point moved for the following mathematical calculations in the metric system.
    a. Division
    b. Multiplication

29. Fill in the correct term and the value relative to the basic unit of metric measurement.

    a. dl _____ = _____ L

    b. mg _____ = _____ g

    c. cm _____ = _____ m

    d. kl _____ = _____ L

30. Fill in the apothecary measurement units for each abbreviation or symbol.

    a. gr _____

    b. ℥ _____

    c. f℥ _____

    d. m _____

    e. ℨ _____

31. Write the appropriate abbreviation for 4 grains.

32. Complete the table of measurement equivalents.

Metric	Apothecary	Household
1 ml	_____ minims	_____ drops
_____ ml	_____ fluid drams	1 tablespoon
30 ml	_____ fluid ounce(s)	_____ tablespoon
_____ ml	_____ fluid ounce(s)	1 cup
_____ ml	1 pint	_____ pint
_____ ml	_____ quart	1 quart

33. Describe what is meant by the following descriptions of a solution concentration.
    a. 5% dextrose in water
    b. 1:1000
    c. 250 mg/ml

34. Complete the following conversions:

    a. 100 mg = _____ g

    b. 2.5 L = _____ ml

    c. 500 ml = _____ L

    d. 60 ml = _____ f℥

    e. 15 mg = _____ gr

    f. 30 gtt = _____ ml

    g. gr $^1/_6$ = _____ mg

35. Write out the formula applied to determine the correct dose when preparing solid or liquid forms of medications.

36. Write out the formula applied to most accurately calculate pediatric dosages.

37. The physician's order reads "digoxin, 0.125 mg POqAM." The drug available is digoxin, 0.25-mg tablets.
    a. What would the nurse administer?
    b. How would this be prepared?

38. The physician's order reads "morphine sulfate, gr ⅛ IM q4h prn pain." The drug available is morphine sulfate, 10 mg/ml.
    a. What would the nurse administer?
    b. How would this be prepared?

39. The physician's order reads "erythromycin suspension, 200 mg PO q6h." The drug available is erythromycin suspension, 400 mg/5 ml.
    a. What would the nurse administer?
    b. How would this be prepared?

40. A 3-year-old is to receive the antibiotic cephalothin (Keflex). The normal single adult dosage is 500 mg. The child's body surface area, according to the standard chart, is 0.40m². How many milligrams of cephalothin should the child receive?

41. Match the common type of medication order with the corresponding example.

Example

    a. Colace, 1 capsule PO qAM _____

b. NPH insulin, 12 units SC at 0800, 5/7 _____

c. Morphine sulfate, 10mg IM now _____

d. Acetaminophen grx PO q4h for headache _____

Order

1. Stat order
2. prn order
3. One-time order
4. Standing order

42. Identify the primary responsibilities of the following health care team members in giving medications to clients:
    a. Physician
    b. Pharmacist
    c. Nurse

43. The medication distribution system that most effectively reduces the number of medication errors and reduces dispensing time is:
    a. stock supply.
    b. individual client supply.
    c. unit-dose system.

44. List at least seven areas for nursing assessment and the rationale for obtaining this information before medication administration.

    a.

    b.

    c.

    d.

    e.

    f.

    g.

45. A nurse who administers an incorrect drug or dose because of a transcription error is legally responsible for the medication error. (True or false?)

46. List five guidelines to ensure proper use and storage of drugs in the home.

    a.

    b.

    c.

    d.

    e.

47. Mr. Williams is very unhappy about the medications he is receiving to prevent seizures. Each time he takes the medication he states that he he feels "different and very uneasy." Mr. Williams has all of the following rights except:
    a. to be informed of the drug's action and potential undesired results.
    b. to request that the nurse reduce the prescribed dose to decrease side effects.
    c. to request that the physician assess for drug allergies.
    d. to refuse to take the medications that are preventing seizures.

48. List the "five rights" of medication delivery.
    a.
    b.
    c.
    d.
    e.

49. Describe the three checks that the nurse performs to ensure that the client receives the right drug.
    a.
    b.
    c.

50. In which situation may the nurse correctly administer a medication?
    a. When the drug is prepared by another nurse
    b. When the drug label is not clear but confirmed by another nurse
    c. When a scored tablet is broken unevenly but administered for two successive doses
    d. When a second nurse validates the dose prepared in the syringe

51. What two steps must be taken by the nurse to ensure that the client is correctly identified before receiving the prescribed medication?
    a.
    b.

52. A routine medication is ordered for 9 AM. The medication may be administered:
    a. between 8 and 9 AM.
    b. between 8:30 and 9:30 AM.
    c. only between 8:45 and 9:15 AM.
    d. only at 9 AM.

53. What nursing action would be appropriate in administering medications to an infant or child?
    a. Allowing the parent to give the medication to the child with the nurse's supervision
    b. Providing detailed explanations to the child before administering the medication
    c. Giving the child the option of taking or refusing the medication
    d. Avoiding any explanation that might increase the child's anxiety before administering the injection

54. Which of the following would be an acceptable guideline for administration of medications through a nasogastric tube?
    a. Crush sustained-release, enteric-coated tablets into a fine powder.
    b. Dissolve the powder in 20 to 30 ml of cold water.
    c. Administer medications over 30 to 60 minutes.
    d. Follow medications with at least 60 ml of water.

55. Number the following steps for preparation of an oral medication in their proper order.
   a. Assist the client to a sitting position. _____
   b. Pour or place the unit-dose medication into a medicine cup. _____
   c. Chart medication in the medicine record. _____
   d. Check accuracy and completeness of information on medication ticket or record with physician's order. _____
   e. Compare medication ticket or record with the prepared drug and its container. _____
   f. Check client identification band and ask client's name. _____
   g. Calculate correct dosage. _____
   h. Offer preferred or recommended liquids with drugs to be swallowed. _____

56. When the nurse prepares unit-dose tablets or capsules, the package or wrapper should be removed before placing the medication into the medicine cup. (True or false?)

57. Powdered liquids and effervescent powders or tablets should be prepared with the appropriate liquids at the bedside. (True or false?)

58. Label the parts of the syringe shown in the diagram at the bottom of the page.
   a.
   b.
   c.
   d.
   e.

59. What three factors must be considered in selecting the needle for an injection?
   a.
   b.
   c.

60. When preparing small amounts of potent medication for injection (less than 1 ml) the nurse would select which type of syringe?
   a. 5-ml syringe
   b. 3-ml syringe
   c. Insulin syringe
   d. TB syringe

61. What does it mean when an insulin bottle is labeled U-100?

62. From the list provided, select the needle most appropriate for the specified injection.
   a. Intramuscular injection _____
   b. Subcutaneous injection _____
   c. Intravenous injection _____
   d. Intradermal injection _____
      (1) 26 gauge, ¼ in.
      (2) 21 gauge, 1½ in.
      (3) 18 gauge, 1 in.
      (4) 25 gauge, ⅝ in.

63. A glass container that must be broken to remove medication for injection is a (an) _____

64. A glass container that has a rubber seal at the top to maintain a closed system for medication storage is a (an) _____

65. When a nurse mixes diluent with a powder in a multidose vial, what two pieces of information must be placed on the label.
   a.
   b.

66. The nurse is preparing a medication from a multidose vial.
   a. Which key step is missing from the process?
      (1) Wipe the top of the vial with an alcohol swab.
      (2) Pull back on the plunger to draw air into the syringe equivalent to the drug volume.
      (3) Insert the needle tip into the vial.
      (4) Invert the vial.
      (5) Withdraw the medication from the vial.
   b. Where should the missing step be inserted into the process?

67. Briefly describe how the nurse would avoid contamination of one medication with another when mixing medications from one single-dose vial (vial A) and one multidose vial (vial B).

68. What technique will prevent medication contamination when mixing medications from two multidose vials (vial A and vial B)?

69. When mixing medications from an ampule and a vial, which medication should be prepared first?
   a. Medication in the vial
   b. Medication in the ampule
   c. Either

70. Which statement about insulin preparations is correct?
   a. An insulin vial must be shaken to properly distribute particles.

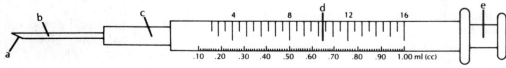

b. Insulin must be kept refrigerated at all times.

c. The only insulin for intravenous use is regular (short acting).

d. Slower-acting, modified insulins appear clear.

71. When preparing insulin from two vials, the nurse:

a. shakes each vial to properly distribute the particles.

b. injects air into the clear, unmodified (regular) vial first.

c. uses separate syringes to draw the dose from each vial.

d. withdraws the cloudy (modified) insulin last.

72. List six techniques to minimize client discomfort associated with injections.

a.

b.

c.

d.

e.

f.

73. Using the diagrams below, shade in the areas of the body suitable for subcutaneous injections.

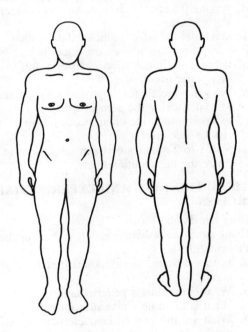

74. The site most frequently recommended for subcutaneous heparin injection is the _____

75. The maximal volume of water-soluble medication that may be administered subcutaneously to an adult is:

a. 0.5 ml.

b. 1.0 ml.

c. 1.5 ml.

d. 2.0 ml.

76. State the rule that may be followed to determine whether a subcutaneous injection should be given at a 90- or 45-degree angle.

77. The angle of needle insertion for an intramuscular injection is:

a. 15 degrees.

b. 45 degrees.

c. 60 degrees.

d. 90 degrees.

78. Indicate the maximal volume of medication for intramuscular injection in each of the following groups.

a. Well-developed adults

b. Older children, older adults, or thin adults

c. Older infants and small children

79. The preferred sites for intramuscular injections in the adult or child are the:

a. vastus lateralis and ventrogluteal.

b. dorsogluteal and deltoid.

c. ventrogluteal and dorsogluteal.

d. vastus lateralis and deltoid.

80. The injection site that poses the greatest risk of contamination and potential client injury is the:

a. vastus lateralis.

b. ventrogluteal.

c. dorsogluteal.

d. deltoid.

81. The deltoid injection site:

a. is an acceptable injection site for infants and children.

b. is the preferred site for older adults.

c. lacks major nerves and blood vessels.

d. is acceptable only for small volumes of medication.

82. Describe the method for accurately locating the following injection sites.

a. Deltoid

b. Ventrogluteal

c. Vastus lateralis

d. Dorsogluteal

83. The Z-track method for administering an intramuscular injection is used when the:

a. amount injected is greater than 3 ml of fluid.

b. drug is extremely irritating to subcutaneous tissue.

c. drug is extremely potent or has many side effects.

d. client is incontinent or cachexic.

84. Describe the procedure used in administering an intramuscular injection using the Z-track technique.

85. Number the following steps for preparing and administering an intramuscular injection in the correct sequence.

a. Aspirate medication by pulling back on the plunger. _____

b. Discard the needle and syringe into the appropriate receptacle. _____

c. Cleanse the injection site with an alcohol swab. _____

d. Quickly inject the needle at a 90-degree angle. _____

e. Explain the procedure to the client; assist the client to the proper position. _____

f. Massage the injection site slowly. _____

g. Inspect and palpate the injection site for proper landmarks, masses, and tenderness. _____

h. Spread the skin tightly across the injection site. _____

i. Withdraw the needle quickly from the site. _____

j. Inject the medication slowly. _____

86. A skin test will not be valid if a bleb does not appear at the injection site. (True or false?)

87. All of the following actions are appropriate to medication administration. Which is specific to the nurse giving intravenous drugs?

  a. Know the five rights of safe drug administration
  b. Have the antidote available during administration.
  c. Monitor the client's vital signs.
  d. Observe the client for adverse reactions.

88. The most dangerous method of drug administration is:

  a. dorsogluteal intramuscular injection.
  b. large-volume intravenous infusion.
  c. intravenous bolus injection.
  d. piggyback infusion.

89. When no specific rate of administration is recommended for an intravenous bolus medication, what is the recommended injection rate?

  a. 1 mg/minute
  b. 1 ml/minute
  c. 10 mg/minute
  d. 100 ml/minute

90. After administering an injection, the nurse carefully recaps the needle before discarding it in the designated container. (True or false?)

91. What precaution should the nurse take when administering locally applied medications such as lotions or ointments?

92. As long as the tip of the applicator remains clean, it is acceptable for a person to use another individual's eyedrops. (True or false?)

93. Which action is appropriate when administering eye medications?

  a. Cleanse eye of any crusts or drainage by wiping from outer to inner canthus.
  b. Instill eye drops onto the cornea from approximately 1 to 2 cm.
  c. Apply gentle pressure to the nasolacrimal duct for 30 to 60 seconds after medication administration.
  d. Instruct the client to squeeze the eyelids closed after instilling the eyedrops.

94. Lisa is a 4-year-old client with an infection of the right ear. The nurse observes a collection of cerumen in the ear canal. Which of the following measures would the nurse not use while administering ear drops to Lisa?

  a. Pull the pinna upward and backward.
  b. Assist Lisa to lie on her left side.
  c. Remove ear wax gently with an applicator.
  d. Instill drops at least 1 cm above the ear canal.

95. Which statement about instillation of vaginal medications is correct?

  a. The client should be instructed to remain on her back for at least 10 minutes after administration.
  b. The pointed end of the vaginal suppository should be inserted into the vagina.
  c. Disposable gloves need not be worn if an applicator is used.
  d. Suppositories need to be inserted approximately 2.5 to 5 cm.

96. Which statement about administration of rectal suppositories is correct?

  a. Suppositories should reach room temperature before insertion.
  b. Suppositories must pass the anus and internal sphincter.
  c. The client should be in the prone position.
  d. Asking the client to bear down assists in relaxing the sphincters.

97. To maximize the effect of metered dose inhaler medications, the nurse advises the client to:

  a. depress the medication canister fully, immediately after exhalation.
  b. hold the breath for approximately 10 seconds after delivering the aerosol spray.
  c. exhale through the open mouth to minimize the risk of side effects.
  d. wait 1 to 2 minutes between inhalations to maximize the therapeutic effect.

CRITICAL THINKING AND EXPERIENTIAL EXERCISES

1. Drug names and forms
   Using a nursing pharmacology text, look up the drug Prostaphlin.
   a. Is this a trade, proprietary, official, or generic name?
   b. What is the drug's generic name?
   c. What is the drug's classification?
   d. What are the general characteristics of medications in this classification?
   e. What are the nursing implications of administering medications in this classification?
   f. What forms of this medication are available?

2. Legislation and drug control
   a. Review your state's nurse practice act as it pertains to the nurse's role and responsibilities in medication administration.
   b. Review your institution's policies and procedures about drug administration.

c. In a small group, invite a hospital pharmacist to discuss narcotic control in your institution.

d. Compare the guidelines for safe narcotic administraton and control listed in your text on p. 615 with your institution's policies and procedures.

e. Observe a nurse's procedure for signing out and counting narcotics at the change of shift.

3. Medication orders

In any client care setting, examine the physician's orders for specific client.

a. Identify each of the following types of orders in the client's record.
   (1) Standing orders
   (2) prn orders
   (3) Single (one-time) orders
   (4) Stat orders

b. Examine one medication order and identify each of the seven essential parts.
   (1) Client's full name
   (2) Date of order
   (3) Drug name
   (4) Dosage
   (5) Route of administration
   (6) Time and frequency of administration
   (7) Signature of physician or nurse

c. Examine the medication record for the specified client. Compare the medication orders to the information recorded on the medication record.

4. Medication assessment

Perform a medication assessment on an assigned client or peer. Formulate nursing diagnoses and interventions related to medication administration based on the information obtained in each of the designated areas. Submit your written work to your instructor for feedback.

a. Pertinent medical history
b. History of allergies
c. Client's current condition
d. Diet history
e. Client's perceptual and coordination abilities or limitations
f. Client's knowledge and understanding of drug therapy
g. Client's attitude about the use of drugs

5. Drug data

Review a client's medication record. Identify at least two drugs the client is receiving routinely. Prepare a drug card or sheet that includes the following information. Submit your written work to your instructor.

a. Generic and tradenames
b. Classification
c. Action
d. Purpose
e. Normal dosages
f. Routes
g. Side effects
h. Toxic effects

i. Nursing implications for administration and monitoring

(Medication cards summarizing this information may be purchased. Your instructor can best advise you about the use of published cards as a quick reference.)

6. Clinical situation: narcotic administration

Mr. Towns is a 50-year-old client who has suffered a traumatic injury to his right leg. His physician ordered codeine, 60 mg PO q4h prn, for pain.

a. To what procedure must the nurse adhere when administering the controlled drug to Mr. Towns?

b. While the nurse assists Mr. Towns to sit up on the side of the bed, the medicine cup is overturned and the codeine tablets fall onto the floor. What responsiblities are involved with the proper disposal of the contaminated codeine.

c. When the nurse returns to the room with the codeine tablets, Mr. Towns requests that the nurse give him only half of the dose (30 mg instead of the 60 mg ordered). What should the nurse do?

7. Clinical situation: nature of drug action

Mrs. Post is a 32-year-old mother of three with metastatic breast cancer. She is requesting pain medication for intense pain. The physician has ordered morphine, 8 mg SQ q3-4h.

a. You review the medication record and find that Mrs. Post received her last morphine injection an hour ago. Would would you do?

b. Discuss the differences between the mechanism of action of morphine and its pharmacokinetics (absorption, distribution, metabolism, and excretion). Which factors associated with drug action might be contributing to Mrs. Post's lack of response to her most recent morphine injection?

c. The physician changes the route of administration to intravenous.
   (1) Why would a different route make the same dose of morphine more effective?
   (2) What risks are associated with the use of the intravenous route for morphine administration?
   (3) What nursing actions should be taken before, during, and after intravenous administration of morphine?
   (4) Describe each of the following effects of morphine that might be expected.
       (a) Therapeutic effect
       (b) Side effects
       (c) Toxic effects
       (d) Idiosyncratic reactions
       (e) Allergic reactions

d. In addition to the intravenous morphine prn, the physician orders enteric-coated aspirin, 650 mg PO qid, for Mrs. Post. Why would the physician prescribe two different medications for pain?

e. What could the nurse do to maximize the pain-relieving action of Mrs. Post's analgesic medications?

8. Clinical situation: intravenous medications
   Mr. Martin has an intravenous medication infusing.
   a. List three methods that can be used to administer a drug intravenously to Mr. Martin.
   b. Discuss the nurse's responsiblities when administering Mr. Martin's drug intravenously.
   c. Mr. Martin has 500 mg of ampicillin ordered q6h IV. Describe how you would add this drug to a 100 ml bag of intravenous solution. What supplies and equipment do you need? Would this 100-ml bag be considered a primary or secondary intravenous infusion? Why?
   d. Mr. Martin's physician has ordered the continuous intravenous infusion to be discontinued and a heparin lock inserted. What nursing implications are involved when administering drugs through a heparin lock? What nursing responsibilities are involved when caring for Mr. Martin while this heparin lock is in place?
9. Clinical situation: medication errors
   A student is caring for two clients, Mr. Roth and Mr. Evans, who are roommates. The student is to administer Mr. Roth's 10 PM medications, which have already been checked in the medicine room by the student's clinical instructor. The student enters the room and administers the medication to Mr. Evans.
   a. What should the student do?
   b. Which of the five rights have been violated in this situation?
   c. How could this error have been prevented?
   d. Using your institution's guide, determine what information should be included on the incident report.
   e. What information should be charted in Mr. Evans' medication record and chart.
10. Clinical situation: client education and compliance
    a. Ms. Owens is a 32-year-old client who lives with her parents. She has diabetes complicated by renal disease and blindness. Ms. Owens requires regular insulin injections, an antihypertensive medication given 4 times a day, and a daily iron supplement. Develop a care plan that will enable Ms. Owens to maintain her independence and ensure that she takes her prescribed medication at the right times each day.
11. Clinical situation: medications and the older adult
    a. Mr. Win is an 84-year-old client admitted to your nursing unit. The physician has ordered three different oral medications for Mr. Win. Considering the physiological changes that accompany aging, identify the factors that should be addressed to determine the likelihood that the drugs can be administered effectively.
12. Clinical situation: medications and the toddler
    Bryan is an 18-month-old toddler who is hospitalized for croup. His medications include an oral antibiotic suspension to be taken q6h and an intramuscular injection twice a day.
    a. What resources would you consult before attempting to administer Bryan's medications?
    b. What psychological preparation would be appropriate for Bryan?
       (1) Before giving his antibiotic?
       (2) Before giving his injection?
    c. What techniques would you use in administering the antibiotics?
    d. What techniques would you use in administering the injection?

SKILL AND TECHNIQUE ACTIVITIES

1. Dosage calculations
   Answer each of the following medication administration problems. Submit your answers to your instructor for validation.
   a. Pronestyl, 500 mg, is ordered qid for Mrs. Adams. The drug is dispensed in 250-mg tablets. Mrs. Adams is going home on a weekend pass, leaving the hospital at 9 AM Saturday and returning at 8 PM Sunday. How many tablets will Mrs. Adams require at home?
   b. Dr. Rose has ordered codeine gr ½ for Wendy Smith. The stock on the unit is codeine gr ⅙. How many tablets would you use?
   c. Convert 250 mg to grams.
   d. 1½ f℥ = F_____ ml
   e. Mr. Cox has Demerol (meperidine), 35 mg, ordered. The supply on the unit is meperidine, 50 mg/ml.
      (1) How many milliliters would you administer?
      (2) How many minims would you administer?
   f. What is the estimated child's dose of morphine sulfate for a 5-year-old weighing 20 kg (45 pounds) who is 109 cm (43 inches) tall? The adult dose is 10 mg. (Refer to the West nomogram in your text.)
   g. The physician's order reads "ampicillin, 50 mg IM q6h." Stock available is a 125-mg vial of ampicillin that requires reconstitution. When 1.2 ml of normal saline is added, the resulting solution strength is 125 mg/ml. How many milliliters would you administer?
   h. The physician's order reads "5000 U heparin SQ q12h." Stock available is a 10,000 U/ml or 1000 U/ml. Both strengths come in a 5-ml multidose vial.
      (1) Which strength would you use and why?
      (2) How many milliliters would you administer?
   i. Joe Williams has a preoperative sedation order as follows: Meperidine, 100 mg IM on call and atropine, 0.2 mg IM on call. Stock available is meperidine, 50 mg/ml; and atropine 0.4 mg/ml. (Meperidine and atropine are compatible.)
      (1) Which strength of meperidine would you use and why?
      (2) How many milliliters of meperidine would you draw into the syringe?

(3) How many milliliters of atropine would you draw into the syringe?

(4) How many milliliters (total) would be in the syringe when both medications have been drawn?

2. Oral medication administration

In a laboratory, practice each of the following techniques:

a. Prepare tablets or capsules (any over-the-counter medication such as aspirin or acetaminophen or a simulated medication provided by your instructor) from a bottle by pouring it into the bottle cap and transferring it into a medicine cup without touching the tablet or capsule with your fingers.

b. If available, prepare tablets or capsules dispensed in a unit-dose package. Over-the-counter medications such as cold capsules are available in this form.

c. Prepare 650 mg of aspirin for administration through a nasogastric tube.

d. Prepare 10 ml of a liquid medication from a bottle.

e. Prepare ½ teaspoon of a liquid medication from a bottle. (Be sure that this dose is accurately measured using equipment available in the hospital.)

3. Preparing injections

In a laboratory, with the materials and equipment provided by your instructor or laboratory assistant:

a. Examine the various types of disposable syringes and needles available in your institution.

b. Identify the following parts of a syringe: bevel, barrel, needle shaft, plunger, hub, milliliter scale, and minim scale.

c. Identify the syringe and most appropriate needle size for each of the following activities.

(1) Insulin injection in an obese adult

(2) Intramuscular injection of 2.5 ml in a well-developed adult

(3) Intramuscular injection of 0.5 ml in an infant

(4) Subcutaneous injection of 1.0 ml in an emaciated adult

(5) Intradermal skin testing with 0.1 ml of prescribed solution

d. Practice handling the syringes, capping and recapping the needle, and changing needles while maintaining aseptic technique. (Remember that once a needle has been used for an injection, it is *never* recapped but discarded immediately into the appropriate receptacle.)

e. Examine a Tubex or Carpuject syringe and cartridge system. Practice loading, handling, and unloading the cartridge.

f. Examine ampules and vials.

g. If available, practice drawing up each of the following volumes. Have a peer or instructor critique your performance and validate the accuracy of your measurement.

(1) 1.5 ml from a multidose vial

(2) 1.8 ml from an ampule

(3) Mixing 1 ml from an ampule and 0.5 ml from a vial

(4) Mixing 0.75 ml from one vial and 0.5 ml from another vial

4. Locating injection sites

With a partner, practice locating each of the following injection sites. Have an instructor validate the accuracy of your site identification.

a. Intramuscular sites

(1) Right and left ventrogluteal

(2) Vastus lateralis

(3) Dorsogluteal

(4) Deltoid

b. Subcutaneous sites

(1) Arms

(2) Legs

(3) Abdomen

(4) Scapular area

c. Intradermal sites

(1) Arms

(2) Scapular areas

5. Administering injections

In the laboratory, using an injection pad, grapefruit, injection hip, or mannequin designed for injection practice, perform each of the following tasks. Have a peer or instructor critique your performance based on the steps presented in your text.

a. Prepare and administer 0.5 ml of sterile saline for subcutaneous injection.

b. Prepare and administer 1.0 ml of sterile saline for intramuscular injection.

c. Prepare and administer 1.5 ml of sterile saline using the Z-track technique.

6. Eye applications

a. In the laboratory, using a mannequin, practice administering eyedrops. Have a peer or instructor critique your performance based on the steps presented in your text.

7. Ear instillations

a. In the laboratory, using a mannequin, practice administering ear drops to an adult and a child. Have a peer or instructor critique your performance based on the steps presented in your text.

8. Insulin preparations

In the laboratory:

a. Examine the variety of insulin syringes available for clients in your institution.

b. If available, examine a variety of insulin preparations. Practice preparation of insulin for injection, including:

(1) 8 units of regular insulin.

(2) 13 units of NPH insulin.

(3) 15 units of NPH and 7 units of regular insulin.

ADDITIONAL READINGS

Beecroft PC, Redick S: Possible complications of intramuscular injections in the pediatric unit, *Pediatr Nurs* 15:333, 1989.

Describes survey findings regarding pediatric nurses' intramuscular injection techniques and complications. Outcomes indicate careful location of anatomical landmarks and use of the ventrogluteal site in adolescents as a means to reduce injection complication.

Clayton M: The right way to prevent medication errors, *RN* 50(6):30, 1987.

Explores the five "rights" of medication administration. Presents several helpful hints and examples to assist in maintaining client safety.

Dunn DL, Lenihan SF: The case for the saline flush, *Am J Nurs* 89:1285, 1989.

Describes a study comparing the cost and efficacy of saline and heparin solutions in maintaining heparin locks.

Hahn K: Brush up on your injection technique, *Nurs 90* 20(9):54, 1990.

Provides recommendations for injection administration. Includes several illustrations.

Keen MF: Get on the right track with Z-track injections, *RN* 20(8):59, 1990.

Outlines the basic steps for administration of intramuscular injections using the Z-track technique.

Keen MF: Comparison of intramuscular injection techniques to reduce site discomfort and lesions, *Nurs Res* 35(4):207,1986.

Describes research examining injection methodology and client comfort. Suggests that the use of the Z-track technique reduces the discomfort experienced after injection.

LeSage J: Polypharmacy in geriatric patients, *Nurs Clin North Am* 26(2):273, 1991.

Discusses the problem of "over-prescription" of medications in older adults. Describes reasons for the phenomenon, its effect on clients, and the potential health risks.

Miyares MV: Medication aids your elderly patient will love, *RN* 48(11):44, 1985.

Pictorial presentation of devices to increase medication compliance in clients with motor or sensory impairments.

Schwertz D: Basic principles of pharmocologic action, *Nurs Clin North Am* 26(2):245, 1991.

Discusses pharmacokinetics and pharmacodynamics. Highlights physiological alterations increasing the probability of reactions.

Statz E: Hand strength and metered dose inhalers, *Am J Nurs* 84:800, 1984.

Presents research findings of a study measuring hand strength associated with 2- and 3-point position using metered dose inhalers. Recommends evaluation of hand strength as a critical element in determining the efficacy of metered dose inhalers. Suggests most appropriate method based on hand strength.

Williams PJ: How do you keep medicine from clogging feeding tubes? *Am J Nurs* 89:181,1989.

Provides guidelines for medication administration via feeding tubes. Includes solution compatibility, viscosity, and tube patency.

Chapter 22
Documentation and Reporting

PREREQUISITE READING
Chapter 22, pp. 694 to 725.

OBJECTIVES
Mastery of content in this chapter will enable the student to:
- Define selected terms associated with documentation and reporting.
- Describe guidelines for effective documentation and reporting.
- Discuss the relationship between documentation and health care financial reimbursement..
- Identify ways to maintain confidentiality of records and reports.
- Describe the purpose of change-of-shift report.
- Present a change-of-shift report on a client.
- Explain how to verify telephone orders.
- Identify seven purposes of a health care record.
- Discuss legal guidelines for recording.
- Describe the different methods in record keeping.
- Discuss the advantages and disadvantages of standardized documentation forms.
- Identify elements to include when documenting a client's discharge plan.
- Identify computerized applications for documentation.

REVIEW OF KEY CONCEPTS
1. Documentation and reporting are less important nursing activities than providing client care. (True or false?)
2. List six guidelines that must be followed to ensure quality documentation and reporting.

   a.

   b.

   c.

   d.

   e.

   f.
3. Record your signature as you would for an entry in the client's record.

4. Which of the following nursing activities does not need to be recorded immediately?
   a. Administering a medication
   b. Providing a back rub
   c. Applying a pressure dressing for bleeding
   d. Transporting a client to the x-ray department
5. What is the military time that corresponds to 10:05 PM civilian time?
6. Which statement concerning confidentiality is inaccurate?
   a. A legal suit can be brought against nurses who disclose information about clients without their consent.
   b. Nurses are responsible for protecting their clients' records from unauthorized readers.
   c. Nurses may only use a client's records for activities directly related to the client's health care management.
   d. Nurses are legally and ethically obligated to keep information about a client confidential.
7. The major purpose of a change-of-shift report is to:
   a. communicate care delivered.
   b. provide an opportunity for nurses to share concerns.
   c. inform the physician of a client's progress.
   d. provide continuity of client care.
8. The basis for a change-of-shift report is the communication of:
   a. the client's health needs.
   b. routine nursing orders.
   c. information on the Kardex.
   d. prescribed medical care.
9. All of the following are examples of information to include in a verbal report except:
   a. Mr. Jones has been started on ampicillin, 500 mg every 6 hours.
   b. Mrs. Smith stated that the heating pad decreased her leg pain.
   c. Ms. Carter has been uncooperative most of the morning.
   d. Mr. Boylan's pulse was 80 at 0800 and 102 at 1200.

10. Identify the eight major areas for inclusion in a change-of-shift report.

    a.

    b.

    c.

    d.

    e.

    f.

    g.

    h.

11. a. Why is it particularly important that information in a telephone report is clear, accurate, and concise?

    b. How does the nurse ensure that information conveyed in a telephone report is accurate?

12. When a physician gives a verbal order over the telephone, the only way for the order to be legal is:

    a. a registered nurse must accept the order.

    b. the physician must give his or her name over the phone.

    c. the physician must sign the order within a prescribed time.

    d. the nurse must record the order in the medical record.

13. List six major information areas in a transfer report.

    a.

    b.

    c.

    d.

    e.

    f.

14. Define incidents.

15. All information documented in an incident report should be duplicated in the client's medical record. (True or false?)

16. What is the purpose of an incident report?

17. Match the purpose of health care records with the best example provided.

    a. Client's records are reviewed to determine whether the standards of care have been met. _____

    b. Student reviews client's charts to assist in planning care. _____

    c. Nurse reviews charts of 10 clients to examine the effects of a preoperative teaching class. _____

    d. Nurse describes client's response to a medication given in error. _____

    e. Client's record is available to all health team members caring for the client. _____

    f. Student reviews the records of two clients with the same nursing diagnosis as a class assignment. _____

    1. Assessment
    2. Education
    3. Legal documentation
    4. Auditing
    5. Research
    6. Communication

18. Briefly describe the relationship between accurate documentation and health care financial reimbursement.

19. Clients have the right to review their medical records. (True or false?)

20. The client's record is confidential and cannot be used in court. (True or false?)

21. Which of the following is a recording error?

    a. Refusing to chart someone else's assessment data

    b. Erasing any errors completely

    c. Beginning each entry with the time

    d. Ending each entry with your signature and title

22. The medical record that is organized into separate sections for data from each discipline is known as a:

    a. source record.

    b. problem-oriented record.

    c. modified problem-oriented record.

    d. SOAP record.

23. Identify one advantage and one disadvantage of a source record:

    a. Advantage:

    b. Disadvantage:

24. List three advantages of the POMR charting method.

    a.

    b.

    c.

25. Briefly describe the information to be included in each of the sections of the SOAP note.

    S:

    O:

    A:

    P:

26. Briefly describe the information to be included in each of the sections of the PIE note.

    P:

    I:

    E:

27. The documentation approach based on standards of practice and predetermined interventions is:

    a. focus charting.

    b. graphic charting.

    c. charting by incident.

    d. charting by exception.

28. Information needed for the daily nursing care of clients is readily accessible in:

    a. the nursing Kardex.

    b. the client order sheets.

c. the nurse's notes.

d. the admission assessment.

29. Describe a critical pathway.

30. All of the following characteristics are important reasons for accurate, complete client documentation. Which one is of particular importance in home health care?

    a. Continuity of care

    b. Eligibility for home health care reimbursement

    c. Client response to home health care

    d. Needs of the family

31. a. What is a standardized care plan?

    b. Identify three advantages of a standardized care plan.

    c. What nursing responsibilities are related to the use of standardized care plans?

CRITICAL THINKING AND EXPERIENTIAL EXERCISES

1. Medical records

    Review a client's medical record.

    a. Locate each of the major pieces of information

        (1) Demographic data

        (2) Consent forms

        (3) Admission nursing histories

        (4) Medical history

        (5) Reports of physical examinations

        (6) Reports of diagnostic studies

        (7) Medical diagnosis (diagnoses)

        (8) Therapeutic orders

        (9) Progress notes

        (10) Nursing care plans

        (11) Record of care and treatment

        (12) Discharge plan and summary

    b. Determine whether your client's medical record is a source, problem-oriented, or modified problem-oriented record.

    c. Identify the characteristics that led you to reach this determination.

2. Standards of practice

    a. Review a copy of your institution's standards of nursing practice. Compare them with the examples of the JCAHO nursing service standards cited in your text on p. 708.

3. Standardized care plans

    a. Review the nursing assessment and medical record of an assigned client.

    b. Identify the priority nursing diagnosis.

    c. Obtain a standardized care plan for the identified diagnosis from those available in your institution or from a textbook of nursing care plans.

    d. Individualize the standardized care plan to meet the unique needs of your client.

    e. What are the advantages of using the standardized care plan for your client?

    f. What are the limitations of using the standardized care plan for your client?

4. Computerized communication systems

    a. Arrange for an orientation to the computer system at your institution. Identify specific computer applications that directly affect client care.

5. Clinical situation: criteria for reporting and recording

    Mr. Knowles enters the hospital with nausea and abdominal pain. His abdomen is distended, tense, slightly tender to touch, with hypoactive bowel sounds in all four quadrants. Mr. Knowles states that he feels jittery and becomes lightheaded when rising to a sitting position. The physician orders codeine, 30 mg intramuscularly at 1425. An endoscopy has been scheduled for the following day, and the primary nurse has provided the client with the standardized endoscopy teaching plan information.

    a. Identify Mr. Knowles' signs and symptoms that should be described in the medical record.

    b. For each of the signs and symptoms you have identified, give examples of at least four criteria that the nurse might use to describe them.

    c. Identify four criteria that the nurse should use to describe the administration of codeine to Mr. Knowles.

    d. Identify three criteria the nurse may use to describe the client teaching that occurred.

6. Clinical situation: confidentiality

    You have been caring for Mrs. Clark, a 39-year-old woman with terminal cancer, for several days. While Mrs. Clark is visiting with her family in the lounge and you are straightening the room, Ms. Olsen, her roommate, begins talking with you. Ms. Olsen tells you that it is so sad to see such a nice young woman (Mrs. Clark) so sick and that it must be hard for you too. She asks you about the nature of Mrs. Clark's diagnosis and her prognosis.

    a. How would you handle this situation?

    b. Specifically, what could you say to Ms. Olsen?

7. Clinical situation: incident reports

    Mr. Neal is an 88-year-old client who underwent surgery for repair of a fractured femur. He returned to the nursing unit after surgery and is in stable condition. During the night, he becomes confused. While attempting to crawl out of bed, over the side rails, he falls to the floor.

    a. What actions should the nurse take?

    b. Using your institution's incident policies as a guide, identify the information needed to complete the incident report. (Or, if feasible, complete a sample incident report form using the information from the simulated clinical situation.)

    c. What information should appear in the client's medical record?

SKILL AND TECHNIQUE ACTIVITIES

1. Change of shift report

    a. Observe or listen to an audiotape of a change-of-shift report. Analyze the report based on the guidelines discussed in your text. Identify positive characteristics of the report. Determine strategies that may be used to improve the report.

    b. Before a client care experience, or in a simulated

situation, practice receiving and presenting an intershift report with a group of peers. Identify areas in which additional information may be required and formulate appropriate questions. Critique personal and peer performance.

   c. Following a client care experience, formulate an intershift report on your client. Practice presenting this report to a peer, or audiotape it for self-evaluation or instructor feedback. Request feedback on your report from the staff nurse to whom you have reported.

2. Kardex forms

   a. Review the Kardex form used in your institution.

   b. Review the Kardex information on an assigned client. Compare the information that appears with data from the medical record.

   c. Complete the Kardex form used in your institution (or the one provided at the end of this chapter) with the information from the following hypothetical postoperative situation.

   Ms. Gina Ross
   Date of birth: June 12, 1970
   Graduate student
   Attending physician: Dr. Wilbur
   Medical diagnosis: appendicitis, appendectomy 1/6/93
   Condition: fair
   Allergies: A.S.A. (aspirin), adhesive tape
   Fluids as tolerated
   IV fluids—1000cc D5NS q8′
   Change abdominal dressing prn
   Up in chair qid
   I & O
   Vital signs q4h × 48 hours
   Obtain CBC 1/7/93
   Portable chest film 1/7/93
   Turn, cough, and deep breaths q2h while awake

3. Charting

   a. Review your institution's policies on nurses' charting. Clarify the responsibilities of nursing students in charting nurse's notes with your instructor or head nurse.

   b. Review the charting forms used by nurses in your institution.

   c. Locate the list of approved charting abbreviations for your institution. With the assistance of your instructor or head nurse, identify the most frequently used abbreviations and write them on a file card for reference when reviewing charts or memorize the list to facilitate chart review.

   d. During a client care experience, complete all appropriate flow sheets and formulate a nurse's note. Submit your written work to your instructor for review before entering it in the medical record.

4. Alternative nurse's note formats

   a. SOAP notes: rewrite the following nurse's note in a SOAP note format.

Client's skin over the sacral area has a 4 cm reddened area, without breakdown, tender to palpation. Client states, "I can't seem to stay off my back." Client's immobility increases risk of skin breakdown. Sacral area cleansed, barrier cream applied. Continue turning every 1 to 2 hours.

   b. Narrative notes: rewrite the following SOAP note in a narrative format.
   S—Client states, "The pain is unbearable when I cough."
   O—Abdominal incision well approximated, without drainage, tender on palpation. Morphine sulfate, 10 mg, given at 10:40 AM for incisional pain, with moderate relief after 30 minutes. Client grimaces during turning. Coughing is shallow and nonproductive.
   A—Alteration in comfort related to abdominal incision
   P—Instruct client on method for splinting incision during coughing. Assist with turning by log rolling. Offer pain medication 30 minutes before ambulation or breathing exercise.

   c. PIE notes; rewrite the above SOAP note in a PIE format.

ADDITIONAL READINGS

Albarado R, McCall V, Thrane J: Computerized nursing documentation, *Nurs Management* 21(7):64,1990.
   Discusses critical elements in the development of a computerized nursing documentation system. Also addresses areas of confidentiality.

Blake P: Incident investigation: a complete guide, *Nurs Management* 15(11):37,1984.
   Comprehensively discusses the nurse's role and responsibilities when incidents occur.

Collins HL: Legal risks of computer charting, *RN*, 53:81, 1991.
   Presents strategies to protect nurses from legal liability related to computerized charting systems.

Edelstein J: A study of nursing documentation, *Nurs Management* 21(11):40,1990.
   Examines problems associated with nursing documentation, and ways to improve quality of charting. Concludes that improvement is needed in nurses' knowledge and attitude about documentation.

Hoke JL: Charting for dollars, *Am J Nurs*, 85:658, 1985.
   Emphasizes the importance of documentation in financial reimbursement through the prospective payment system (DRGs). Illustrates how nursing documentation can affect reimbursement through a case study of a client with peripheral vascular disease.

Miller P, Pastorino C: Daily nursing documentation can be quick and thorough, *Nurs Management* 21(11):17, 1990.
   Describes the use of flow sheets to standardize routine elements of client assessment and care.

Thielman DE: Report: how to say it all in a few words, *RN* 50:15, 1987.
   Provides explicit guidelines for organizing and delivering concise verbal reports.

Medical Diagnosis and other pertinent medical information:

Condition

Allergies (Drugs, food, other)

Adm. Date	Age	Religion		Mode of Travel	
Service	Doctor		Resident	Intern	Stamp Addressograph Plate Here

FREQUENTLY ORDERED ITEMS		Date	Specimens/Daily Lab	Date	Treatments
Temp.					
Pulse & Resp.					
BP					
I & O					
Weights					
Spot Checks					
Chest P.T.					
Incentive Spirometer					
P.T.					

ACTIVITIES	NUTRITION			
Ad lib	Diet			
Ambulate				
Chair		Date	Diagnostic Procedures	
BRP				
Bedrest				
Bath	Feedings			
Self				
Tub	Assist c̄ meals			
Shower	FLUID BALANCE			
Bed	Force			
Assist.	D E N			
	Restrict			
	D E N			
Orderlies Needed				
Family:				

NURSING CARE PLAN

Date	Nursing Diagnosis	Expected Outcomes	Nursing Plan/Orders

Discharge Planning: Destination: | Transportation: | Probable Date: | Referral Agencies: | Appointment:
Supplies:

Patient Name

Chapter 23
The Family

PREREQUISITE READING

Chapter 23, pp. 729 to 745

OBJECTIVES

Mastery of content in this chapter will enable the student to:

- Define selected terms used to describe families.
- Discuss the way family members influence one another's health.
- Describe current trends in the American family.
- Define the family in terms applicable to all family forms.
- Describe four common family forms and discuss the relevant health concerns of each.
- Explain the way family structure and patterns of functioning affect the health of family members and the family as a whole.
- Compare family as context to family as client and explain the way these perspectives influence nursing practice.
- Describe the family nursing process in terms of assessment, nursing diagnosis, planning, intervention, and evaluation.
- Describe the attributes of effective and ineffective families.
- Describe how the health of the family is influenced by its position in society.

REVIEW OF KEY CONCEPTS

1. Identify the definition of family that would be most helpful in providing effective nursing care.
   a. A biological entity, legal unit, or social network
   b. Two or more individuals related by blood, marriage, or adoption
   c. A mother, father, and their children
   d. A set of relationships that the client identifies as family or a network of influence
2. James and Jane Smith are husband and wife. They have an eight-year old daughter named Sally.
   a. James, Jane, and Sally Smith would be considered a (an):
      (1) extended family.
      (2) nuclear family.
      (3) blended family.
      (4) family of origin.
   b. For Sally, this family would be considered her:
      (1) extended family.
      (2) family of procreation.
      (3) family of origin.
      (4) primary support system.
   c. For James and Jane, this family would be considered their:
      (1) family of procreation.
      (2) family of origin.
      (3) blended family.
      (4) extended family.
3. The nuclear family is the dominant family form in North America. (True or false?)
4. The adjustment period experienced by members of a blended family may take as long as:
   a. 6 to 8 weeks.
   b. 6 to 12 months.
   c. 2 years.
   d. 5 years.
5. The key to healthy stepfamily functioning is the establishment of:
   a. very flexible structures within the family.
   b. traditional roles within the family unit.
   c. friendly sibling relationships.
   d. a strong couple bond.
6. Departures from the traditional form of family result in added stress and threatened family health. (True or false?)
7. List at least four characteristic processes necessary for family functioning.

   a.

   b.

   c.

   d.
8. Match the family developmental stage with the task described.

Stage

- **a.** Between families: unattached young adult _____
- **b.** Newly married couple _____
- **c.** Family with young children _____
- **d.** Family with adolescents _____
- **e.** Family launching children and moving on _____
- **f.** Family in later life _____

Task

1. Development of adult-to-adult relationships
2. Life review and integration
3. Refocus on marital and career issues
4. Development of intimate peer relationships
5. Taking on parenting roles
6. Realignment of relationship with extended family and friends

9. Behaviors within a family influence the health of each family member. (True or false?)
10. List at least six strengths of the resilient, effective family.

   a.

   b.

   c.

   d.

   e.

   f.

11. Briefly compare the family as *context* and the family as *client* in relation to the nurse's role in providing care.
12. Mr. Cohen is a client in the ambulatory care clinic. He is 45 years old, married, and the father of three children. When providing care for Mr. Cohen in the ambulatory care clinic, the nurse views the Cohen family as:
   a. dysfunctional.
   b. the context (environment).
   c. the client.
   d. non-traditional.
13. When working with families, the nurse attempts to change the structure to meet the needs of the client requiring care. (True or false?)
14. When formulating a plan of care for a family as client, it is imperative that all members understand and agree to the plan. (True or false?)
15. Identify at least one evaluative measure for each of the following goals of family care:
   a. The client uses appropriate family resources.
   b. The family successfully accomplishes its appropriate developmental task.
   c. The family members understand the client's health problem.
   d. The client returns to a functional state within the family environment.

CRITICAL THINKING AND EXPERIENTIAL EXERCISES

1. Family forms and health concerns
   Compare the types of health concerns or problems typically faced by each of the following family forms.
   a. Single-parent
   b. Extended
   c. Blended
2. The concept of family
   a. Describe your concept of family.
   b. Identify how your perception and values may positively influence your care of families.
   c. Identify how your perception and values might create conflict in caring for families. Discuss how you might address this dilemma to ensure quality client care.
3. Family nursing process
   a. Review the sample family assessment form in your text on p. 740. Consider any additional data you believe are important for a complete data base, and modify the form accordingly. Share your revisions with your instructor.
   b. Using the sample assessment form in your text, with or without modifications, conduct a family assessment of your family or an assigned client's family.
   c. Formulate nursing diagnoses that address the needs of the family.
   d. Based on your assessment and diagnoses, determine whether you will intervene with family as client or context.
   e. Develop a nursing care plan to address the priority nursing diagnosis.
   f. Share your nursing diagnoses, approach, and care plan with your instructor before implementation.
4. Clinical situation: family assessment
   Mrs. Godinez is a 40-year-old Mexican American who recently divorced. She has a 3-year-old son, a 5-year-old daughter, and a 16-year-old daughter. A referral was made to a community health nurse from the school nurse because of increased absenteeism of the 16-year-old daughter.
   a. What type of family form is this unit?
   b. What three major areas of function should the nurse evaluate in this family form?
   c. What resources could the nurse and client pursue to address these three areas of concern?
   d. In addition, Mrs. Godinez's 70-year-old mother has now moved into the household. What family form is created by this change?
   e. Mrs. Godinez's mother has a chronic respiratory condition requiring frequent medical treatment. How will this influence the health of the family members and the family as a whole?
   f. What is the developmental stage of this family, and what are the specific tasks during this stage? How may the nurse facilitate family developmental task achievement?

g. When you visit the home, you note that Mrs. Godinez, her mother, and her 16-year-old daughter are obese. Would you intervene in this situation with the family as client or as environment? How would you approach the problem?

ADDITIONAL READINGS

Ballie V, Norbeck JS, Bares LE: Stress, social support, and psychological distress of the family caregivers of the elderly, *Nurs Res* 37(4):217, 1988.

Reports on a study of family members caring for elderly at home. Results indicate high risk for distress and/or depression when caring for a mentally retarded relative, providing care for an extended period, or experiencing minimal social support.

Friedman M: *Family nursing: theory and assessment*, ed 2, New York, 1986, Appleton-Century-Crofts.

Discusses dynamics of family structure and functions. Includes family case study and analysis to reinforce theoretical concepts.

Leavitt M, editor: Symposium on family nursing in acute care, *Nurs Clin North Am* 19(1):83, 1984.

Series of articles focusing on care of the family unit. Although articles address a variety of acute care situations, principles are applicable to any practice setting. Includes discussion of unique needs of families in specialized areas of nursing practice including mental health, maternal-child care, pediatrics, oncology, and cardiology.

Mercer RT, Ferketich SL: Predictors of family functioning eight months following birth, *Nurs Res* 39(2):76,1990.

Compares the stress perceived by families experiencing high-risk and low-risk pregnancies. Findings indicate long-term effects of stress in families experiencing high-risk pregnancies.

Romanzuk A: Helping the stepparent parent, *MCN* 12:1096, 1987.

Attempts to dispel myths associated with stepparenting. Discusses assessment and care planning to facilitate family adjustment. Includes helpful annotated bibliography of books and audiovisual media for parents and children in reconstituted or blended families.

Sund K, Ostwald SK: Dual-earner families' stress levels and personal and life-style-related variables, *Nurs Res* 34(6):357, 1985.

Identifies stressors and stress levels experienced by dual-earner families in the preschool stage of family development. Information presented may be helpful in counseling dual-earner families in other developmental stages.

Chapter 24
Conception Through Preschool

PREREQUISITE READING

Chapter 24, pp. 746 to 781

OBJECTIVES

Mastery of content in this chapter will enable the student to:

- Define selected terms relevant to human growth and development.
- Describe three commonalities in human development and the seven principles of growth and development related to them.
- Discuss the major factors influencing growth and development.
- Compare and discuss theories used by nurses to understand the development of children.
- Describe nursing strategies for maternal support during pregnancy.
- Discuss physiological and psychosocial health concerns during the transition of the child from intrauterine to extrauterine life.
- Explain the concept of critical periods of development and identify factors that can disturb or promote optimal development of the child.
- Describe characteristics of the physical growth of the unborn child, infant, toddler, and preschooler.
- Describe cognitive and psychosocial development from birth to 6 years.
- Explain the bonding that occurs between parent and child, its development into a deep attachment, and the factors that may impede or facilitate it.
- Describe variables influencing how children learn about and perceive their health status.
- Identify areas in which the parents of well and hospitalized children can benefit from the nurse's anticipatory guidance.
- Use knowledge of growth and development to assess and plan appropriate nursing care of hospitalized children between birth and first grade.
- Describe the use of the nursing process to individualize the nursing care plan for the hospitalized child.

REVIEW OF KEY CONCEPTS

1. Which statement about human growth and development is accurate?
   a. Growth and development processes are unpredictable.
   b. Growth and development begins with birth and ends after adolescence.
   c. All individuals progress through the same phases of growth and development.
   d. All individuals accomplish developmental tasks at the same pace.
2. An individuals' health may be influenced by the ability to progress through each developmental phase. (True or false?)
3. The process of becoming fully developed and grown through physical and behavioral change is _____ .
4. Behavioral change promoting progressive adaptation to the environment is _____ .
5. The quantitative change reflecting an increase in physical measurement is _____ .
6. List three commonalities of growth and development applicable to all people.

   a.

   b.

   c.
7. List the seven basic principles of growth and development.

   a.

   b.

   c.

   d.

   e.

   f.

   g.
8. A critical period of development is:
   a. cephalocaudal and proximodistal growth.
   b. the 9-month prenatal period of neurological development.
   c. the time between conception and medical confirmation of a pregnancy.
   d. a specific time during which the environment has its greatest effect on the individual.

9. The use of a developmental framework for nursing care is only necessary when working with infants and children. (True or false?)

10. List the two internal forces and the five external forces influencing growth and development. By using an asterisk, indicate the four forces considered most influential in human development.
    a. Internal forces/forces of nature
       (1)
       (2)
    b. External forces
       (1)
       (2)
       (3)
       (4)
       (5)

11. Match the theorist with the appropriate development focus.

Theorist

   a. Piaget _____
   b. Erikson _____
   c. Maslow _____
   d. Freud _____
   e. Kohlberg _____

Focus

   1. Psychosexual theory
   2. Psychosocial development
   3. Human needs
   4. Cognitive development
   5. Moral reasoning

12. List the two most common causes of intrauterine health problems.
    a.
    b.

13. Define teratogen.

14. What is meant by the phrase *the fetus is viable*?

15. The cheese-like protective substance covering the skin of the fetus is _____ .

16. The fine hair covering most of the body of the fetus is _____ .

17. When is the mother most likely to become aware of fetal movement?
    a. First trimester
    b. Second trimester
    c. Third trimester

18. The two most common causes of damage to the fetal central nervous system during the third trimester are:
    a. noxious agents and poor maternal nutrition.
    b. viral infection and maternal stress.
    c. bacterial infection and maternal drug abuse.
    d. maternal tobacco and alcohol abuse.

19. It is believed that the biochemical environment of the uterus and postpartum emotional status of the mother can influence the psychosocial development of the child. (True or false?)

20. List the three priority physical health needs of the neonate.
    a.
    b.
    c.

21. Immediately after birth, the neonate receives an instillation of erythromycin 0.5% into the eyes to prevent _____ .

22. Common care of the umbilical cord stump includes all of the following except:
    a. application of antibacterial agent such as triple dye.
    b. application of alcohol with each diaper change.
    c. application of sterile dressing or bandage.
    d. folding the diaper to avoid contact with the stump.

23. List the five physiological parameters evaluated through the Apgar assessment.
    a.
    b.
    c.
    d.
    e.

24. A neonate receives an Apgar score of 4 one minute after birth and a score of 6 five minutes after birth. These Apgar scores indicate that the neonate is:
    a. adjusting well to extrauterine life.
    b. experiencing little difficulty adjusting to extrauterine life.
    c. experiencing moderate difficulty adjusting to extrauterine life.
    d. experiencing severe distress.

25. What two factors are most important in promoting closeness of the parents and the neonate?

26. Define bonding.

27. Which neonatal assessment finding would be considered abnormal?
    a. Cyanosis of the hands and feet during activity
    b. Palpable anterior and posterior fontanels
    c. Soft protuberant abdomen
    d. Sporadic asymmetrical limb movements

28. Infants normally double their birth weight by:
    a. 3 months.
    b. 6 months.
    c. 9 months.
    d. 1 year.

29. Which statement about guidelines for infant feeding is accurate?
    a. There is a standard diet plan appropriate for all infants.
    b. Solid foods are usually introduced before the sixth month.
    c. The nurse should encourage all mothers to breast feed.
    d. Fluoride supplements are necessary for breast-fed infants.
30. Which statement about infant cognitive development is accurate?
    a. Sensory stimuli are less important than food for healthy development.
    b. Hospitalized infants require continuous stimuli to enhance cognitive development.
    c. By 12 months, infants are able to comprehend simple commands.
    d. By 12 months, infants continue to have difficulty localizing and discriminating sounds.
31. To promote optimal stimulation, it is appropriate to assign several nurses to provide daily care for a hospitalized infant. (True or false?)
32. Why does the toddler frequently demonstrate temper tantrums?
33. The mother of a 2-year-old expresses concern that her son's appetite has diminished and that he seems to prefer milk to other solid foods. Which response by the nurse reflects knowledge of principles of communication and nutrition?
    a. "Oh, I wouldn't be too worried; children tend to eat when they're hungry. I just wouldn't give him dessert unless he eats his meal."
    b. "That is not uncommon in toddlers. You might consider increasing his milk to 2 quarts per day to be sure he gets enough nutrients."
    c. "Have you considered feeding him when he doesn't seem interested in feeding himself?"
    d. "A toddler's rate of growth normally slows down. It's common to see a toddler's appetite diminish in response to decreased calorie needs."
34. The preschool years are characterized by:
    a. the development of autonomy.
    b. rapid physical growth.
    c. slowed psychosocial development.
    d. beginning intuitive thought.
35. The preschooler tells his parent that his toy car is sad because the wheel fell off. The child is demonstrating:
    a. artificialism.
    b. imminent justice.
    c. animism.
    d. egocentricity.
36. The preschooler demonstrates concrete thinking and interprets words literally. (True or false?)
37. Define regression.
38. Fill in the expected age of children and the characteristic play pattern.

Play Pattern	Age Span	Characteristic Behaviors
Cooperative		
Parallel		
Associative		

39. Indicate the age span and average heart and respiratory rate for each age group.

Stage	Age Span	Heart Rate	Respiratory Rate
Fetus			
Neonate			
Infant			
Toddler			
Preschooler			

40. List four factors influencing a child's reaction to illness and hospitalization.
    a.
    b.
    c.
    d.
41. What standardized test may the nurse use in determining a child's developmental level?
42. Fear of body injury and pain reactions occurs in all children, including neonates. (True or false?)
43. List four goals to include when planning care for a hospitalized child.
    a.
    b.
    c.
    d.
44. List at least five actions that may mimimize a child's separation anxiety.
    a.
    b.
    c.
    d.
    e.
45. Identify at least four actions that may facilitate establishing trust with the child and family.
    a.
    b.
    c.
    d.
46. Match the age group with the most commonly experienced fears.

Age group

a. Birth to 3 months _____

b. 4 to 12 months _____

c. 1 to 3 years _____

d. 3 to 6 years _____

Fears

1. Dark, being alone, separation from parent, and loud machines
2. Body mutilation, supernatural beings, monsters, ghosts, separation from trusted adults and familiar routines, and abandonment
3. Sudden movements, loud noises, and loss of physical support
4. Strangers, strange objects, heights, and anticipation of previous uncomfortable situations

47. List four nursing actions to minimize fear in the hospitalized child.

    a.

    b.

    c.

    d.

48. List at least five guidelines to minimize children's physical discomfort associated with hospitalization.

    a.

    b.

    c.

    d.

    e.

49. List at least four guidelines to foster normal growth and development in the hospitalized child.

    a.

    b.

    c.

    d.

50. List at least six guidelines when planning play for the hospitalized child.

    a.

    b.

    c.

    d.

    e.

    f.

CRITICAL THINKING AND EXPERIENTIAL EXERCISES

1. Stages of growth and development

    a. Observe children in any setting (such as home, community, or health care facility). Identify physical and psychosocial behaviors of the children and match them to the milestones expected at each stage of growth and development. When possible, attempt to confirm the actual chronological ages of children with the individual supervising the activity.

    b. Conduct a developmental assessment of an assigned client, friend, or relative. Identify the individual's stage of growth and development and determine the developmental tasks that have been accomplished. Formulate nursing interventions to promote the individual's developmental task achievement.

    c. Observe a skilled nurse perform a Denver Developmental Screening Test (or examine the materials in a DDST kit.) Attempt to perform the DDST on a healthy child and plot the development levels on a DDST graph. Identify play activities for the child appropriate to the developmental level displayed.

2. Promoting fetal growth and development

    Structure a teaching plan for a pregnant woman and her partner that is directed toward maintenance of fetal health in each of the following areas.

    a. Physical development

    b. Cognitive development

    c. Psychosocial development

3. Transition from intrauterine to extrauterine life

    a. Arrange to talk with a nurse or clinical specialist working in the area of maternal-child care. Ask the nurse to discuss how the staff promotes the neonate's physical and psychosocial health and facilitates family acquaintance and attachment.

    b. Ask your instructor to arrange for an observational experience in any setting in which prenatal, intrapartal, or postpartal care is provided. Identify actions by the nurse promoting physical health and psychosocial development of the mother, father, and child as individuals and as a family.

4. Clinical situation: developmental theories

    Timmy Johnson is a 24-month-old child with recurrent ear infections (otitis media and serous otitis). He lives with his mother (age 21), his stepfather (age 35) and his stepbrother (age 14). He and his mother have a well-child appointment with the pediatric nurse practitioner.

    a. What physical developmental milestones should the nurse evaluate in Timmy? (Name at least five.)

    b. According to Freud, what is Timmy's developmental stage, and what developmental skills are affected by this stage?

c. According to Erikson, what conflict is commonly experienced by children Timmy's age, and what anticipatory guidance can the nurse offer?

d. According to Erikson, what are the psychosocial tasks for the other members of Timmy's family, and what anticipatory guidance can the nurse offer?

e. According to Maslow, what is Timmy's developmental stage or category? What needs must Timmy and his family meet to progress?

f. Identify the major external forces presenting opportunities for Timmy's growth and development. What are the relevant influences of each of these forces?

5. Clinical situation: the hospitalized child
Jeffrey is a 4-year-old admitted to the hospital for a tonsillectomy. He is accompanied by his mother, who will remain with him throughout the entire hospitalization. His father lives in another state and will not be available to the family except by telephone. Jeffrey's grandmother lives nearby and will be caring for his 6-year-old brother, Brian.

a. Identify factors to assess during the admission interview. Describe why each of these factors will be important in planning care.

b. Formulate at least four nursing diagnoses that might be applicable to Jeffrey.

c. State four goals for care during Jeffrey's hospitalization.

d. Identify at least one outcome criterion and three interventions to achieve each of the stated goals. Be sure the interventions are developmentally appropriate for Jeffrey.

e. How will Brian's perceptions of this event differ from his brother's? What anticipatory guidance should be provided for the family about Brian's needs?

ADDITIONAL READINGS

Behrman RE, Vaughan, VC, editors: *Nelson textbook of pediatrics,* ed 13, Philadelphia, 1987, Saunders.
A comprehensive pediatric textbook. Includes detailed discussion of growth and development from the prenatal period through adolescence. A superior reference for information related to physical and psychological disorders found in neonates, infants, children, and adolescents. Describes in detail the pathology, diagnostic tests, sympto-mology, and usual medical treatment of pediatric disorders.

Craft MJ, Wyatt N: Effect of visitation of siblings on hospitalized children, *MCN* 15(1):47, 1986.
Describes a study to evaluate the effect of sibling visitation on the hospitalized child. Findings suggest visitation produces age-related changes in sibling feelings and behaviors. Identifies needs of siblings of hospitalized children. Well referenced to assist in accessing related readings.

Dole JC: A multidimensional study of infant's response to painful stimuli, *Pediatr Nurs* 12(1):27, 1986.
Study to identify common behaviors of infants in response to acute pain. Points to the need for multisystem assessment for accurate pain assessment.

Garot PA: Therapeutic play: work of both child and nurse, *J Pediatr Nurs* 1(2):111, 1986.
Discusses therapeutic play as a valuable nursing intervention.

Hauck, MR: Cognitive abilities of preschool children: Implications for nurses working with young children, *J Pediatr Nurs* 6(4): 230, 1991.
Describes thought processes and comprehension levels of preschool children. Suggests that Piaget's theory of cognitive development is limited and that preschoolers are more cognitively competent than the theory implies.

Kennedy, CM, Gyr, PM, Garst, KF: A nursing tool to assess children upon hospital admission, *MCN* 16(2): 78. 1991.
Presents a precise format to guide admission interviewing and subsequent care planning.

Kramer, NA: Comparison of therapeutic touch and casual touch in stress reduction in hospitalized children, *Pediatr Nurs* 16(5): 483, 1990.
Examines children's response to Krieger's steps of therapeutic touch. Findings reveal that consistent use of therapeutic touch, when compared with casual touch, reduced the time needed to calm hospitalized children after a stressful experience.

Schepp, KG: Factors influencing coping effort of mothers of hospitalized children, *Nurs Res* 40 (1): 42, 1991.
Study of maternal response to child's hospitalization. Identifies that anxiety is consistently reduced in mothers who remain well informed about the plan of care.

Whaley, LF, and Wong, DL: *Nursing care of infants and children,* ed.4, St. Louis, 1991, Mosby–Year Book.
A comprehensive pediatric nursing text. Detailed description of normal growth and development, physical and developmental assessment, and common and unusual health problems (and related treatment) from infancy through adolescence. Describes the nurse's role in pediatric care from the perspective of traditional and expanded practice roles.

Chapter 25
School Age Through Adolescence

PREREQUISITE READING
Chapter 25, pp. 782 to 807

OBJECTIVES
Mastery of content in this chapter will enable the student to:
- Define selected terms relevant to growth and development of children and adolescents.
- Describe the normal physical changes that occur during the school-age years and adolescence.
- Discuss behaviors reflecting psychosocial and cognitive development of the school-age child and adolescent.
- Contrast the cognitive abilities of the school-age child and adolescent.
- Identify factors that contribute to a sense of self-esteem in youth.
- Describe the influence of the school environment on the development of the school-age child and adolescent.
- Discuss ways in which the nurse can help parents meet their children's developmental needs.
- Compare and contrast the ways by which a school-age child and adolescent develop moral values.
- Discuss the development of identity in the adolescent.
- Explain the significance of Erikson's psychosocial moratoriums to the adolescent.
- Identify health concerns of the school-age child and adolescent.
- Describe nursing interventions to promote optimal health in the school-age child and adolescent.
- Describe the use of the nursing process to individualize the nursing care of youth.

REVIEW OF KEY CONCEPTS
1. Match the developmental behavior with the typical age group.

Behavior
- a. Potential for nutritional deficiencies increases. _____
- b. There is desire for increased independence and autonomy. _____
- c. Feelings of competence regarding task mastery are key in formation of self-esteem. _____
- d. Peer group is critical for recognition and acceptance. _____
- e. Defense mechanisms include regression, denial, aggression, and suppression. _____
- f. Defense mechanisms include rationalization and intellectualization. _____
- g. Fears are related to school, family, and death. _____
- h. There are frequent conflicts with siblings at home and strong sibling alliance outside of home. _____

Age group
1. School-age child
2. Adolescent

2. Which statement about physical development in the school-age child is accurate?
- a. The rate of growth during early school years is more rapid than during the preschool period.
- b. Fine motor skills are more refined than gross motor skills.
- c. Girls begin changes associated with puberty as early as age 9.
- d. Regular measurement of height and weight are less important than during other developmental stages.

3. List the average heart rate, respiratory rate, and blood pressure for the typical school-age child.
- a. Heart rate
- b. Respiratory rate
- c. Blood pressure

4. The most common nutritional deficiencies during the school-age period include:
- a. calcium, vitamin C, and B complex vitamins.
- b. iron, calcium, and vitamin A.
- c. iron and vitamin K.
- d. calcium, vitamin D, and vitamin C.

5. What is the best way to ensure adequate nutrition intake for the school-age child?

6. Match the description of cognitive behavior with the appropriate term.

Description

a. Recognition that the amount of a substance remains the same even when the shape or appearance changes _____

b. Ability to use symbols to carry out mental activities _____

c. Ability to place objects in order according to increasing or decreasing size _____

d. Ability to trace thought processes back to point of origination _____

e. Ability to concentrate on more than one aspect of a situation _____

Term

1. Concrete operations
2. Decenter
3. Reversibility
4. Conservation
5. Seriation

7. The leading cause of death in school-age children is:
   a. accident.
   b. infectious disease.
   c. cancer.
   d. suicide.

8. The transition period between childhood and adolescence is:
   a. pubescence.
   b. late childhood.
   c. transescence.
   d. all of the above.

9. The period of psychological maturation of the individual is _____ .

10. The period of biological maturation, making reproduction possible, is _____ .

11. Describe the differences between primary and secondary sex characteristics.

12. List the four major physical changes associated with sexual maturation (according to Tanner, 1974).

   a.

   b.

   c.

   d.

13. The time of onset of pubertal changes may have an effect on psychosocial development. (True or false?)

14. Which statement about pubertal growth changes is correct?
   a. The timing of pubertal growth changes is the same in most females.
   b. The time when sexual changes begin is more significant than their pattern of onset.
   c. The sequence of pubertal growth changes is the same in most individuals.

d. Growth changes result from pituitary secretion of gonadotropin-releasing hormones.

15. Teenagers have the ability to think as well as adults. (True or false?)

16. Adolescents have mastered age-appropriate sexuality when they feel comfortable with their sexual:
   a. behaviors.
   b. choices.
   c. relationships.
   d. all of the above.

17. The strong need for group identity often conflicts with the adolescent's quest for personal identity. (True or false?)

18. Define Erikson's "psychological moratorium."

19. The leading cause of death in adolescents is:
   a. motor vehicle accidents.
   b. drug abuse.
   c. suicide.
   d. infectious disease.

20. List the six warning signs of suicide in adolescents.

   a.

   b.

   c.

   d.

   e.

   f.

21. The most common communicable diseases among adolescents are _____ .

22. List five areas for nursing assessment of the school-age child and adolescent.

   a.

   b.

   c.

   d.

   e.

23. Briefly describe the differences between internal and external support systems.

CRITICAL THINKING AND EXPERIENTIAL EXERCISES

1. Stages of growth and development
   a. Observe school-age children and adolescents in any setting. Identify physical and psychosocial behaviors and match them to expected characteristics of the designated stage of growth and development.
   b. Conduct a developmental assessment of a school-age child or adolescent. Determine the developmental tasks that have been accomplished. Formulate nursing interventions to promote individual developmental task achievement.

2. School-related stressors
   For each of the designated age groups, identify at

least two school-related stresses and an appropriate nursing intervention to assist the child in stress reduction.
   a. Age 6 to 8
   b. Age 8 to 10
   c. Age 10 to 12
3. Developmental health concerns and health education
   a. Identify a major health problem/health education need for school-age children or adolescents.
   b. Identify the target audience and formulate a developmentally appropriate teaching plan to address the health problem/educational need.
4. Clinical situation: developmental theories, growth and development
   Chip Brown is a 7-year-old who fractured his right arm while climbing a tree. He lives with his parents and his 4-year-old brother. The pediatric nurse practitioner is responsible for Chip's follow-up care.
   a. What physical characteristics should be evaluated (based on Chip's age)?
   b. According to Freud, what is Chip's developmental stage and what developmental skills are affected by his injury?
   c. According to Erikson, what conflict is commonly experienced by children Chip's age, and what anticipatory guidance can the nurse offer?
   d. According to Erikson, what are the psychosocial tasks for other members of Chip's family? What anticipatory guidance can the nurse offer for family health?
   e. According to Maslow, what is Chip's developmental category or stage? What needs must Chip and his family meet to progress?
   f. Identify the major positive and negative forces influencing Chip's growth and development. What actions can the nurse take to promote his normal growth and development?
5. Clinical situation: care of the hospitalized adolescent
   Barry Dobbs is a 15-year-old boy hospitalized for a fractured jaw resulting from a motorcycle accident. After surgery, he experiences postoperative pain and swelling. He is very concerned about his appearance.

His jaw is wired, impairing his ability to speak clearly. He is receiving his meals in a semiliquid form through a small feeding tube.
   a. Identify factors to assess before planning Barry's care.
   b. What major task would concern Barry during the adolescent stage of development? What areas of developmental adjustment should the nurse consider when formulating a plan of care?
   c. Based on the information provided, formulate at least four nursing diagnoses that might apply to Barry.
   d. State four goals for Barry's care during hospitalization.
   e. Identify at least one criterion and three interventions to achieve each of the stated goals. Be sure that your interventions are appropriate to the adolescent developmental level.

ADDITIONAL READINGS

Please refer to additional readings cited in Chapter 24 that apply to school-age children and adolescents. References previously cited are not repeated in this chapter.
Antwerp CV, Paniolo AM: Checking out children's lifestyles, *MCN* 16(3):144, 1991.
   Presents an excellent lifestyle assessment tool directed at health promotion, injury prevention, and expression of feelings. Useful in designing plans for health maintenance and illness prevention in children.
Lee E et al: Stressful life events and accidents at school, *Pediatr Nurse* 15(2):140, 1989.
   Relates high levels of adolescent stress with school accidents and injuries. Emphasizes that school teachers, nurses, and counselors must be alert to life events that place students at particular risk for physical injury and must take appropriate action to maintain physical and psychological health.
Oldaker S: Identity confusion: nursing diagnosis for adolescents, *Nurs Clin North Am* 20(4):763, 1985.
   Describes research investigating developmental health and psychological symptoms among high school adolescents. Explores potential causes of identity confusion and explores critical diagnostic criteria. Correlates etiology and diagnostic criteria with developmental tasks.

Chapter 26
Young and Middle Adult

PREREQUISITE READING
Chapter 26, pp. 808 to 827

OBJECTIVES
Mastery of content in this chapter will enable the student to:
- Define selected terms relevant to the young- and middle-adult years.
- Discuss developmental theories of the young and middle adult.
- List and discuss major life events of the young and middle adult and the childbearing family.
- Describe developmental tasks of the young adult, the childbearing family, and the middle adult.
- Discuss the significance of family in the life of the adult.
- Describe normal physiological changes in young and middle adulthood and in pregnancy.
- Discuss cognitive and psychosocial changes occurring during the adult years.
- Describe health concerns of the young adult, the childbearing family, and the middle adult.
- List nursing diagnoses appropriate for the young and middle adult.
- Use the nursing process to administer care to young and middle adults.

REVIEW OF KEY CONCEPTS
1. Briefly describe the characteristics of the mature adult.
2. List and briefly describe the five phases of young- and middle-adult development described by Levinson.

   a.

   b.

   c.

   d.

   e.

3. Theorists propose that intellectual and moral development is gender specific. (True or false?)
4. According to Gilligan, what constitutes women's primary developmental issue?

5. Describe the five developmental tasks of the young adult proposed by Diekelmann.

   a.

   b.

   c.

   d.

   e.

6. According to Erikson's developmental theory, the primary developmental task of the middle years is to:
   a. achieve generativity.
   b. achieve intimacy.
   c. establish a set of personal values.
   d. establish a sense of personal identity.
7. Identify Havighurst's proposed seven developmental tasks for the middle adult.

   a.

   b.

   c.

   d.

   e.

   f.

   g.

8. List the four phases of the childbearing cycle in their appropriate sequence.

   a.

   b.

   c.

   d.

9. Describe four tasks that should ideally be completed by a couple before marriage.

   a.

   b.

c.

d.

10. Describe four tasks to be accomplished by the married couple establishing a household and family.

    a.

    b.

    c.

    d.

11. List six hallmarks of emotional health indicating that the young adult has successfully mastered the developmental stage.

    a.

    b.

    c.

    d.

    e.

    f.

12. Lifestyle patterns during the young adult years may place the individual at risk for development of illnesses or disabilities during middle or older adult years. (True or false?)

13. The greatest cause of illness and death in the young adult population is:
    a. sexually transmitted disease.
    b. violence.
    c. cardiovascular disease.
    d. substance abuse.

14. Define infertility.

15. Pregnancy produces cognitive and psychosocial changes affecting not only the mother but also the father, siblings, and grandparents. (True or false?)

16. An overweight woman attempting to become pregnant would be advised to begin a weight reduction diet. (True or false?)

17. Match the physiological changes of pregnancy with the trimester when they most commonly occur.

Change

    a. Increased colostrum _____

    b. Fatigue _____

    c. Quickening _____

    d. Hypertrophy of gums _____

    e. Breast enlargement _____

    f. Nausea or vomiting _____

Trimester

    1. First trimester
    2. Second trimester
    3. Third trimester

18. Define puerperium.

19. Psychosocial changes of pregnancy commonly involve all of the following areas except:
    a. body image.
    b. anxiety and depression.
    c. role changes.
    d. sexuality.

20. Which physiological change would be a normal assessment finding in a middle adult?
    a. Increased breast size
    b. Abdominal tenderness and organomegaly
    c. Increased anteroposterior diameter of thorax
    d. Reduced auditory acuity

21. Define menopause.

22. Define climacteric.

23. A man remains capable of fathering a child after andropause. (True or false?)

24. List four risk factors for depression in the middle adult.

    a.

    b.

    c.

    d.

25. State three health maintenance goals that would be appropriate for the young or middle adult.

    a.

    b.

    c.

26. Which statement about behavior and habits is incorrect?
    a. Habits often meet a basic need for the person.
    b. Any change in habits or behavior patterns creates stress.
    c. Habits can be stress-reduction mechanisms.
    d. Nurses are able to change clients' habits.

27. Identify at least two external and two internal barriers to change.
    a. External

       (1)

       (2)

    b. Internal

       (1)

       (2)

CRITICAL THINKING AND EXPERIENTIAL EXERCISES

1. Stages of marriage
    a. Interview at least one married couple from each stage of marriage: establishment, family orientation, and postparental family.
    b. For each couple interviewed, attempt to have the husband and wife identify the primary focus of their work as a couple, the major stressors they encounter, and the coping mechanisms they use to deal with the stressors.

c. Compare the information given with the tasks and goals of married couples described in your text.

2. Psychosocial assessment

   a. In collaboration with your instructor, develop a questionnaire or structure interview questions for assessment of a young adult's emotional health. Be sure to refer to the 10 hallmarks of emotional health described in your text as a guide.

   b. Interview a young adult based on the questionnaire or interview questions developed.

   c. Analyze the data obtained to determine whether the young adult has successfully matured in this developmental stage. Identify specific behaviors that reflect the individual's ability or inability to meet the developmental tasks.

   d. Formulate goals and related nursing interventions supporting or promoting successful maturation of the individual at the current specific developmental stage.

3. Lifestyle habits and illness risk

   a. Develop a 10- to 20-minute teaching session identifying common lifestyle habits increasing the risk of illness in the young and middle adult. Be sure to include a brief overview of methods of illness prevention related to each lifestyle habit.

   b. Present the teaching session to a group of peers or submit the plan to your instructor; request feedback.

   c. If feasible, identify a target audience in your community and, with your instructor as resource, present this information in a formal or informal teaching session.

4. Assessment of the middle adult

   a. Conduct an assessment of a middle adult using any comprehensive assessment tool (sample tool in your text, tool used in your institution, or tool you have developed or revised).

   b. Identify the developmental tasks for the middle adult and determine whether the individual is working toward or has achieved the tasks identified.

   c. Identify assessment findings reflecting expected physiological changes occurring in the middle adult years.

   d. Describe positive and negative health behaviors identified in the assessment.

   e. Identify risk factors for:
      (1) cancer.
      (2) cardiovascular disease: hypertension, heart attack, stroke.
      (3) depression.

5. Clinical situation: marriage and family development Jim and Joanna Hammer (both age 35) have been married for 2 years and are struggling with the decision to begin a family. They describe their marriage as "good" and frequently state that "our biological clock is running out." They have requested an appointment with the nurse at the neighborhood family-planning clinic to discuss their concerns and questions.

   a. What behaviors would indicate that Jim and Joanna have successfully worked through the establishment stage of their marriage?

   b. Several factors influence the decision to start a family. List and briefly describe the factors that the nurse would explore with the Hammers.

   c. If the Hammers decide to begin a family, what advice would the nurse give to Mrs. Hammer about her health practices before conception?

   d. What anticipatory guidance could the nurse offer to the Hammers at this time?

6. Clinical situation: nursing process for the middle adult Grace Charis, 53 years old, is admitted to the hospital for a hysterectomy to treat cervical cancer. Mrs. Charis has been married for 30 years and has three children, 17 to 24 years old. She describes her husband as her "best friend" and tells the nurse she is preparing to send her youngest child to college this fall. Mrs. Charis has smoked approximately five cigarettes per day for the past 35 years.

   a. What major task would concern Mrs. Charis as an individual in her middle years? What effect could her current health status have on task achievement?

   b. What stage of family development are the Charises experiencing? What feelings might parents experience during this stage? What behaviors or activities are characteristic of this stage? What influence could Mrs. Charis' status have on this stage of family development?

   c. Formulate at least four nursing diagnoses applicable to Mrs. Charis.

   d. State four goals for Mrs. Charis' care during hospitalization.

   e. Identify at least one outcome criterion and three interventions to achieve each of the stated goals. Be sure your interventions are appropriate to middle adult developmental tasks.

ADDITIONAL READINGS

Please refer to readings cited in Chapters 24 and 25 that apply to young and middle adults. References previously cited are not repeated in this chapter.

Beck CM, Rawlins RR, Williams SR: *Mental health–psychiatric nursing: a holistic life-cycle approach*, , ed 2, St Louis, 1988, Mosby–Year Book.

Comprehensively explores psychosocial development and mental health throughout the life span. Presents detailed discussion of theoretical foundations for practice. Uses physical, emotional, intellectual, social, and spiritual dimensions of mental health and illness as organizational frameworks for the study of normal development, behavior, and psychopathology. Presents nursing care using the nursing process format.

Bobak IM, Jensen MD: *Essentials of maternity nursing*, ed 3, St Louis, 1991, Mosby–Year Book.

Comprehensive maternity nursing text with a strong orientation to client education from a female perspective.

Brown MA: Social support, stress, and health: a comparison of expectant mothers and fathers, *Nurs Res* 35:72, 1986.

Examines the influence of social support and stress on the

health of expectant mothers and fathers. Identifies differences in social supports valued by mothers and fathers.

Gilligan C: *In a different voice*, Cambridge, Mass, 1982, Harvard University Press.

A frequently referenced discussion of female thought and moral development. Emphasizes the significant differences between male and female perspectives.

Laffrey SC: Normal and overweight adults: perceived weight and health behavior characteristics, *Nurs Res* 35:173, 1986.

Concludes that there is no difference in the perception of health in comparative groups of normal and overweight adults. Emphasizes the importance of understanding the clients' perception of health and individualized approaches to health practices.

Chapter 27
Older Adulthood

PREREQUISITE READING

Chapter 27, pp. 828 to 857

OBJECTIVES

Mastery of content in this chapter will enable the student to:
- Define selected terms relevant to the older adult and the aging process.
- Describe common myths and stereotypes about older adults.
- Discuss nurses' attitudes toward older adults.
- Discuss biological and psychosocial theories of aging.
- State and discuss developmental tasks of the older adult.
- Describe physiological changes of aging.
- Describe cognitive changes of dementia and delirium found in some older adults.
- Describe common causes of dementia and delirium.
- Discuss psychosocial changes of retirement, social isolation, sexuality, housing, and death to which older adults must adjust.
- Discuss physical and psychosocial health concerns of older adults and related nursing interventions.
- Describe community and institutional health care services available to older adults.
- Formulate a plan of care and interventions for an older adult with selected nursing diagnoses.
- Evaluate the plan of care and interventions for an older adult with selected nursing diagnoses.

REVIEW OF KEY CONCEPTS

1. Define geriatrics.
2. Define gerontology.
3. Which statement about older adults is accurate?
   a. Most older adults are institutionalized.
   b. Most older adults live on a fixed income.
   c. Most older adults cannot learn to care for themselves.
   d. Most older adults have no sexual desire.
4. Define ageism.
5. It is important to incorporate routines or rituals of the older adult into the plan of care. (True or false?)
6. Match the theory of aging with the most accurate description.

Description

a. Chemical reactions cause collagen to become rigid and less permeable with age. _____
b. Aging people withdraw from customary roles and engage in introspective, self-focused activities. _____
c. Extracellular changes create a reaction altering the structure or function of the cell membranes. _____
d. Older adults need to maintain physical, mental, and social activities. _____
e. Personality remains the same and behavior becomes more predictable as people age. _____
f. Erratic cellular mechanisms attack body tissues through autoaggression or immunodeficiency. _____

Theory

1. Free radical theory
2. Cross-link theory
3. Immunological theory
4. Continuity theory
5. Disengagement theory
6. Activity theory
7. List five developmental tasks of the older adult.

   a.

   b.

   c.

   d.

   e.

8. Indicate whether the physical assessment finding is expected (E) or pathological (P) in the older adult.

   a. Melanoma _____

   b. Presbyopia _____

   c. Absent bowel sounds _____

   d. Decreased lung expansion _____

   e. Diminished light reflex on tympanic membrane _____

   f. Enlarged prostate _____

   g. Diminished pedal pulses _____

   h. Positive ankle clonus _____

   i. Positive guaiac stools _____

9. Structural and physiological changes in the brain associated with the aging process will affect adaptive and functional abilities of the older adult. (True or false?)

10. Preexisting behavioral tendencies are magnified as a person ages. (True or false?)

11. Define dementia.

12. What is the most frequent cause of irreversible dementia?

13. List three common causes of reversible dementia in the older adult.

   a.

   b.

   c.

14. Which statement describing delirium is correct?
   a. Illusions and hallucinations may be experienced by persons with delirium.
   b. The onset of delirium is slow and insidious.
   c. Symptoms of delirium are stable and unchanging.
   d. Symptoms of delirium are irreversible.

15. Cognitive changes are expected outcomes of the aging process. (True or false?)

16. List three signs of the early stages of Alzheimer's disease.

   a.

   b.

   c.

17. Jack Waycome is a 56-year-old business executive showing behavioral changes over the past few years. Mr. Waycome is hesitant in responding to questions posed by his co-workers. He misses regularly scheduled weekly meetings. His secretary must constantly remind him about scheduled appointments and must find his reading glasses, pens, papers, and briefcase. Lately he has come to work without showering, shaving, or changing clothes from the previous day. Mr. Waycome's behaviors are characteristic of which stage of irreversible dementia (Alzheimer's disease)?
   a. Final or terminal
   b. Later
   c. Advanced
   d. Early

18. Multiinfarct dementia is associated primarily with:
   a. substance abuse.
   b. infectious processes.
   c. cardiac disorders.
   d. vascular disorders.

19. Long-term abuse of alcohol and drugs can produce permanent damage to the nervous system. (True or false?)

20. Individuals who plan their retirement activities generally make a better adjustment during the older adult years. (True or false?)

21. List at least four areas to be addressed when counseling an older adult for retirement.

   a.

   b.

   c.

   d.

22. Briefly describe the four types of social isolation experienced by older adults.
   a. Attitudinal isolation
   b. Presentational isolation
   c. Behavioral isolation
   d. Geographical isolation

23. Decreased libido is frequently associated with the aging process. (True or false?)

24. List four factors to assess when assisting older adults with housing needs.

   a.

   b.

   c.

   d.

25. By the time adults reach old age, they are emotionally prepared to die. (True or false?)

26. List the four major causes of death in older adults.

   a.

   b.

   c.

   d.

27. Confusion regularly occurring during the evening or night is _____

28. Nutritional needs of the older adult:
   a. are exactly the same as those of young and middle adults.
   b. include increased amounts of vitamin C, vitamin A, and calcium.
   c. include increased kilocalories to support metabolism and activity.
   d. include increased proteins and carbohydrates.

29. What advice should the nurse give to an older adult before the adult begins a formal exercise program?

30. List and briefly describe four techniques used to maintain psychosocial health of the older adult.

a.

b.

c.

d.

31. Recalling the past to assign new meaning to experiences is:
a. validation therapy.
b. reminiscence.
c. body image therapy.
d. confabulation.

32. The following are examples of nursing interventions useful in reality orientation. Label each example with the characteristic principle of reality orientation illustrated.
a. Give directions in clear, simple, short statements. _____
b. Encourage client to perform tasks and make decisions without assistance from other people. _____
c. Reward correct behavior with verbal praise, touch, or smiles. _____
d. Use time, date, place, and name in conversations. _____
e. Maintain continuity of care by assigning the same personnel to care for the client. _____
f. Repeat information, directions, statements, and questions when necessary. _____
g. Allow clients to keep familiar treasures and objects. _____

33. List four guidelines for conducting discussion sessions with older adults.

a.

b.

c.

d.

34. Identify the type of community or institutional care facility appropriate for the older adult based on the primary health care service described.
a. Services focusing on self-care and maintenance of activities of daily living _____
b. Services to meet the needs of the terminally ill client and family _____
c. Health services for a client able to remain home during the evening _____
d. Service enabling the care taker of a dependent adult to be away from home for a few days _____
e. Extended residential, intermediate, or specialized health care _____

35. List three factors to be considered when establishing goals of care for the older adult client.

a.

b.

c.

CRITICAL THINKING AND EXPERIENTIAL EXERCISES

1. Values clarification: aging
a. Imagine that you are the sole care giver for a newborn. How do you feel about feeding, bathing, diapering, touching, talking to, cuddling, and maintaining safety for a newborn 24 hours a day? Now imagine that you are the sole care giver for an older, bedridden client. How do you feel about feeding, bathing, touching, talking to, cuddling, and maintaining safety for the client, as well as dealing with incontinence, 24 hours a day? Were your feelings the same or different? Why?
b. Describe your attitudes toward older adults in your family and community. Discuss how you would like to be viewed and treated as an older adult.
c. In a small group of peers, select one of the following "limitations of aging" and experience it for at least one hour in or out of class. Each "aging peer" should be supervised by a "nonaging peer" to ensure safety and observe responses of others. Discuss your perceptions and feelings with the group after the experience.
  (1) Wear disposable gloves.
  (2) Wear dark sunglasses or sunglasses smeared with petroleum jelly.
  (3) Use a walker or tripod cane while walking, getting out of a chair, or going to the restroom.
  (4) Gently plug ears with cottonballs.
  (5) Splint several fingers together with gauze wrap and tape.

2. Assessment of the older adult
a. Conduct an assessment of an older adult using any comprehensive assessment tool (sample tool in your text, tool used in your institution, or tool you have developed or revised).
b. Identify the developmental task for the older adult, and determine whether the individual is working toward or has achieved the tasks identified.
c. Identify assessment findings reflecting expected physiological changes occurring in the older adult years.
d. Formulate a list of nursing diagnoses based on your assessment findings.

e. Identify the priority nursing diagnosis, and formulate a plan of care. Be sure that interventions reflect the developmental stage of the client.

3. Clinical situation: retirement

Mr. and Mrs. Jones have been married for more than 40 years. Mr. Jones works with a company that has an employee health nurse. Before his annual physical, Mr. Jones tells the nurse that he plans to retire after his next birthday.

   a. What issues should the nurse discuss with Mr. Jones?
   b. Mr. Jones tells the nurse that he and his wife anticipate that Mrs. Jones' mother, who recently suffered a stroke, will join their household. Assuming that the Joneses are living in your neighborhood, what community services would be available to assist them in adapting to this change? (Include at least five services or agencies.)
   c. What formal or informal contacts could Mr. and Mrs. Jones use to increase their social network after retirement? (Include at least five formal and five informal contacts.)

4. Clinical situation: reversible dementia

Margaret Hutchinson is an older client who has been independently caring for herself at home. She was hospitalized for treatment of congestive heart failure and has become confused every night.

   a. What factors may be contributing to Miss Hutchinson's confusion?
   b. What is the name given to the episodes of confusion Miss Hutchinson has been experiencing?
   c. Identify at least five nursing interventions to reduce the incidence of Miss Hutchinson's confusion at night.

5. Clinical situation: client with senile dementia, Alzheimer's type (SDAT)

Anna Mueller is a 58-year-old housewife in the advanced stages of Alzheimer's disease. Her husband continues to work outside the home but is increasingly concerned about leaving Mrs. Mueller alone at home during the day. The Muellers have two adult children living in the area, but they both work full time and have their own families.

   a. What symptoms would Mrs. Mueller most likely display during this stage of irreversible dementia?
   b. Identify at least four care objectives that would be particularly important for Mrs. Mueller at this time. Formulate at least three interventions for each objective.

   c. What health care services (i.e., community based or institutional) might be appropriate for the Muellers at this time?

ADDITIONAL READINGS

Please refer to readings cited in Chapters 24 through 26 that apply to older adults. References previously cited are not repeated in this chapter.

Abraham IL, Buckwater KC, Neundorfer M, editors: Alzheimer's disease, *Nurs Clin North Am* 23(1):1, 1988.
   Series of articles addressing issues and comprehensive approaches to care of the client and family experiencing Alzheimer's disease.

Chang BL et al: Adherence to health care regimens among elderly women, *Nurs Res* 34:27, 1985.
   Reports about a study to determine factors that contributed to the intent of elderly women to adhere to a plan of care. Illustrates the significance of psychosocial care on client intent. Identifies individual characteristics associated with high intent to adhere to care.

Ebersole P, Hess P: *Toward healthy aging: human needs and nursing responses,* ed 2, St Louis, 1990, Mosby–Year Book.
   Comprehensive gerontological nursing text. Approaches care of the older adult in the context of Maslow's hierarchy of needs. Identifies needs of the older client and describes appropriate nursing interventions. Includes theoretical foundations, roles, functions, and practice issues of gerontological nursing.

Falmer T: Mistreatment of elders: assessment, diagnosis, and intervention, *Nurs Clin North Am* 24(3):707, 1989.
   Describes growing problem of elder abuse. Provides parameters for assessment and suggests possible interventions.

Foreman MD: Acute confusional states in hospitalized elderly: a research dilemma, *Nurs Res* 35:34, 1986.
   Reviews the literature on acute confusional states. Includes information about classification, incidence. Uses tables to summarize information comparing acute confusional states with dementia.

Gropper-Katz EI: Reality orientation research, *J Gerontol Nurs* 13(8):13, 1987.
   Review of five articles addressing reality orientation as an intervention for elderly persons with moderate to severe degrees of confusion.

Lappe JM: Reminiscing: the life review therapy, *J Gerontol Nurs* 13(4):12, 1987.
   Describes research study examining the use of reminiscing in older adults. Suggests that life review is essential for adjusting to older adulthood and accepting death.

Rempusheski VF: The role of ethnicity in elder care, *Nurs Clin North Am* 24(3):717, 1989.
   Emphasizes the importance of culturally sensitive care for the older adult.

Chapter 28
Loss, Death, and Grieving

PREREQUISITE READING
Chapter 28, pp. 858 to 885

OBJECTIVES
Mastery of content in this chapter will enable the student to:
- Define selected terms associated with loss, death, and the grieving process.
- Identify the nurse's role in assisting clients with problems related to loss, death, and grief.
- Describe and compare the phases of grieving from Engel, Kübler-Ross, and Martocchio.
- Discuss five basic categories of loss and six dimensions of hope.
- Assess a client's reaction to loss and ability to cope.
- Describe the characteristics of a person experiencing grief.
- Compare and contrast grief after loss, anticipatory grief, and resolved grief.
- Develop a care plan for a client or family experiencing grief.
- Implement interventions for grieving clients to provide therapeutic communication, maintain self-esteem, and promote return to normal activities.
- Describe how the nurse helps meet the dying client's needs for comfort.
- Explain ways for the nurse to assist a family in caring for a dying client.
- Discuss the purposes of a hospice.
- List and discuss important factors in caring for the body after death.
- Discuss the role of the nurse's own loss experience as it influences care of grieving clients.
- Identify two ways nurses can meet their self-care needs related to loss.

REVIEW OF KEY CONCEPTS
1. Which statement about loss is accurate?
   a. Loss is only experienced when there is an actual absence of something valued.
   b. The more an individual has invested in what is lost, the less the feeling of loss.
   c. Loss may be maturational, situational, or both.
   d. The degree of stress experienced is unrelated to the type of loss.

2. List and briefly describe the five categories of loss.
   a.
   b.
   c.
   d.
   e.

3. The state of thought, feeling, and activity after a loss is:
   a. grief.
   b. mourning.
   c. bereavement.
   d. anticipatory grief.

4. List four tasks to be accomplished by the grieving person to facilitate effective adjustment.
   a.
   b.
   c.
   d.

5. The grieving process may promote personal growth. (True or false?)

6. In the table below, list the phases of the grieving process proposed by each theorist.

Engle	Kübler-Ross	Martocchio
a.	a.	a.
b.	b.	b.
c.	c.	c.
	d.	d.
	e.	e.

7. Individuals experiencing loss will progress through each phase of the grieving process sequentially. (True or false?)

8. It is common for people to be engaged in the mourning process for 3 to 5 years. (True or false?)

9. Match the behaviors described to the stage of dying identified by Kübler-Ross.

Behavior

    a. Becomes quiet, noncommunicative, and inattentive to personal appearance _____

    b. Becomes fearful of losing body functions or control _____

    c. Gives away personal possessions and reminisces about the past _____

    d. Becomes demanding and anxious with low self-esteem _____

    e. Fails to comply with medical therapy and is unable to deal with treatment decisions _____

Stage

    1. Anger
    2. Depression
    3. Denial
    4. Acceptance
    5. Bargaining

10. Recognition and reaction to loss are age-dependent. (True or false?)

11. The developmental stage at which the child is first able to understand logical explanations about death is:

    a. toddler years.
    b. preschool age.
    c. school age.
    d. adolescence.

12. Match the developmental stage with the most characteristic description.

Stage

    a. Infant _____
    b. Toddler _____
    c. Preschooler _____
    d. School-age child _____
    e. Adolescent _____
    f. Young adult _____
    g. Middle adult _____
    h. Older adult _____

Description

    1. Is the least likely of any age group to accept loss of life
    2. Perceives that death is associated with destruction
    3. Derives concept of death primarily from religious or cultural beliefs.
    4. Has difficulty separating fact from fantasy, which prevents comprehension of death
    5. Often fears events surrounding death more than death itself

    6. Must first develop attachment before responding to death
    7. Perceives death as a kind of sleep or temporary departure
    8. Recognizes life as finite and considers options to gain personal fulfillment

13. List five needs of a spouse when attempting to cope with a mate's impending death.

    a.
    b.
    c.
    d.
    e.

14. Which statement about bereavement is accurate?

    a. Recovery occurs more rapidly when the death is sudden and unanticipated.
    b. Persons experiencing grief consistently use the support provided by others.
    c. Resolution depends on the meaning of the loss and the situation surrounding the loss.
    d. Persons experiencing less visible or invisible losses tend to receive greater social support.

15. List and briefly define the six dimensions of hope described by Dufault and Martocchio.

    a.
    b.
    c.
    d.
    e.
    f.

16. List five risk factors increasing a person's potential for suffering psychological or physical illness during bereavement.

    a.
    b.
    c.
    d.
    e.

17. Persons experiencing loss may display physical symptoms of grief. (True or false?)

18. Define anticipatory grief.

19. List four goals appropriate to the client or family engaged in the grieving process.

    a.
    b.
    c.
    d.

20. List five goals of care appropriate for terminally ill clients and their families.

a.

b.

c.

d.

e.

21. What are the three most crucial needs of the dying client?

a.

b.

c.

22. Donna Kane has just been told that she has cancer and requires extensive surgery and chemotherapy. Ms. Kane tells the nurse, "I know that the tests are wrong. I feel just fine." The best response by the nurse at this time would be to:

a. convey a willingness to be available to talk to Ms. Kane.

b. assure Ms. Kane that cancer can be successfully treated when intervention begins promptly.

c. tell Ms. Kane that the tests are very reliable and accurate.

d. acknowledge that Ms. Kane looks healthy and should request a second opinion.

23. Identify one nursing strategy to promote hope in each of the dimensions listed.

a. Affective

b. Cognitive

c. Behavioral

d. Affiliate

e. Temporal

f. Contextual

24. Refusal to die or accept the feeling of helplessness is a motivator for the terminally ill client. (True or false?)

25. Describe four ways that the nurse or family can provide spiritual comfort to the dying client.

a.

b.

c.

d.

26. What is the purpose of a hospice program?

27. A hospice program emphasizes:

a. curative treatment and alleviation of symptoms.

b. palliative treatment and control of symptoms.

c. hospital-based care.

d. prolongation of life.

28. Identify the physiological changes after death that the stated nursing interventions are intended to minimize.

a. Remove tape and dressings gently. _____

b. Elevate head. _____

c. Position body in normal alignment. _____

CRITICAL THINKING AND EXPERIENTIAL EXERCISES

1. Personal loss experiences
Identify a situation in which you have experienced a personal loss.

a. Determine the category or type of loss that was experienced.

b. Identify the physical and emotional responses that you experienced.

c. Describe strategies that you used in coping with your loss.

d. Share this information, verbally or in writing, with a friend, another student, or your instructor.

2. Experiences of other health care professionals
Talk with one or more of the following individuals about their experiences with dying clients and their families: social worker, clinical specialist, hospice volunteer, hospice staff member, hospital staff nurse, student nurse, or instructor. Include in your discussion:

a. interventions used to assist clients and families.

b. personal coping strategies used to assist clients and their families.

c. the individual's belief about self-assessment as the first step in assisting client's experiencing loss.

3. Losses associated with chronic illness

a. Interview a client with a chronic illness.

b. Identify actual and potential losses faced by the individual as a result of chronic illness.

c. Determine the meaning of each loss to the client.

d. Describe the potential effect of the loss on physical and psychological function.

e. Identify nursing interventions to minimize loss and maximize physical and psychological function in the presence of the chronic illness.

f. Share your conclusions with your instructor for feedback.

4. Nursing assessment of the client experiencing loss

a. Perform a nursing assessment of a grieving client using any comprehensive assessment tool.

b. Based on your assessment, describe how each of the following variables are influencing the client's grief reaction.

(1) Age

(2) Personal relationships

(3) Nature of loss or death

(4) Cultural and spiritual beliefs

(5) Sex roles

(6) Socioeconomic status

c. Based on identified client behaviors, identify the client's stage of grieving according to:

(1) Engle.

(2) Kübler-Ross.
(3) Martocchio.
d. Identify at least one intervention the nurse may use to support the client in each of the following dimensions.
(1) Affective
(2) Cognitive
(3) Behavioral
(4) Affiliate
(5) Temporal
(6) Contextual

5. The Dying Person's Bill of Rights
a. Select three of the dying person's rights that you consider to be most important.
b. Discuss why you value these rights.
c. Identify at least three nursing interventions to assist in preserving each of these rights.
d. Share the information individually with a peer or instructor during small group discussion.

6. Nursing care of the terminally ill client
Observe or assist a nurse caring for a terminally ill client or independently provide nursing care to a dying client.
a. Perform a nursing assessment using a comprehensive assessment tool.
b. Formulate and prioritize three nursing diagnoses for the client.
c. Develop a nursing care plan for the client that includes the following goals. For each goal, state at least one expected outcome and two individualized nursing interventions.
(1) Promote comfort.
(2) Maintain independence.
(3) Maintain hope.
(4) Achieve spiritual comfort.
(5) Gain relief from loneliness and isolation.

7. Clinical situation: needs of spouses; survivor's risks
Mr. and Mrs. Merton have been married for 54 years. Mrs. Merton has been admitted to the hospital in the terminal phase of congestive heart failure. The physician has informed Mr. and Mrs. Merton of the seriousness of the illness and its very grave prognosis.
a. Identify five needs that Mr. Merton may have in attempting to cope with his wife's impending death. Describe at least two nursing interventions to assist in meeting each of the identified needs.
b. Mr. Merton is at risk for psychological and physical illness during bereavement. Identify six risk factors to assess and describe at least two nursing interventions to minimize the identified risk.
c. The Mertons' daughter, Caroline, tells the nurse about Mr. Merton's anger and frequent emotional outbursts before Mrs. Merton's admission. She expresses concern that Mr. Merton will never recover from his wife's death.
(1) What explanation could the nurse provide about Mr. Merton's anger and emotional outbursts?

(2) How long a period should Caroline expect her father to need to resolve his loss?
(3) What behaviors should be considered normal for Mr. Merton during his bereavement?
(4) What behaviors would alert Caroline to the fact that her father is experiencing dysfunctional grief?

ADDITIONAL READINGS

Engle GL: Grief and grieving, Am J Nurs 64(9):93, 1964.
Discusses the experience of the grieving process and behaviors characteristic during each stage. Offers potential interventions for assisting the grieving client.
Hampe SO: Needs of the grieving spouse in a hospital setting, Nurs Res 24:113, 1975.
Study that identified common needs of grieving spouses. May be helpful in designing family-centered care of the dying client and fostering improved coping for spouses of the terminally ill.
Johnson SH: 10 ways to help the family of a critically ill patient, Nurs 86 16:50, 1986.
Describes strategies for working with families of the critically ill. Cites examples that clearly illustrate the application of strategies to actual clinical practice.
Martocchio B, Dufault K: Symposia of (1) hospice and (2) compassionate care and the dying experience, Nurs Clin North Am 20(2), 1985.
Two separate but related symposia. "Hospice" symposium presents comprehensive overview of issues and practices associated with hospice programs. "Compassionate Care and the Dying Experience" symposium explores the physical and psychosocial needs of dying clients and their families.
Miles JS, Hays DR: Widowhood, Am J Nurs 75: 280, 1975.
Summarizes common problems facing the newly widowed spouse. Discusses the nursing role in supporting the grieving spouse.
Musgrave CF: The ethical and legal implications of hospice care: an international overview, Cancer Nurs 10:183, 1987.
Analyzes the basic rights of the dying client. Discusses unique religious beliefs and their effect on care of the terminally ill. Compares laws related to terminal care in the United States, Great Britain, and Israel.
O'Connor AP: Understanding the cancer patient's search for meaning, Cancer Nurs 13:167, 1990.
Provides insight into the cancer patient's psychosocial response to terminal illness. Concepts presented may be applied to clients experiencing other terminal illnesses.
Strickney SK, Garnder ER: Companions in suffering, Am J Nurs 84:1491, 1984.
Discusses grief experienced by family members and nurses caring for dying clients. Proposes approaches to increase coping abilities of family members and care givers.
Taylor PR, Gideon MD: Holding out hope to your dying patient, Nurs 82 12:42, 1982.
Discusses clinical situations in which nurses fostered hope to support dying clients. Redefines the concept of hope in relation to unique client situations. Contends that hope may be honest and realizable even in the final stages of illness.

Chapter 29
Basic Human Needs

PREREQUISITE READING
Chapter 29, pp. 888 to 903

OBJECTIVES
Mastery of content in this chapter will enable the student to:
- Define selected terms associated with basic human needs.
- Discuss each component of Maslow's hierarchy of needs.
- Describe assessment techniques for identifying unmet needs.
- Identify actual or potential conditions that threaten fulfillment of a client's needs.
- Identify nursing diagnoses appropriate for unmet basic needs.
- Describe the basic nursing implications of unmet needs.
- Describe relationships among the different levels of needs.
- State factors that influence the individual client's need priorities.

REVIEW OF KEY CONCEPTS
1. What are basic human needs?
2. Build the hierarchy of human needs by writing in the five levels of basic needs identified by Maslow.

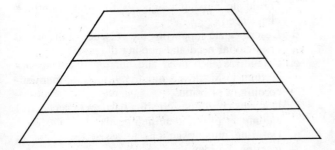

3. Which statement about the hierarchy of basic needs is incorrect?
   a. Priorities assigned to basic human needs are the same in all individuals.
   b. Unmet needs place the individual at risk for illness.
   c. Environmental and social factors may influence the ability to meet needs.
   d. Hospitalized clients have basic needs that are actually or potentially unmet.
4. List the eight physiological needs in Maslow's hierarchy. Using an asterisk, indicate the need that has highest priority.

   a.

   b.

   c.

   d.

   e.

   f.

   g.

   h.
5. List four client groups frequently requiring assistance in meeting physiological needs.

   a.

   b.

   c.

   d.
6. List the two age groups at greatest risk for unmet needs.

   a.

   b.
7. Clients with appropriate body weight may still have nutritional deficits. (True or false?)
8. Sexual need refers exclusively to an individual's need for physical sex. (True or false?)
9. Nancy Williams is an 18-year-old nursing student assigned to care for a 20-year-old man with a spinal cord injury. Nancy identifies that the client's sexual needs may be unmet because of his paralysis but recognizes that she is very uncomfortable discussing this topic. Which action would be most appropriate for Nancy to take at this time?

a. Ignore the subject because the client has not mentioned any concerns about sex.

b. Design a plan of care that addresses physical needs that have higher priority.

c. Try to talk to the client about sexual matters, no matter how uncomfortable it may be.

d. Identify another health care worker who can talk to the client about sexual matters.

10. Safety needs may take precedence over a physiological need. (True or false?)

11. Which factor is of greatest importance in determining the effect of a body image change on self-esteem?

a. Magnitude of the change

b. Nature of the illness precipitating change

c. Person's self-perception after the change

d. Extent to which changes can be seen by others

12. List six characteristics indicating that an individual has achieved self-actualization.

a.

b.

c.

d.

e.

f.

13. It is appropriate for the nursing care plan to address needs in more than one level of the hierarchy at a time. (True or false?)

14. List four factors that influence need priorities.

a.

b.

c.

d.

15. Match the description or term with the most closely associated basic need.

Term

a. Cyanosis _____

b. Edema _____

c. Self-confidence _____

d. Privacy with spouse _____

e. Skin breakdown _____

f. Activity patterns _____

g. Glucose _____

h. Community resources _____

i. Body image _____

j. Oliguria _____

k. Fear of the unknown _____

l. Significant others and peers _____

m. Shivering _____

Need

1. Oxygen
2. Fluids
3. Nutrition
4. Temperature
5. Elimination
6. Shelter
7. Rest
8. Sex
9. Physical safety
10. Psychological safety
11. Love and belonging
12. Esteem
13. Self-actualization

CRITICAL THINKING AND EXPERIENTIAL EXERCISES

1. Personal needs

a. Formulate a list of your personal needs and classify them in relation to Maslow's hierarchy.

b. Determine relationships among your identified needs.

c. Identify those needs you consider to be priorities and describe factors that influence your ranking.

d. Identify available resources to assist you in meeting these needs (for example, personal strengths, family, friends, colleagues, educational setting, health care institution, community).

e. Identify ways in which needs from different levels may be met simultaneously.

f. Share the results of this exercise with a friend, peer, family member, or instructor.

2. Assessment of client needs

a. Conduct a comprehensive nursing assessment of a client in any health care setting.

b. Identify actual and potential client needs.

c. Formulate nursing diagnoses for each identified client need.

d. Describe data supporting the presence of the actual or potential need and nursing diagnosis.

e. Categorize each need and nursing diagnosis according to Maslow's hierarchy, ranking them according to priorities.

f. Describe conditions creating barriers to successful attainment of the identified needs.

g. Describe nursing actions to assist the client in meeting the identified needs.

ADDITIONAL READING

Ellis JR, Nowlis EA: Homeostasis and human needs. In Ellis JR, Nowlis EA: *Nursing: a human needs approach*, ed 4, Boston, 1989, Houghton Mifflin.

Describes human needs in the context of Maslow's hierarchy and relates these needs to major nursing theories. Presents nursing diagnoses associated with physiological, psychological, and safety needs. Includes discussion of the human needs of nurses.

Sorenson KC, Luckmann J: Meeting human needs through the nursing process, *Basic nursing: a psychophysiologic approach*, ed 2, Philadelphia, 1986, Saunders.

Describes basic human needs and discusses their importance in maintaining health. Explores role of nursing in meeting needs of client through the nursing process.

Chapter 30
Adaptation to Stress

PREREQUISITE READING
Chapter 30, pp. 904 to 925

OBJECTIVES
Mastery of content in this chapter will enable the student to:
- Define selected terms associated with stress and adaptation to it.
- Discuss the limitations of homeostatic control.
- Discuss four models of stress as they relate to nursing practice.
- Describe how adaptation occurs in each of the five dimensions.
- Describe two forms of local physiological adaptation.
- Describe the three phases of the general adaptation syndrome.
- List and discuss behaviors that are responses to stress.
- List and discuss the most common ego-defense mechanisms that are responses to stress.
- Discuss the effects of prolonged stress on each of the five dimensions of a person's function.
- Describe stress-management techniques that nurses can help client use.
- Discuss techniques of crisis intervention.
- Describe stress-management techniques that can benefit nurses.

REVIEW OF KEY CONCEPTS
1. Which definition does not characterize stress?
   a. Any situation in which a nonspecific demand requires an individual to respond or take action
   b. A phenomenon affecting social, psychological, developmental, spiritual, and psychological dimensions
   c. A condition eliciting an intellectual, behavioral, or metabolic response
   d. Efforts to maintain relative constancy within the internal environment
2. Which statement about homeostasis is inaccurate?
   a. Homeostatic mechanisms provide long-term and short-term control over the body's equilibrium.
   b. Homeostatic mechanisms are self-regulatory.
   c. Homeostatic mechanisms function through negative feedback.
   d. Illness may inhibit normal homeostatic mechanisms.

3. Match the descriptions with the characteristic model of stress.

Description
   a. Stress is demonstrated by a specific physiological reaction, the general adaptation syndrome, without consideration of cognitive influences. _____
   b. Four factors determine whether a situation is stressful: ability to cope with stress, practice and norms of the peer group, effect of the social environment, and resources used to deal with the stressor. _____
   c. Model examines disturbing or disruptive characteristics within the environment. It views life-change events as normal and dismisses individual perceptions of events as irrelevant in reaching the threshold causing illness. _____
   d. Model views the person and environment in a dynamic, reciprocal, bidirectional relationship and stress as a result of the individual's perception between self and the environment. _____

Model
   1. Transaction-based model
   2. Adaptation model
   3. Response-based model
   4. Stimulus-based model
4. Which nursing intervention is best used when applying the adaptation model of stress?
   a. Interventions to improve or stabilize blood pressure
   b. Interventions to reduce anxiety
   c. Interventions to maintain fluid balance
   d. Interventions to promote reality orientation
5. List the four characteristics of a stressor that influence a person's response.

   a.

   b.

   c.

   d.

6. List the four requirements for successful family adaptation.

    a.

    b.

    c.

    d.

7. List the five human dimensions and briefly describe how adaptation occurs in each.

    a.

    b.

    c.

    d.

    e.

8. Define local adaptation syndrome (LAS).

9. Define general adaptation syndrome (GAS).

10. Describe the four common characteristics of the local adaptation response.

    a.

    b.

    c.

    d.

11. The body's response to localized stress could include all of the following except:
    a. blood clotting.
    b. wound healing.
    c. inflammatory response.
    d. fever.

12. List the five characteristic signs and symptoms of the inflammatory response.

    a.

    b.

    c.

    d.

    e.

13. The body systems primarily involved in GAS are the:
    a. central nervous system and cardiovascular system.
    b. endocrine system and respiratory system.
    c. autonomic nervous system and endocrine system.
    d. musculoskeletal system and immunological system.

14. List (in sequence) and briefly describe the three stages of GAS.

    a.

    b.

    c.

15. Match the physiological response to the stage of GAS.

Response

    a. Death _____
    b. Release of epinephrine, norepinephrine _____
    c. Homone levels returning to normal _____
    d. Increased blood glucose level _____
    e. Diminished physiological regulation _____
    f. Vital signs returning to normal _____
    g. Increased blood volume _____
    h. Dilated pupils _____

Stage

    1. Alarm
    2. Resistance
    3. Exhaustion

16. Psychological adaptive behaviors may be constructive or destructive. (True or false?)

17. List and briefly describe the two general types of psychological adaptive behaviors (coping mechanisms).

    a.

    b.

18. Nancy recently had a disagreement with her friend about a class assignment. To avoid interacting with her friend, she comes to class late and sits in the back of the room. This task-oriented form of coping is called:
    a. attack behavior.
    b. withdrawal behavior.
    c. compromise behavior.
    d. regressive behavior.

19. List and briefly describe six common ego-defense mechanisms.

    a.

    b.

    c.

    d.

    e.

    f.

20. List at least eight physical indicators of stress.

    a.

    b.

    c.

    d.

    e.

    f.

g.

h.

21. Identify at least one indicator of stress for each developmental stage.
    a. Infant
    b. Toddler
    c. Pre-school age
    d. School age
    e. Adolescent
    f. Young adult
    g. Middle adult
    h. Older adult

22. List 10 behavioral and emotional indicators of stress.

    a.

    b.

    c.

    d.

    e.

    f.

    g.

    h.

    i.

    j.

23. List four intellectual indicators of stress.

    a.

    b.

    c.

    d.

24. List two spiritual indicators of stress.

    a.

    b.

25. Identify stress-reduction methods for each stress management goal.

Reducing Stressful Situations	Decreasing Physiological Responses	Improving Responses to Stress
a.	a.	a.
b.	b.	b.
c.	c.	c.
d.	d.	
e.	e.	

26. List three factors essential to crisis resolution.

    a.

    b.

    c.

CRITICAL THINKING AND EXPERIENTIAL EXERCISES

1. Concepts of stress
   Identify and analyze a recent situation in which you felt stressed. After your analysis, respond to the following questions.
   a. What did you perceive as the primary stressor?
   b. From which human dimension did the stressor arise?
   c. Would the stressor be classified as internal or external? Why?
   d. Identify your response to the stressor in each human dimension.
      (1) Physical-developmental
      (2) Emotional
      (3) Intellectual
      (4) Social
      (5) Spiritual
   e. Describe the nature of the stressor in each of the following areas and analyze how each influenced your response
      (1) Intensity of the stressor
      (2) Scope of the stressor
      (3) Duration of the stressor
      (4) Number and nature of other stressors
   f. Which stress model did you use in coping with the stressor? How was this helpful?
   g. Would a different model have been more helpful in understanding and responding to the stressor? Which would it have been and why?

2. Nursing process and adaptation to stress
   Perform a comprehensive nursing assessment of a client in any health care setting.
   a. Identify indicators of stress in each dimension of adaptation.
   b. List nursing diagnoses directly associated with the client's stress.
   c. For the primary diagnoses, identify two goals for care.
   d. For each goal, describe one expected outcome and three specific, individualized nursing interventions.

3. Stress management
   Nursing school, like any educational environment, presents students with multiple stressors. Because it is impossible to eliminate all stressors, it is important to develop strategies to manage stress.
   a. Formulate at least three strategies for each major goal of stress management. Be sure that the strategies you select are realistic for your and your situation.
      (1) Reducing stressful situations
      (2) Decreasing physiological response to stress
      (3) Improving behavioral and emotional response to stress
   b. Select a deadline for implementation of your strategies and write the date selected on your paper.

c. Photocopy your paper and share your strategies and deadline with a friend, relative, peer, or instructor.

d. Set a time and date, after the identified deadline, to review, evaluate, and (if necessary) revise your strategies.

4. Clinical situation: LAS, GAS, crisis intervention
John Trout, a sales representative for a local pharmaceutical company, enters the emergency room after an automobile accident. He has several lacerations and a fractured left arm.

His admission assessment includes the following: temperature, 37.2°C; pulse, 106 beats/min; respirations, 26 breaths/min; blood pressure, 140/90 mm Hg; pupils large, equal, and reactive to light; speech rapid. Mr. Trout is asking many questions about medical and nursing care, is requesting the same information from different care givers, and is extremely angry and critical about the "inefficiency" of the hospital staff.

No one else was injured in the accident. Mr. Trout's car was totaled, and he is very concerned about business losses that will occur because of the accident and his injuries. He tells the staff that he is the "best sales representative in the midwest" and requests the opportunity to come to speak to the staff about his company's products.

a. Which stage of GAS is Mr. Trout experiencing?

b. Based on the data provided, identify the indicators of stress that Mr. Trout displays and categorize them into each of the human dimensions.

c. Based on the situation, describe each of the localized stress responses Mr. Trout may experience. (Name at least five.)

d. The trauma of the lacerations will precipitate the inflammatory response.

(1) What signs and symptoms should Mr. Trout expect to have as a result of inflammation?

(2) Identify and describe each of the three phases of this response.

e. What type of crisis does the accident represent for Mr. Trout?

f. Based on principles of crisis intervention, describe interventions you would use in caring for Mr. Trout in the emergency room.

ADDITIONAL READINGS

Aguilera DC: *Crisis intervention: theory and methodology,* ed 6, St Louis, 1989, Mosby–Year Book.
    A classic, comprehensive text that presents the theoretical concepts and practical helping techniques related to crisis intervention. Information from this text is frequently cited in nursing literature addressing care of the client in crisis.

Foxall JH, Zimmerman L, and Bene B: A comparison of frequency and sources of nursing job stress perceived by intensive care, hospice, and medical-surgical nurses, *J Adv Nurs* 15:77, 1990.
    Identifies similarities and differences in stress perceived in a variety of practice settings. May be helpful in identification and management of nurses' stressors.

Luczun ME, editor: Stress in sickness and health, *J Adv Med Surg Nurs* 1(4), 1989.
    Journal volume entirely dedicated to stress and related nursing implications. Examines specific diseases states, posttraumatic stress disorder, and culture as they are affected by and affect client stress. Also describes use of relaxation, imagery, and music in contemporary nursing practice.

Robinson L: Stress and anxiety, *Nurs Clin North Am* 25(4):935, 1990.
    Examines stress in different theoretical constructs: biological, psychosomatic, life-events, and interactionistic/transactional. Describes specific responses to stress. Includes implications for nursing research and practice.

Skipper JK, Jung JD, Coffey LC: Nurses and shiftwork: effects on physical health and mental depression, *J Adv Nurs* 15:835, 1990.
    Examines the relationship between physical health and mental depression of nurse shiftworkers. Found that other factors were of greater consequence than shiftwork in levels of health and depression.

Chapter 31
Self-Concept

PREREQUISITE READING
Chapter 31, pp. 926 to 957

OBJECTIVES

Mastery of content in this chapter will enable the student to:
- Define selected terms associated with self-concept.
- Discuss factors that influence each component of self-concept, including identity, body image, self-esteem, and roles.
- Describe the five processes of socialization.
- Identify stressors that affect each component of self-concept.
- Explain the processes that can lead to role conflict, role ambiguity, and role strain.
- Discuss identity confusion as a developmental aspect of adolescence and as a problem of self-concept.
- Describe development of self-concept, relating Erikson's psychosocial stages and cognitive stages.
- Discuss ways in which the nurse's self-concept and nursing activities can affect the client's self-concept.
- Describe behaviors or defining characteristics that may indicate identity confusion, disturbed body image, low self-esteem, and role conflict.
- List, for each component of self-concept, a common nursing diagnosis related to self-concept disturbance and related factors.
- Describe goals of care, specific nursing interventions, and outcome and evaluation measures for a client with self-concept disturbance.

REVIEW OF KEY CONCEPTS

1. Define self-concept.
2. List five sources from which self-concept is derived.

    a.

    b.

    c.

    d.

    e.
3. Define body image.
4. A person's body image is always consistent with the actual body structure or appearance. (True or false?)

5. Define self-esteem.
6. List the four components of self-concept.

    a.

    b.

    c.

    d.
7. Which developmental stage is particularly crucial for identity development?
    a. Infancy
    b. Preschool age
    c. Adolescence
    d. Young adult
8. A person's sense of identity, once developed, will not change in response to life circumstances. (True or false?)
9. Define sexual identity.
10. Which of the following statements about body image is correct?
    a. Physical changes are quickly incorporated into a person's body image.
    b. Body image refers only to the external appearance of a person's body.
    c. Body image is a combination of the person's actual and perceived (ideal) body.
    d. Perceptions by other persons have no influence on the person's body image.
11. Extreme disparity between ideal self and self-concept is characteristic of many persons with mental illness. (True or false?)
12. The process by which a person acquires values, behaviors, skills, and roles from social norms and significant others is _____
13. List and briefly describe the five methods through which children learn socially approved behaviors.

    a.

    b.

    c.

    d.

    e.

14. Robert, 2 years old, is praised for using his potty instead of wetting his pants. This is an example of learning a behavior by:
  a. identification.
  b. imitation.
  c. substitution.
  d. reinforcement-extinction.
15. Identify the role stressor category for each example provided.
  a. Mr. Jones is admitted to the hospital with symptoms of a myocardial infarction (heart attack). _____
  b. Jean Wallace, 15 years old, experiences menarche. _____
  c. Ms. Hamet receives a job promotion requiring a cross-country move. _____
16. Define role conflict.
17. Match the most characteristic type of role conflict with the situation described.

Situation
  a. A college student wishes to study all weekend, but his parents expect him to participate in a family reunion. _____
  b. A nurse who believes that life is sacred must care for a teenager who has made repeated suicide attempts. _____
  c. A woman who is a wife, mother of three school-age children, and part-time grocery clerk returns to college to earn a degree. _____
  d. A client expects the nurse to let him sleep during the night. The doctor writes orders to arouse the client every 2 hours. _____

Role conflict
  1. Interpersonal
  2. Interrole
  3. Person-role
  4. Role overload
18. Unclear role expectations and an inability to predict the reactions of other persons to one's behavior are characteristic of _____
19. In which developmental stage is role ambiguity most common?
  a. Older adult
  b. Middle adult
  c. Young adult
  d. Adolescence
20. A feeling of frustration associated with perceived inadequacy in a role is _____
21. Match the developmental stage with the most characteristic aspect of self-concept or body image described.

Characteristic
  a. Self-concept is expanded through games. _____
  b. Person is unable to differentiate self from environment. _____
  c. Self-concept is complicated by societal confusion in gender behavior, meaning of sexuality, and role conflicts. _____
  d. Person considers distal body parts as separate from self and other parts, such as hair, as permanent. _____
  e. Changes in appearance and function negatively affect self-concept. _____
  f. Body acts as primary source for acceptance or rejection by others. _____
  g. Hormonal changes produce physical alterations and self-concept realignment. _____
  h. Body boundaries and gender become defined. _____

Stage
  1. Infant
  2. Toddler
  3. Preschool age
  4. School age
  5. Adolescent
  6. Young adult
  7. Middle adult
  8. Older adult
22. At which developmental level do children usually establish a positive or negative self-concept?
  a. Toddler years
  b. Preschool age
  c. School age
  d. Adolescence
23. Sensory changes associated with the aging process may produce negative personality changes. (True or false?)
24. Describe three messages to be conveyed by the nurse to provide an environment supporting the client's self-concept.
  a.
  b.
  c.
25. List five behaviors involved in establishing rapport with a client.
  a.
  b.
  c.
  d.
  e.

26. List the five sequential levels of intervention for assisting a client to attain a positive self-concept or adapt to changes in self-concept.

    a.

    b.

    c.

    d.

    e.

27. What action would be taken by the nurse when the client experiences a severe alteration in self-concept?
28. After a major life change, adjustment of self-concept requiring more than one year should be considered maladaptive. (True or false?)
29. A minor change in function, appearance, or role can create a severe self-concept problem. (True or false?)

CRITICAL THINKING AND EXPERIENTIAL EXERCISES

1. Personal role stressors
   Identify a personal situation in which you experienced role transition.
   a. Categorize the type of role transition you experienced as developmental, situational, or health-illness.
   b. Role transitions frequently affect self-concept and result in role conflict, role ambiguity, or role strain. Describe which of these reults you may have experienced. Be sure to relate the theoretical concept described in your text with the feelings you experienced.
   c. Identify coping strategies you used in adapting to the role transition. Did you think these were adaptive or maladaptive.
   d. Describe alternative strategies you believe could be implemented in future role conflict, ambiguity, or strain.
   e. If desired, seek assistance from a counselor, teacher, or nursing instructor in clarifying alterative coping strategies to address role stress.
2. Clinical situation: self-concept stressors
   Andy Sawchuck, a 44-year-old professional golfer, has developed a severe back problem that will require spinal surgery. He has reduced sensation in his left leg and is developing a limping gait.
   Mr. Sawchuck is a highly valued golf professional at the most respected country club in the city. He is accustomed to entering several national tournaments each year and finishing in the top five. His physician has informed him that he will not be able to resume golfing for at least 1 year after surgery, and then it should be restricted to nine holes weekly.
   Mr. Sawchuck has recently remarried. He has two teenage children from a former marriage. These children visit him frequently during the school year and live with him during the summer months. His back

problem has altered his sexual relationship with his wife, who has been very supportive. Mr. Sawchuck is very depressed and worried about his future. Golf is his and his family's sole means of financial support.
   a. What normal developmental events are expected at Mr. Sawchuck's present age? What effect could the situation described have on his normal developmental tasks.
   b. Describe at least two stressors and the dynamics that are affecting or that could affect each component of Mr. Sawchuck's self-concept. (Keep in mind the client's normal developmental tasks and the information presented about the situation.)
      (1) Body image
      (2) Self-esteem
      (3) Role
      (4) Identity
   c. What factors should the nurse examine and attempt to understand before assisting Mr. Sawchuck? Why is this step crucial to Mr. Sawchuck's care?
   d. Describe how the nurse can create a therapeutic environment that will facilitate Mr. Sawchuck's self-concept adaptation.
3. Clinical situation: altered self-concept and the nursing process
   Mrs. Cruz, a 30-year-old mother of a 6-year-old son and an 8-year-old daughter, is recovering from a motor vehicle accident. She suffered severe facial lacerations and will require several surgical procedures to reconstruct her face. She will be left with some permanent facial scarring.
   Mrs. Cruz avoids eye contact with people talking to her, including her husband and children. She seems very quiet and stays in her bed sleeping most of the time. She refuses to look in a mirror.
   One day after visiting hours, the nurse sees Mr. Cruz sitting in the lounge with his head buried in his hands. The nurse talks to him for 30 minutes. She learns that Mr. Cruz is very worried about his wife because she says she wishes she would have died in the accident. He tells the nurse that he does not know what to do to help his wife. He says she seems to ignore her children and tells him not to bring them to visit anymore. He says that when he tells his wife that the children miss her, she just turns away from him.
   a. Based on the information provided, write three nursing diagnoses related to altered self-concept.
   b. Which of the adaptation continuums would you consider the most appropriate for Mrs. Cruz? Provide a rationale to support your answer.
   c. Using the five levels of interaction as a guide:
      (1) Write two short-term goals and one long-term goal consistent with the priority nursing diagnosis you previously stated.
      (2) Identify the sequential level of intervention for self-concept disturbance that each goal represents.

(3) For each goal, identify one expected outcome and evaluative measures you would use to determine goal achievement.

(4) Formulate three nursing interventions for each goal.

(5) State the rationale for the interventions you selected.

ADDITIONAL READINGS

Manglass L: Self-concept. In Flynn JB, Heffron PB: *Nursing from concepts to practice,* ed 2, Norwalk, Conn, 1988, Appleton & Lange.

Presents self-concept in the framework of adaptation. Provides assessment parameters and nursing interventions for client care.

Molla PM: Self-concept in children with and without physical disability, *J Psych Nurs* 19(6):22, 1981.

Discusses self-concept and body image in the context of the developmental process. Explores the effect of physical disability on children's self-concept. Based on research findings, makes recommendations for nursing approaches to promote more positive self-concept in children with physical disabilities.

Norris J, Kunes-Connel M: Self-esteem disturbance, *Nurs Clin North Am* 20(4):745, 1985.

Examines self-esteem disturbance as a nursing diagnosis in detail. Describes a study conducted to support clinical validation of nursing diagnosis. Identifies defining characteristics and explores potential contributing factors of self-esteem disturbance.

Oldaker S: Identity confusion: nursing diagnosis for adolescents, *Nurs Clin North Am* 20(4):763, 1985.

Describes research investigating developmental health and psychological symptoms among high school students. Explores potential causes of adolescent identity confusion, identifies diagnostic criteria, and correlates this information with developmental task achievement.

Schroeder MA: Theories of personhood. In Flynn JB, Heffron PB: *Nursing from concepts to practice,* ed 2, Norwalk, Conn, 1988, Appleton & Lange.

Provides basic definitions and descriptions of major theories of personality and personhood. Gives specific examples to illustrate application of concepts to practice.

Chapter 32
Sexuality

PREREQUISITE READING

Chapter 32, pp. 958 to 999

OBJECTIVES

Mastery of content in this chapter will enable the student to:

- Define selected terms associated with sexuality.
- Identify personal attitudes, beliefs, and biases related to sexuality.
- Discuss the nurse's role in maintaining or enhancing a client's sexual health.
- Define sexuality as a component of personality.
- Describe key concepts of sexual development during infancy, childhood, adolescence, and adulthood.
- Identify male and female genitalia and describe functions related to sexual stimulation, response, and reproduction.
- Describe the sexual response cycle (Masters and Johnson model).
- Describe physical, therapeutic, and psychological issues affecting sexuality.
- Identify potential causes of sexual dysfunction.
- Assess a client's sexuality.
- Define appropriate nursing diagnoses on sexuality.
- Identify and describe nursing interventions to promote sexual health.
- Evaluate a client's sexual health.
- Identify sexual concerns outside the nurse's level of expertise and identify potential referral resources.

REVIEW OF KEY CONCEPTS

1. Compare the meaning of the terms sex and sexuality.
2. An individual's sense of being feminine or masculine is known as _____ .
3. The way a person acts as male or female is _____ .
4. The clear, persistent, erotic preference of a person for one sex or the other is _____ .
5. An individual whose inner sense of sexual identity does not match the biological body is known as a:
   a. lesbian.
   b. homosexual.
   c. transsexual.
   d. transvestite.

6. List four major factors influencing an individual's sexual attitudes and behaviors.
7. What is the most common concern people have about their sexuality?
8. Complete the table below, outlining the physiology of the female reproductive system.

Structure/Organ	Function(s)
Vulva	
Labia minora	
Labia majora	
Clitoris	
Vestibule	
Introitus	
Bartholin's glands	
Hymen	
Vagina	
Uterus	
Cervix	
Body	
Myometrium	
Endometrium	
Fallopian tubes	
Ovaries	
Breasts	

9. Fill in the name of the hormone or hormones responsible for the menstrual cycle beside the anatomical component of the feedback loop.

   a. Hypothalamus _____
   b. Pituitary _____
   c. Pituitary _____
   d. Ovaries _____
   e. Corpus luteum _____

10. The follicular phase of the menstrual cycle is characterized by:
    a. increasing levels of progesterone.
    b. reduction in ovarian production of estrogen.
    c. inhibition of follicle-stimulating hormone.
    d. rupture of the Graafian follicle.

11. Which statement about the uterine secretory phase of the menstrual cycle is accurate?
    a. The secretory phase is the time before ovulation.
    b. The uterus is under the influence of high levels of estrogen.
    c. Cervical mucus becomes more clear, slippery, and stretchable.
    d. In the absence of pregnancy, the endometrium begins to slough.

12. List four signs or symptoms experienced by women with premenstrual syndrome (PMS).

    a.

    b.

    c.

    d.

13. Complete the table below, outlining the physiology of the male reproductive system.

Structure/Organ	Function(s)
Penis	
Scrotum	
Testis	
Seminiferous tubules	
Epididymis	
Vas deferens	
Ampulla	
Seminal vesicles	
Prostate gland	
Bulbourethral (Cowper's) glands	

14. The removal of the foreskin or prepuce from the penis is _____ .

15. At what age is it particularly important for children reared in single-parent families to be exposed to same-sex adults?
    a. Infancy
    b. Toddlerhood and preschool years
    c. School age
    d. Adolescence

16. In the school-age child, learning and reinforcement of gender-appropriate behaviors are most commonly derived from:
    a. parents.
    b. teachers.
    c. siblings.
    d. peers.

17. The onset of the menstrual cycle is _____ .

18. Adolescent females experiencing menarche and males experiencing first ejaculations should assume that they are fertile. (True or false?)

19. List four sexual issues that should be addressed with adolescents.

    a.

    b.

c.

d.

20. The capacity for sexuality is lifelong. (True or false?)

21. List four areas of concern that affect sexual functioning in the older adult.

    a.

    b.

    c.

    d.

22. Sequentially list and briefly describe the four phases of the sexual response cycle (according to Masters and Johnson).

    a.

    b.

    c.

    d.

23. Which statement about sexual response in the older adult is correct?
    a. The resolution phase is slower.
    b. The orgasm phase is prolonged.
    c. The plateau phase is prolonged.
    d. The refractory phase is more rapid.

24. Normal pregnancy presents no physiological contraindications to sexual intercourse. (True or false?)

25. Why is it important for a woman, during the second half of pregnancy, to select intercourse positions other than lying flat on her back.

26. Describe two ways in which sexual intercourse or nipple stimulation may accidently or therapeutically stimulate or accelerate labor.

    a.

    b.

27. Which of the following statements about sexuality during the postpartum period is incorrect?
    a. Couples should restrain from sexual intercourse until vaginal bleeding has stopped and discomfort subsides.
    b. In the early postpartum period, breastfeeding couples need not be concerned about using contraceptives.
    c. The demands of the baby may negatively influence sexual desire in both partners.
    d. Hormonal changes will decrease the amount of vaginal lubrication, necessitating the use of water-soluble lubricants during intercourse.

28. List seven questions to explore with a client when clarifying values and providing information about contraconception.

29. In the following outline, identify examples of contraception methods for each classification listed.
    a. Biological
       (1)
       (2)

    (3)
    (4)
  b. Chemical
    (1)
    (2)
  c. Chemical-mechanical
    (1)
  d. Mechanical
    (1)
    (2)
    (3)
    (4)
  e. Surgical
    (1)
    (2)

30. The most effective means of preventing pregnancy is _____ .

31. The least effective means of preventing pregnancy is:
   a. coitus interruptus.
   b. calendar (rhythm) method.
   c. body temperature method.
   d. mucus method.

32. A client wishes to use the rhythm method for contraception. She reports cycles between 24 and 32 days in length. Which days of the cycle should she refrain from intercourse?

33. A client wishes to use the basal body temperature (BBT) as a method of preventing conception. Client education should include which of the following points?
   a. BBT rises 0.4° to 0.8° just before ovulation.
   b. Schedule changes and illness will not affect the use of BBT.
   c. BBT is most accurately measured in the late afternoon or early evening.
   d. Conception is possible if intercourse occurs several days before BBT elevation.

34. How can cervical mucus be used to predict ovulation?

35. Which contraceptive method is most effective in protecting men and women against sexually transmitted diseases?
   a. Spermicide
   b. Condom
   c. Diaphragm
   d. Oral contraceptive

36. Males may remain fertile for 6 to 8 weeks after a vasectomy. (True or false?)

37. Infertility is primarily a female problem. (True or false?)

38. Which statement about abortion is correct?
   a. Women who decide to abort an unwanted fetus will not experience any guilt.
   b. Nurses are obliged to participate in abortion, even if it conflicts with personal values.
   c. The male partner may experience loss and grief, requiring professional support.
   d. Women who abort a deformed fetus will not experience any loss or grief.

39. Sexually transmitted diseases (STDs) infect and are transmitted only through genital organs. (True or false?)

40. Match the characteristics described with the sexually transmitted diseases.

Characteristics

   a. May be asymptomatic or present with soft, flesh-colored lesion _____
   b. Treatable but not curable _____
   c. Painless chancre _____
   d. Incurable and usually fatal _____
   e. Cluster of painful blisters _____
   f. Dysuria, genital discharge _____
   g. Fever, diarrhea, weight loss, and fatigue _____
   h. Sterility if untreated _____
   i. Central nervous system damage in the tertiary stage _____
   j. Linked to increased incidence of cancer _____

Disease

   1. Gonorrhea, Chlamydia
   2. Syphilis
   3. Herpes simplex II
   4. Human papilloma virus (HPV)
   5. Human immunodeficiency virus (HIV)

41. List five measures to promote safer sex.
   a.
   b.
   c.
   d.
   e.

42. The only 100% effective method to avoid contracting a disease through sex is:
   a. using condoms.
   b. avoiding sex with partners at risk.
   c. knowing the sexual partner's health history.
   d. abstinence.

43. Potential sexual abuse provides a strong rationale for assessing sexuality in all age groups. (True or false?)

44. List the three body systems that must be intact for sexual behavior to occur.
   a.
   b.
   c.

45. Illnesses that do not affect systems directly involved in sexual behavior may still influence feelings of desirabilty and arousal. (True or false?)

46. List two simple ways in which the nurse may assist clients in learning to meet sexual needs in the hospital.

    a.

    b.

47. Mr. James has demonstrated persistent sexual acting out since he was admitted for a myocardial infarction. This behavior has occurred with several female nurses. Which action by the head nurse would be most appropriate at this time?
    a. Tell Mr. James that his behavior is inappropriate and unacceptable.
    b. Assign only male nurses to Mr. James.
    c. Tell the nurses to avoid interacting with Mr. James.
    d. Obtain a consultation from a psychiatric nurse specialist.

48. List six general psychological factors that may contribute to sexual dysfunction.

    a.

    b.

    c.

    d.

    e.

    f.

49. Which sexual dysfunction in females is most often associated with physiological factors.
    a. Primary orgasmic dysfunction
    b. Secondary orgasmic dysfunction
    c. Dyspareunia
    d. Vaginismus

50. List four physiological conditions contributing to sexual dysfunction.

    a.

    b.

    c.

    d.

51. List and briefly describe the four major factors affecting sexuality.

    a.

    b.

    c.

    d.

52. List two general sex-related questions that may be used to initially determine whether the client has any sexual concerns.

    a.

    b.

53. List two general sex-related questions that may be used to initially determine whether a child's parents have any concerns related to the child's sexuality.

    a.

    b.

54. State one general sex-related question that may be used to initially determine whether the adolescent client has any sexual concerns.

55. Mary Webb visits the postpartum clinic 4 weeks after delivering her first child. When the nurse begins to talk about contraception, Ms. Webb looks away and changes the subject. How should this behavior be interpreted?
    a. Ms. Webb is not interested in talking about contraception.
    b. Ms. Webb does not want to use contraception.
    c. Ms. Webb may have a problem or concern related to her sexuality.
    d. Ms. Webb probably understands contraception because her pregnancy was planned.

56. Identify six interview strategies to enhance the client's and nurse's comfort when eliciting a sexual history.

    a.

    b.

    c.

    d.

    e.

    f.

57. List five questions that the nurse could use in eliciting a brief sexual history from a client.

    a.

    b.

    c.

    d.

    e.

58. Kegel exercises minimize problems with urinary incontinence in men and women. (True or false?)

59. Describe Kegel exercises.

60. What major factor determines whether the nurse diagnoses sexual dysfunction or altered patterns of sexuality?

61. List four general goals appropriate for the client experiencing actual or potential alterations in sexual functioning.

    a.

    b.

    c.

    d.

62. What action should the nurse take when sexual dysfunctions such as ongoing premature ejaculation, vaginismus, or concerns about transsexual dressing are identified?

CRITICAL THINKING AND EXPERIENTIAL EXERCISES

1. Sexual history
  a. Examine nursing assessment and health history forms used in your institution. Identify information elicited through the tool that would be useful in evaluating a client's sexuality.
  b. Formulate two general sex-related questions that you could routinely use in determining whether a client has any sexual concerns.
    (1) Practice asking these questions by standing in front of a mirror, audiotaping or videotaping, or asking another person.
    (2) Repeat this exercise until you feel comfortable asking your questions.
  c. Using guidelines described in your text, structure a questionnaire to be used in eliciting a brief sexual history for an adult. Try to limit the tool to 10 or fewer questions.
  d. Practice taking a sexual history by answering the questions in a self-developed questionnaire.
    (1) If any concerns were identified, determine the resources you could contact to receive needed assistance. (Your instructor, counselor, or personal health care provider could assist you in making any needed contacts.)
    (2) Identify questions with which you were comfortable and those that were more difficult to ask or answer. Attempt to analyze your feelings and consider whether an alternative approach or another health care provider would be needed to address these questions when you are working with a client. (If you found questions difficult to ask, it might be helpful to discuss this matter with your instructor.)
    (3) Use the tool to elicit a sexual history from a peer, friend, or family member. The assessment could be realistic and factually based, or your "client" could simulate a fictitious client situation. If possible, audiotape or videotape the interaction. Analyze the interaction, including your comfort, the client's comfort, and alternative approaches that might be used.
2. Aging and sexual response
  a. Design an in-service or community informational program on "Sexuality and the Older Adult." Limit your presentation to approximately 15 to 20 minutes. Include a discussion of common concerns that older adults have that may affect sexual functioning.
  b. Present your program to a peer group or group of students or staff nurses. If possible, audiotape or videotape or have an instructor or experienced

staff nurse monitor the presentation to provide feedback for evaluation.
  c. If possible, using your instructor as a resource person, present your program to a selected community group or clients in a health care setting.
3. Safer sex and STDs
  a. Design an informational presentation on "safer sex" for college-age students. Include in the presentation what is meant by safer sex, the nature of transmission and signs of sexually transmitted diseases, and how one can engage in responsible sexual practices.
  b. Practice presenting this information to a peer group. Request peer and instructor feedback or videotape the session.
  c. If feasible, using an instructor as a resource person, present this information to a selected college-age student population.
4. Sexual dysfunction
  a. Conduct a comprehensive nursing assessment or review the medical records of a client in any health care setting.
  b. Describe physical or psychological conditions that could actually or potentially contribute to sexual dysfunction.
  c. Review the actions and side effects of the medications that have been prescribed for the client. Identify any medications that could contribute to sexual dysfunction and describe their effect on the client's sexuality or sexual function.
5. Clinical situation: sexual development
  For each of the following situations, discuss the information you would share with the client based on the stage of sexual development described.
  a. Mrs. Williams is very concerned because her 5-year-old son Robert frequently touches or holds his genitalia. Mrs. Williams tells the nurse that this is very embarrassing, particularly when they are out in public. What information would you include in discussing Mrs. Williams' concerns?
  b. Mrs. McArthur, 47 years old, is experiencing difficulty sleeping at night and has frequent "hot flashes." She realizes she is "going through the change of life." As her nurse, what information could you provide to assist her in adjusting to the physiological changes she is experiencing?
  c. John Dempsey, 12 years old, visits his pediatrician for a well-child visit. John's mother, a single parent, is concerned because John seems much more withdrawn and is easily embarrassed when any sexual issues are brought up for discussion.
    (1) As the nurse, what information would you provide to John's mother?
    (2) What approach or approaches could be effective in meeting John's needs?
    (3) What information would be most important to share with John during this office visit?
    (4) What information about sexuality should be presented to John?

6. Clinical situation: contraception

Miss Atkinson, 18 years old, is planning to be married. She and her fiance do not want to have children until their college educations have been completed. She asks you, a community health nurse, about the best method of contraception.

a. What additional information would be important for you to determine before designing a teaching plan for Miss Atkinson?

b. Prepare a chart or table that lists six of the more effective nonpermanent methods of contraception, including advantages and disadvantages of each method, to use in the client-teaching situation.

c. Should Miss Atkinson's fiance be involved in the educational process? Why or why not? How could you approach the issue?

d. Miss Atkinson tells you that many of her friends use "birth control pills" and have encouraged her to select this contraceptive method. To assist in clarifying Miss Atkinson's values and provide accurate information about this method, what specific questions (and answers) would you address in your teaching plan?

7. Clinical situation: attitudes toward sexuality

Role play each of the following situations with a peer, implementing approprriate communication skills. Audiotape the role-playing situation and critique it to determine your level of effectiveness and assess your comfort level when dealing with sexuality and sensitive nursing procedures. Share your experience and feelings with your instructor for feedback.

a. Mr. Wenzel, a 26-year-old single professional football player, is admitted to the hospital for repair of an inguinal hernia. After surgery, you must frequently assess the scrotal area for bruising and swelling. Role play how you would inform Mr. Wenzel about the need for frequent assessment.

b. Mr. Henry, a 68-year-old retired farmer, has been admitted to the hospital for prostate surgery. After the preoperative teaching session, he says, "I've heard that this operation will prevent me from— performing with my wife, if you know what I mean. Is that true?" Role play your response.

c. Ms. Spooner is a 25-year-old single business woman who has decided to use the diaphragm as a nonpermanent contraceptive method. Role play how you would instruct Ms. Spooner about the technique of diaphragm insertion.

8. Clinical situation: sexuality and the nursing process

Mrs. Livingston, 35 years old, has been admitted to the hospital for a hysterectomy. She has been troubled by heavy menstrual bleeding for the past 6 months. Her physician has informed her that she has uterine fibroids; therefore her uterus must be removed, but her ovaries will be left intact.

Mrs. Livingston has two sons, 10 and 12 years old. She says she is "happily married" and that she and her husband have a "good''relationship, but she asks a lot of questions that allude to her "role as a wife and mother after this surgery." She says, "It's so final, but my doctor says there is no alternative because the fibroids will just get bigger and cause me more problems."

During Mr. Livingston's visit, Mrs. Livingston seems happy, but after her husband leaves, she says, "I wish I knew what my husband will really think of me after my surgery. He always talked about having a big family."

a. Identify two nursing diagnoses related to Mrs. Livingston's sexuality.

b. For each diagnosis, formulate at least one goal related to Mrs. Livingston's actual or potential sexual alteration and describe the expected outcomes that could be used in determining goal achievement.

c. For each goal, describe at least three nursing interventions.

ADDITIONAL READINGS

Boyle CA, Berkowitz, GS, Kelsey JL: Epidemiology of premenstrual symptoms, *Am J Public Health* 77(3):349, 1987.
    Studies a selected population to identify the prevalence of specific premenstrual symptoms and common associated factors. Presents detailed information in a table format.

Fogel CI, Woods NF: *Health care of women: a nursing perspective*, St Louis, 1981, Mosby–Year Book.
    Comprehensively addresses health and health care of women across the life span. Includes special sections on common health problems encountered by women at various developmental stages.

Katsin L: Chronic illness and sexuality, *Am J Nurs* 90(1):54, 1990.
    Discusses the importance of sexuality in adults with chronic illness. Highlights chronic pulmonary disease, arthritis, and diabetes. Describes changes experienced by clients and provides suggestions that clients and partners may use to increase satisfaction with intimacy. Well referenced for additional direction in reading.

McCracken AL: Sexual practices by elders, *J Gerontol Nurs* 14(10):13, 1988.
    Presents information about sexual practices of older adults. Useful for nurses in any setting with older adults.

Muscarei ME: Obtaining the adolescent sexual history, *Pediatr Nurs* 13(5):307, 1987.
    Discusses the importance of self-awareness and interviewing skills in obtaining an adolescent sexual history. Emphasizes the significance of clearly understanding and comfortably articulating information and issues associated with adolescent sexuality.

Rieve JE: Sexuality and the adult with acquired physical disability, *Nurs Clin North Am* 24(1):265, 1989.
    Describes multiple factors influencing sexuality in the physically disabled adult. Presents strategies for assessment, counseling, and intervention. Identifies research topics and area for additional investigation.

Shipes E: Sexual functioning following ostomy surgery, *Nurs Clin North Am* 22(2):303, 1987.
    Addresses physical and psychological effect of ostomy surgery on sexual function. Provides guidelines for counseling clients about sex and sexuality after ostomy or other cancer therapies.

Chapter 33
Spiritual Health

PREREQUISITE READING
Chapter 33, pp. 1000 to 1013

OBJECTIVES
Mastery of content in this chapter will enable the student to:
- Define selected terms associated with spiritual health.
- Discuss the relationship of spiritual health to physiological and psychosocial health.
- Contrast spiritual and religious aspects of health.
- Assess components of spiritual health.
- Describe a spiritually healthy person.
- Describe the signs of unmet spiritual needs.
- List interventions in the nursing plan for spiritual care.
- Evaluate attainment of spiritual health.
- Identify resources that can help clients attain spiritual health.

REVIEW OF KEY CONCEPTS
1. Define spiritual health.
2. Define faith.
3. Spiritual distress can lead to physical or emotional illness. (True or false?)
4. A set of organized beliefs, rituals, and practices taken on by people to understand and worship a deity

   is _____ .
5. The spiritual dimension of health care is limited to the client's religious affiliation and practices. (True or false?)
6. Which faith group is most likely to resist complying to medical treatment?
   a. Hindus
   b. Buddhists
   c. Conservative Muslims
   d. Reformed Jews
7. Match the religion to the religious belief described.

   a. Views illness as a result of misuse of body

   _____

   b. Use faith healing as psychological support

   _____

   c. Consider visiting the sick a religious obliga-

   tion _____

d. Generally are opposed to blood transfusions

_____

e. Family available for physical and emotional

care _____

Religion
1. Jehovah's Witnesses
2. Judaism
3. Islam
4. Hinduism
5. Buddhism

8. Mrs. Smith, in her fourth month of pregnancy, has just aborted the fetus for life-threatening medical reasons. What bearing would the client's religious practice have on the manner in which the fetus should be disposed of if Mrs. Smith is a:
   a. Reformed Jew
   b. Roman Catholic
   c. Follower of Islam
9. Mrs. F. is in the terminal stages of illness and death is imminent. What religious practices or rites would the nurse anticipate occuring before and after Mrs. F. dies if she is a(n):
   a. Hindu?
   b. Moslem?
   c. Roman Catholic?
   d. Orthodox Jew?
   e. Lutheran?
   f. Jehovah's Witness
10. What dietary restrictions might be imposed if a client is a:
   a. Hindu?
   b. Follower of Islam?
   c. Orthodox Jew?
   d. Mormon?
   e. Roman Catholic?
11. List six questions that may provide information about a client's spiritual health.

   a.

   b.

   c.

   d.

e.

f.

12. In the table below, identify client behaviors that reflect spiritual health and spiritual distress.

Spiritual health	Spiritual distress
a.	a.
b.	b.
c.	c.

13. What is the nurse's primary responsiblity in meeting the client's spiritual needs?

14. It is appropriate for a nurse who is comfortable with prayer to pray with a client when requested to do so. (True or false?)

15. List five resources that may be of assistance in maintaining or promoting a client's spiritual health.

a.

b.

c.

d.

e.

16. List five questions the nurse may ask in evaluating interventions directed toward a client's spiritual health.

a.

b.

c.

d.

e.

17. It is appropriate for nurses to seek personal assistance from pastoral care associates to meet spiritual needs of clients. (True or false?)

CRITICAL THINKING AND EXPERIENTIAL EXERCISES

1. The role of pastoral care associates/clergy
   Talk with an associate of the pastoral care department at your institution to determine:
   a. the role of the associate in meeting clients' spiritual needs.
   b. the associate's perception of the role and responsibilities of the nurse in meeting clients' spiritual needs.
   c. the assistance available to clients and nurses through the pastoral care department.
   (If your institution does not have a pastoral care department, you might ask to speak with clergy who are on call for the institution or direct these questions to your own spiritual advisor.)

2. Resources for spiritual health
   Independently, or in a small group:
   a. Identify resources available in your institution to assist clients and health team members in restoring or maintaining spiritual health.
   b. Identify at least four resources available in your community to assist clients and health team members in restoring or maintaining spiritual health.

3. Spiritual assessment
   a. Using suggested questions presented in your text, develop a brief spiritual assessment tool. (validate tool with your instructor.)
   b. Perform a self-assessment of spiritual health. Analyze the data obtained. If spiritual distress is present, make an appointment to talk with you spiritual advisor or member of a pastoral care team.
   c. Perform a spiritual assessment of a peer, friend, or family member. Analyze the data obtained. If spiritual distress is present, encourage the individual to seek assistance from his or her spiritual advisor or other appropriate resource.

4. Clinical situation: spiritual health and the nursing process
   Mr. Samanski, a 38-year old construction worker, has been hospitalized with the diagnosis of acute leukemia. He is aware that his prognosis is poor. Mr. Samanski is married and has two children, 6 and 8 years old. His wife is employed part time as a clerk in a department store. He has listed his religion as Christian but has not stated a specific denomination.
   One day, while the nurse is making Mr. Samanski's bed, he says, as his eyes fill with tears, "You know, I guess I don't really mind dying . . . if that's what He has planned for me. But I really need to stay alive to help my kids grow up. Boy, it really makes me wonder what I've done wrong." The nurse remains silent, quickly finishes the bed, and says, "Is there anything I can get for you?" Mr. Samanski replies, quietly, "No, I . . . I guess I'm fine." The nurse leaves the room.
   a. What information is presented that would support a diagnosis of spiritual distress?
   b. What factors could have influenced the nurse's reluctance to openly respond to Mr. Samanski's comment about his spiritual beliefs?
   c. Formulate possible responses that the nurse could have used to support Mr. Samanski and help him explore his feelings. (If possible, role play this situation with a peer. Analyze your feelings and behaviors orally or in writing.)
   d. Based on the nursing diagnosis of spiritual distress, develop a nursing care plan for Mr. Samanski. Include one short-term goal and three appropriate nursing interventions.
   e. Identify what assistance you as the nurse might need in providing needed spiritual care for Mr. Samanski.
   f. Submit your care plan and analysis to your instructor for feedback.

ADDITIONAL READINGS

Carson VB: *Spiritual dimensions of nursing practice,* Philadelphia, 1989, Saunders.

A comprehensive, indexed, well-referenced text addressing spirituality and its relationship to health care. Western and eastern spirituality, religious beliefs, and legal issues influencing the spiritual dimension are discussed. Integrates the nursing process in meeting spiritual needs of chronically ill and terminally ill clients. Also presents "burnout" as a spiritual issue in nursing practice.

Clark CC, Cross JR, Diane DM, Lowry L: Spirituality: integral to quality care, *Holistic Nurs Pract* 5(3):67, 1991.

Emphasizes the importance of meeting spiritual needs for purpose, love, trust, hope, forgiveness, and creativity. Uses Neuman Systems Model as a structure for exploring the nurse-client relationship and fostering spiritual care.

Charnes LS, Moor PS: Meeting patient's spiritual needs: The Jewish perspective, *Holistic Nurs Pract* 6(3):64, 1992.

Points out the need for increased nursing knowledge and sensitivity in caring for the spiritual and religious needs of the Jewish patient. Presents the unique influence of Jewish culture, religious beliefs, history, and life experience on universal spiritual questions of all religions.

Highfield MF, Cason C: Spiritual needs of patients: are they recognized? *Can Nurs* 6(3):187, 1987.

Study to identify nurses' awareness of clients' spiritual concerns. Data presented indicated nurses were unaware of many behaviors and conditions associated with clients' spiritual needs. Makes recommendations about interventions to more effectively address the spiritual domain of clients' needs.

Miller JF: Inspiring hope, *Am J Nurs* 85(1):22, 1985.

Explores the relationship between hope and client survival. Identifies ways the nurse can inspire hope—even in the face of serious and prolonged illness—by helping the client develop and use personal resources.

Peck ML: The therapeutic effect of faith, *Nurs Forum* 22(2):153, 1981.

Defines faith. Cites research indicating that faith is associated with a psychic energy that has curative power. Validates the belief that traditional customs and faith practices aid in restoring health.

Stoll R: Guidelines for spiritual assessment, *Am J Nurs* 79:1574, 1979.

Provides clear comparison between spiritual and religious beliefs. Offers guidelines for questions to assess the client's state of spiritual health.

Chapter 34
Hygiene

PREREQUISITE READING

Chapter 34, pp. 1016 to 1091.

OBJECTIVES

Mastery of content in this chapter will enable the student to:
- Define selected terms associated with client hygiene.
- Identify common skin problems and related interventions.
- Describe factors that influence personal hygienic practices.
- Discuss conditions that may put a client at risk for impaired skin integrity.
- Describe the types of bathing techniques used for various physical conditions.
- Develop a care plan based on client preferences and hygienic practices.
- Perform a complete bed bath and back rub.
- Discuss factors that influence the conditions of the nails and feet.
- Explain the importance of foot care for the diabetic client.
- Describe the methods used for cleaning and cutting the nails.
- Discuss conditions that may put a client at risk for impaired oral mucous membranes.
- Discuss measures used to provide special oral hygiene.
- Assist with or provide oral hygiene.
- List common hair and scalp problems and their related interventions.
- Offer hygiene for clients requiring eye, ear, and nose care.
- Successfully make an occupied, unoccupied, and surgical hospital bed.

REVIEW OF KEY CONCEPTS

1. List five factors influencing the manner in which a person performs personal hygiene.

   a.

   b.

   c.

   d.

   e.

2. Briefly describe the hygienic care appropriate for each time frame.
   a. Early morning
   b. Morning or after breakfast
   c. Afternoon
   d. Evening or hour of sleep
3. For each of the skin functions listed, describe at least two factors guiding nursing actions when bathing a client.
   a. Protection

      (1)

      (2)
   b. Sensation

      (1)

      (2)
   c. Temperature regulation

      (1)

      (2)
   d. Excretion and secretion

      (1)

      (2)

4. Match the description with the most appropriate term.

Description

   a. Resident skin bacteria _____
   b. Secrete heavy, oily substance to protect ear _____
   c. House glands, hair follicles _____
   d. Secrete oily lubricant for hair and skin _____
   e. Located in axillary and genital areas _____
   f. Replaces cells shed from skin's outer surface _____
   g. Assist in temperature control through evaporation

      _____

h. Responsible for skin pigmentation _____

i. Serves as heat insulator _____

Term

1. Epidermis
2. Melanocyte
3. Dermis
4. Normal flora
5. Eccrine glands
6. Apocrine glands
7. Ceruminous glands
8. Sebaceous glands
9. Subcutaneous tissue

5. Which assessment finding would indicate an abnormal skin characteristic?
   a. Skin intact without abrasions
   b. Skin warm to touch
   c. Skin color variation from body part to body part
   d. Skin slowly returns to resting position after pinching

6. Complete the table below by identifying the skin problem and describing at least two related interventions.

Description	Skin Problem	Inter-ventions
a. Inflammatory, papulopustular skin eruption usually involving bacterial breakdown of sebum	_____	(1) (2)
b. Scraping or rubbing away of epidermis	_____	(1) (2)
c. Excessive growth of body and facial hair	_____	(1) (2)
d. Flaky, rough skin texture on exposed areas	_____	(1) (2)
e. Skin eruptions	_____	(1) (2)
f. Abrupt onset of skin inflammation	_____	(1) (2)

7. For each developmental stage, briefly describe normal conditions creating high risk for impaired skin integrity.
   a. Neonate
   b. Toddler
   c. Adolescent
   d. Older adult

8. List six factors to assess to determine a client's self-care ability to perform personal skin care.
   a.
   b.
   c.
   d.
   e.
   f.

9. List six general conditions placing clients at risk for impaired skin integrity.
   a.
   b.
   c.
   d.
   e.
   f.

10. Larry Noah, a well-nourished 19-year-old, is hospitalized for a fractured right femur. The fracture is being treated with skeletal traction, so Larry is confined to bed. Larry has also had a fever and episodes of diaphoresis. Which risk factor for skin impairment would not be applicable for this client?
    a. Immobilization
    b. Secretions and excretions on the skin
    c. Age
    d. Presence of external devices

11. The purposes of a cleansing bath and skin care include all of the following except:
    a. stimulating circulation
    b. providing exercise
    c. promoting comfort
    d. reducing local inflammation.

12. List three goals for clients requiring skin care.
    a.
    b.
    c.

13. Describe each type of therapeutic bath by completing the table.

Therapeutic Bath	Purpose	Safety Factors to Consider
Sitz bath		
Hot water tub bath		
Warm water tub bath		
Cool water bath (tepid sponging)		
Soak		

14. A physician's order is required for therapeutic baths. (True or false?)

15. Which position of the client and the hospital bed is most appropriate for administering a bed bath?
    a. Move the client away from the nurse and put the bed in low position.

b. Move the client away from the nurse and put the bed in high position.

c. Move the client toward the nurse and put the bed in low position.

d. Move the client toward the nurse and put the bed in high position.

16. When changing the hospital gown of a client with an IV line, remove the gown from the arm with the IV line first. (True or false?)

17. Describe the technique for washing a client's eyes.

18. What nursing action will promote the safety of a client taking a tub bath or shower?
    a. Adjusting the water temperature to 120° F
    b. Checking on the client every 10 minutes
    c. Instructing client to remain in tub 20 to 30 minutes
    d. Draining the tub before the client gets out

19. Describe what is meant by a partial bed bath.

20. As a safety precaution, clients should be instructed to stay in the bathtub no longer than:
    a. 5 minutes
    b. 10 minutes
    c. 20 minutes
    d. 40 minutes

21. When administering a tepid sponge bath to reduce a client's fever, the nurse should assess:
    a. pulse and temperature immediately before and after the procedure
    b. pulse and temperature immediately before and every 15 minutes during the procedure
    c. pulse and temperature before the procedure and 1 hour later
    d. pulse and temperature every 30 minutes for 1 hour after the procedure

22. What is the correct temperature of tepid water?

23. List four guidelines the nurse should follow when assisting or providing a client with any type of bath.

    a.

    b.

    c.

    d.

24. Provide the rationale for each action included in bathing an infant.
    a. Keeping the infant covered as much as possible

    _____

    b. Using plain water (no soaps) for bathing

    _____

    c. Avoiding use of lotions and oils

    _____

    d. Eliminating use of cotton-tipped swabs for cleansing ears or nares _____

    e. Applying alcohol or triple dye to the umbilical cord _____

f. Drying gently but thoroughly _____

25. The grayish-white, cheeselike substance covering the skin of the neonate is _____

26. Which nursing action would be inappropriate for the infant after circumcision?
    a. Frequent tub baths to reduce inflammation
    b. Loose application of the diaper
    c. Gentle removal of blood with clean, moistened cotton balls
    d. Thorough cleansing of the anal area after bowel movements

27. Which statement regarding perineal care is inaccurate?
    a. The nurse should wear disposable gloves during the procedure.
    b. The client should be allowed to perform self-care whenever possible.
    c. Perineal care includes cleansing of external genitalia and surrounding skin.
    d. Perineal care may be omitted when the client and nurse are of opposite genders.

28. Which perineal care procedure is appropriate for a female client?
    a. Separate the labia with a gloved hand and wipe from the pubic area to the rectum using a circular motion.
    b. Separate the labia with a gloved hand and wipe from the pubic area to the rectum in one smooth stroke.
    c. Separate the labia with a gloved hand and wipe from the rectum to the pubic area using a circular motion.
    d. Separate the labia with a gloved hand and wipe from the rectum to the pubic area in one smooth stroke.

29. An effective backrub takes:
    a. 1 to 3 minutes.
    b. 3 to 5 minutes.
    c. 5 to 10 minutes.
    d. 10 to 15 minutes.

30. Which method of massage should be used at the end of a backrub?
    a. Kneading skin by grasping tissue between thumb and fingers
    b. Firm, slow strokes across the width of the back
    c. Light strokes moving in a circular pattern up the back
    d. Long, stroking movements laterally along the sides of the back

31. It is important for nurses to assess pulse and blood pressure after backrub for which of the following clients?
    a. Clients with rib fractures
    b. Clients with dysrhythmias
    c. Clients with vertebral fractures
    d. Clients with burns to the thorax

32. Match the following foot or nail problem with the most characteristic description.

Description

   a. Cone-shaped, round, raised, and often painful

   areas on toes _____

   b. Fungal lesion on sole of foot _____

   c. Unusually long, curved nail _____
   d. Flat, painless, thickened areas, often on under-

   surface of foot _____

   e. Inflammation of tissue surrounding nail _____
   f. Fungal infection of the foot with scaling, crack-

   ing, and blistering _____

Problem

   1. Callus
   2. Corn
   3. Plantar wart
   4. Tinea pedis
   5. Ram's horn nail
   6. Paronychia
33. Why is it important for diabetic clients to carefully inspect their feet on a daily basis?
34. Elderly clients with chronic foot problems should be encouraged to use over-the-counter preparations to provide optimal care for their feet and nails. (True or false?)
35. A client with complex foot and nail problems should

be referred to a _____.
36. List three goals for clients receiving nail and foot care.

   a.

   b.

   c.
37. List four client groups at risk for foot or nail problems.

   a.

   b.

   c.

   d.
38. When caring for a client's feet and nails, the nurse routinely:
   a. checks the femoral pulses.
   b. cuts the nails straight across below the tops of the toes.
   c. soaks the client's feet for 10 to 20 minutes before trimming nails.
   d. trims away calluses with a sterile blade or scissors.
39. List seven guidelines to include when advising clients with diabetes or peripheral vascular disease about foot care.

   a.

   b.

   c.
   d.
   e.
   f.
   g.
40. Deciduous refers to:
   a. baby teeth.
   b. permanent teeth.
   c. changes in teeth associated with dental decay.
   d. changes in teeth associated with the aging process.
41. List six questions to assess a client's oral-hygiene practices.

   a.

   b.

   c.

   d.

   e.

   f.
42. Match the following problems with the most characteristic description.

Description

   a. Bad breath _____
   b. Transparent coating on the teeth composed of

   mucin, carbohydrates, and bacteria _____

   c. Inflammation of the gums _____

   d. Cavities _____

   e. Inflammation of the mouth _____
   f. Cracking of the lips, especially at the corners of

   the mouth _____

   g. Inflammation of the tongue _____
   h. Dead bacteria that collect along the gum line

   _____

Problem

   1. Caries
   2. Plaque
   3. Stomatitis
   4. Halitosis
   5. Glossitis
   6. Cheilosis
   7. Gingivitis
   8. Tartar
43. What are the two best actions to prevent tooth loss?
44. Describe why each of the following clients is at risk for oral problems.
   a. Client receiving radiation therapy
   b. Client with diabetes
   c. Right-handed client with a stroke affecting the right side

d. Client who has had oral surgery
e. Client with a nasogastric tube and continuous nasal oxygen
f. Depressed client

45. List at least three assessment findings associated with oral malignancy.

a.

b.

c.

46. List three goals for clients requiring oral hygiene.

a.

b.

c.

47. Healthy clients of all ages should have a dental checkup at least every:
a. 3 months.
b. 6 months
c. 12 months.
d. 2 years.

48. An effective oral hygiene program involves:
a. brushing the teeth twice each day.
b. using a hard bristle brush to maximize cleaning.
c. holding the toothbrush at a 90-degree angle to the gum surface.
d. flossing at least once each day.

49. Which of the following oral hygiene products would place the client at risk for oral problems?
a. Hydrogen peroxide and water
b. Moi-Stir salivary supplement
c. Lemon-glycerin sponges
d. Fluoride toothpaste

50. Which of the following observations is most important to determine before providing oral hygiene to the unconscious client?
a. Presence of a functioning gag reflex
b. Presence of dental caries or halitosis
c. Color, texture, or bleeding of gums
d. Dryness or discoloration of the tongue

51. Mrs. Crystal is an 18-year-old who is unconscious as a result of a head injury. When providing mouth care, the nurse should:
a. position the client in a semi-Fowler's position to prevent aspiration of secretions.
b. swab the client's mouth with a gloved finger while she is lying in a reverse Trendelenburg position.
c. position the client on her side and have suction equipment available to remove secretions.
d. position the client on her back and use a padded tongue blade to keep the teeth separated.

52. The nurse should wear disposable gloves when providing oral hygiene. (True or false?)

53. Excessive fluoridation can result in discoloration of tooth enamel (True or false?)

54. When caring for a client with dentures, the nurse:
a. stores the dentures in a clean, dry container.
b. uses hot water to ensure thorough cleansing of dentures.
c. rinses dentures in cold water to promote client comfort.
d. assists the client in brushing gums, palate, and tongue.

55. What action should be taken when a tick is found on a client's skin?

56. Fill in the correct term for each of the following parasitic conditions.
a. Tiny, gray-white parasites found in pubic hair

_____

b. Tiny, gray-white parasites that are difficult to see and often cling to clothing _____
c. Tiny, gray-white parasites found on the scalp and attached to hair strands _____

57. List two goals for clients in need of hair and scalp care.

a.

b.

58. Combing the hair helps keep it clean and distributes oil along the hair shafts. (True or false?)

59. The nurse should request the permission of the client to:
a. shave a beard or mustache.
b. braid the hair.
c. cut tangled or matted hair.
d. all of the above.

60. List two groups of clients for whom it is preferable to use an electric razor for shaving.

a.

b.

61. List at least two factors to assess about a client's knowledge and use of each sensory aid.
a. Eyeglasses

(1)

(2)
b. Artificial eye

(1)

(2)
c. Hearing aid

(1)

(2)

62. List at least four factors to assess about a client's knowledge and use of contact lenses.

a.

b.

c.

d.

63. List two goals for clients requiring special hygienic care related to the eyes, ears, or nose.

  a.

  b.

64. Describe the special eye care that may be required for the unconscious client.

65. To safely remove a contact lens from an unconscious or immobilized client, the nurse should first make sure that the lens is placed directly over the:
  a. cornea.
  b. medial aspect of the sclera.
  c. lateral aspect of the sclera.
  d. conjunctiva.

66. A client wearing contact lenses complains of blurred vision. The cause of blurring could include:
  a. dirty or damaged lenses.
  b. lens placed in the opposite eye.
  c. corneal irritation.
  d. all of the above.

67. Identify three situations in which the client's contact lenses should be removed immediately.

  a.

  b.

  c.

68. Describe each of the following techniques necessary in caring for an artificial eye.
  a. Removal
  b. Cleansing
  c. Reinsertion
  d. Storage

69. Excessive or impacted cerumen is most effectively removed by:
  a. gentle use of cotton-tipped applicators.
  b. bulb syringe irrigation with hot water.
  c. Water Pik irrigation with cold water.
  d. mineral oil drops and tepid water irrigation.

70. Draw a simple stick figure diagram to describe each of the following positions.
  a. Fowler's
  b. Semi-Fowler's
  c. Trendelenburg
  d. Reverse Trendelenburg

71. Whenever possible, the nurse should make the bed while it is unoccupied. (True or false?)

72. Which of the following points should the nurse remember when making a client's bed?
  a. Shake and refold used linen.
  b. Place dirty linen directly on the floor.
  c. Place the hem of the bottom sheet "seam up."
  d. Carry the dirty linen away from the body.

73. After making the bed, the nurse should:
  a. lower the bed as close to the floor as possible.
  b. secure the call light within the client's reach.
  c. assist the client to a comfortable position.
  d. all of the above.

CRITICAL THINKING AND EXPERIENTIAL EXERCISES

1. Assisting with client hygiene
  a. After an observational experience or when assigned to provide hygienic care to a client, perform a self-care ability assessment.
  b. Include each of the following areas in your assessment:
    (1) Balance
    (2) Activity tolerance
    (3) Muscle strength
    (4) Coordination
    (5) Vision
    (6) Ability to sit without support
    (7) Hand grasp
    (8) Extremity range of motion
    (9) Cognitive function
  c. Describe modifications in technique that would be required based on your assessment.

2. Bathing an infant
  a. Prepare a teaching plan to instruct a new parent on bathing an infant. Include equipment and supplies needed. (If possible, visit a local store to determine the cost of equipment and supplies.)
  b. Formulate a rationale for each step of the procedure.
  c. Obtain a doll and demonstrate the technique. Have a peer observe and critique your performance, or if possible videotape the simulated session for self-evaluation and/or instructor evaluation.

3. Foot care for the diabetic patient
  a. Develop a teaching booklet addressing foot care for clients in the community with diabetes or peripheral vascular disease.
  b. Practice teaching the basic principles of foot care to a small group of peers based on the information presented in the teaching booklet. If possible, videotape or audiotape the simulated teaching session. Ask your peers to critique the teaching session and formulate your own self-evaluation.
  c. Submit your teaching booklet to your instructor for feedback.
  d. With your instructor as a resource and proctor, present your teaching session or booklet to a group of older adults in the community.

4. Clinical situation: special hygiene needs
Helen Ziegler, a 55-year-old black music teacher, requires total care following a stroke. She is unable to speak or write and unable to move her right arm or leg. She has upper dentures. She has no blink reflex in her left eyelid. She has an indwelling Foley catheter for urinary drainage. Mrs. Ziegler has a history of diabetes mellitus.
  a. What factors must be considered before initiating Mrs. Ziegler's hygiene?
  b. Identify the conditions that currently place Mrs. Ziegler at risk for skin breakdown. Briefly describe the physiological basis for these risks.

c. Identify the conditions that currently place Mrs. Ziegler at risk for oral problems. Briefly describe the physiological basis for these risks.

d. Discuss the procedure and related rationale for providing Mrs. Ziegler with each of the following:

  (1) Oral hygiene
  (2) Eye care
  (3) Perineal care
  (4) Skin care
  (5) Hair care

SKILL AND TECHNIQUE ACTIVITIES

1. Use of hospital room equipment

  a. Arrange to visit an unoccupied room on your assigned nursing unit to examine and practice working with the room equipment including:

  (1) nursing call system.
  (2) room lights.
  (3) overbed table.
  (4) bedside stand.
  (5) shower or tub fixtures.

  b. In your nursing laboratory or on your nursing unit, practice the following activities using an empty hospital bed:

  (1) Unlocking and locking the bed wheels
  (2) Raising and lowering the side rails
  (3) Positioning the bed in Fowler's, semi-Fowler's, Trendelenburg, and reverse Trendelenburg positions

  c. When you have practiced each of the skills using an empty hospital bed, have a peer climb into the bed and perform each of the techniques again.

2. Oral hygiene technique

  a. Examine your institution's procedure for administering oral hygiene.

  b. Write a list of all of the equipment and supplies needed to provide oral hygiene to an unconscious client and locate them on your nursing unit.

  c. Practice administering oral hygiene to a partner while a peer observes and critiques your performance based on the steps described in your text.

  d. Elicit an instructor's evaluation of your technique for administering oral hygiene.

3. Bathing techniques

  a. Examine your institution's procedure for hygienic care.

  b. Write a list of all of the equipment and supplies needed to administer a complete bed bath and locate these items on your assigned clinical area.

  c. Practice giving a bed bath to a demonstration mannequin or a peer in your nursing laboratory. Using the steps listed in your text, critique your performance or have the peer critique your performance.

  d. Volunteer to have another student give you a bed bath. Describe how it feels to have someone give you a bath. Identify actions that made you feel more comfortable. Identify actions that made you feel uncomfortable. Formulate approaches that would reduce your discomfort.

  e. Observe or assist a nurse administering a bed bath to a client. Compare the techniques you observed with those described in your text. Attempt to determine the rationale for modification of the techiques you observed. Discuss your observations with your instructor.

  f. Elicit an instructor's evaluation of your bed bath technique.

4. Sponge bath technique for infant

  a. Examine your institution's procedures for bathing an infant.

  b. Write a list of all of the equipment and supplies needed to bathe an infant.

  c. Practice giving a sponge bath to a doll while a peer observes and critiques your performance. (If you wish, practice bathing a doll independently and perform a self-evaluation.)

  d. Elicit an instructor's evaluation of your infant bathing technique.

5. Shaving technique

  a. Examine your institution's policies for shaving clients using safety razors or electric shavers.

  b. Practice shaving a peer, friend, or family member.

6. Perineal care technique

  a. Examine your institution's procedure for administering perineal care.

  b. Write a list of the equipment and supplies needed to administer perineal care.

  c. Using a demonstration mannequin in your nursing laboratory, practice administering perineal care while a peer observes and critiques your performance based on the steps described in your text.

  d. Independently or in a role-playing situation, practice explaining the steps of perineal care in a simulated setting. Audiotape your explanation. Review and critique your performance.

  e. Elicit an instructor's evaluation of your perineal care technique.

7. Backrub technique

  a. Practice administering a backrub to a partner while a peer observes and critiques your performance.

  b. Elicit an instructor's evaluation of your backrub technique.

8. Bed-making technique

  a. In the nursing laboratory, practice the following bed-making techniques while a peer observes and critiques your performance based on the steps described in your text:

  (1) Open, unoccupied bed
  (2) Closed, unoccupied bed
  (3) Surgical, recovery, or postoperative bed

  b. In the nursing laboratory, practice making an occupied bed with a partner acting as the client.

Ask your partner to observe and critique your performance.

c. Observe or assist another nurse making an occupied bed. Compare the techniques to the steps described in your text. Attempt to determine the rationale for modifications in the nurse's technique. Discuss your observations with your instructor.

d. Elicit an instructor's evaluation of your bedmaking technique.

ADDITIONAL READINGS

Arentsen JJ: A review of complications associated with soft contact lenses, *J Ophthalmic Nurse Technol* 6(6):230, 1987.
Describes proper lens care, potential problems associated with soft contact lenses, and common symptoms for early recognition of these problems.

Harrell JS, Damon JF: Prediction of patient's need for mouth care, *West J Nurse Res* 11(6):748, 1989.
Analysis of data identifying stressors predisposing clients to oral complications. Emphasizes nursing assessment and early interventions to prevent oral complications.

Joyner M: Hair care in the black patient, *J Pediatr Health Care* 2(6):281, 1988.
Explains concepts critical to transcultural health care including sensitivity to cultural values, beliefs, and practices. Presents hair care practices deeply embedded in cultural beliefs and practices of blacks.

Malloy MB, Perez-Woods RC: Neonatal skin care: prevention of skin breakdown, *Dermatol Nurs* 3(5):318, 1991.
Well-referenced discussion of problems of skin care in infants with low birth weights. Emphasizes skin care protocols to decrease skin breakdown and subsequently reduce morbidity and mortality.

Miller CA: Ins and outs of skin care, *Geriat Nurs* 12(3):111, 1991.
Discussion of skin care unique to the elderly client. Practical pointers for care of healthy and chronically ill clients.

Moss SJ: Preventive techniques in infant dental care, *Nurs Practitioner* 13(7):37, 1988.
Presents dental caries as the most prevalent disease among young people in the United States. Overviews preventive dental techniques for infants.

Kelsey L: Mouth care and the intubated patient—the aim of prevention infection, *Intensive Care Nurs* 1(4):187, 1986.
Examines mouth care procedures involving four different mouth care solutions. Study of intubated clients receiving antibiotic therapy revealed that no one mouthwash solution was more effective than tap water and a toothbrush in oral care.

Osguthorpe NC: If your patient has contact lenses, *Am J Nurs* 84:1255, 1984.
Describes how to locate, remove, and protect contact lenses. Describes eye care appropriate for clients with contact lenses. Includes photographs depicting lens removal.

Poland JM: Comparing Moi-Stir to lemon glycerin swabs, *Am J Nurs* 87:422, 1987.
Summarizes a review of the literature addressing use of lemon-glycerin swab sticks for mouth care. Describes a study comparing lemon-glycerin swabs with Moi-Stir swabs (a salivary supplement), which revealed the superiority of Moi-Stir in client satisfaction and dental and gingival health.

Wanich CK: Incontinence care products: non-surgical management of urinary incontinence, *Ostomy/Wound Manage* 34:45, 1991.
Describes current products to facilitate care and maintain skin integrity in incontinent clients. Useful information for institutional and home care.

Winslow EH et al: Oxygen uptake and cardiovascular response in control adults and acute myocardial infarction patients during bathing, *Nurs Res* 34:164, 1985.
Describes a study comparing physiological responses before, during, and after three types of baths (basin, tub, and shower) in a normal adult control group and clients with acute myocardial infarction. Findings revealed similar physiological costs for the various bathing methods, with differences in physiological response related primarily to subject variability.

Chapter 35
Nutrition

PREREQUISITE READING
Chapter 35, pp. 1092 to 1143.

OBJECTIVES
Mastery of content in this chapter will enable the student to:
- Define selected terms associated with nutrition.
- List the six categories of nutrients and explain why each is necessary for nutrition.
- Explain the importance of a balance between energy intake in foods and energy output.
- List the end products of carbohydrate, protein, and lipid metabolism.
- Explain the significance of saturated, unsaturated, and polyunsaturated lipids in nutrition.
- Describe the food guide pyramid and discuss its value in planning meals for good nutrition.
- Explain recommended daily allowances (RDAs).
- List seven dietary guidelines for health promotion.
- Discuss the major areas of nutritional assessment.
- Identify three major nutritional problems and describe clients at risk for these problems.
- State the goals of enteral and total parenteral nutrition.
- Describe the procedure for initiating and maintaining tube feedings.
- Describe methods to avoid complications associated with tube feedings.
- Describe the procedure for initiating and maintaining total parenteral nutrition.
- Discuss the importance of diet counseling in evaluation and client teaching before discharge.

REVIEW OF KEY CONCEPTS
1. Match the following terms with the definition provided.

Definition

a. Biochemical reactions that build body tissues _____

b. Proportion of essential nutrients in relation to total calories _____

c. Foods containing elements needed for body functions _____

d. Resting energy requirements _____

e. Biochemical reactions that break down body tissues _____

f. All biochemical reactions within the body _____

Term
1. Metabolism
2. Nutrients
3. Anabolism
4. Catabolism
5. Nutrient density
6. Basal metabolic rate (BMR)

2. List the six categories of nutrients; using an asterisk, identify the one that is most important.

a.

b.

c.

d.

e.

f.

3. List the two developmental age groups most vulnerable to water deprivation or loss.

a.

b.

4. The preferred energy source for the body is found in:
   a. proteins.
   b. carbohydrates.
   c. lipids.
   d. minerals.

5. Carbohydrates are stored in the body in the form of:
   a. starch.
   b. monosaccharides.
   c. glucose.
   d. glycogen.

6. Indicate the total calories produced by metabolism of each nutrient listed.
   a. 20 g of protein
   b. 15 g of fat
   c. 50 g of carbohydrate

7. What is a complete protein?

8. Complete the following table by listing three food sources for each protein classification.

Complete proteins	Incomplete proteins
a.	a.
b.	b.
c.	c.

9. Briefly describe what is meant by each of the following:
   a. Nitrogen balance
   b. Negative nitrogen balance
   c. Positive nitrogen balance
10. The primary role of protein is to:
    a. provide energy.
    b. promote tissue growth, maintenance, and repair.
    c. serve as a catalyst for the body's metabolic reactions.
    d. store energy.
11. Indicate the effect of ingestion of each of the following lipid forms on blood cholesterol levels.
    a. Polyunsaturated fatty acids
    b. Unsaturated fatty acids
    c. Saturated fatty acids
12. Most animal fats have a higher proportion of:
    a. saturated fatty acids.
    b. unsaturated fatty acids.
    c. polyunsaturated fatty acids.
    d. polyunsaturated and unsaturated fatty acids
13. Identify the essential fatty acid and list three potential dietary sources.

    a.

    b.

    c.
14. The body stores energy as:
    a. fat.
    b. carbohydrate.
    c. amino acid.
    d. protein.
15. USDA Nutritional guidelines recommend the adult dietary lipid intake of no more than:
    a. 45% of total caloric intake.
    b. 30% of total caloric intake.
    c. 20% of total caloric intake.
    d. 10% of total caloric intake.
16. Which statement about water-soluble vitamins is correct?
    a. Vitamins A and K are examples of water-soluble vitamins.
    b. Water-soluble vitamins are stored in the body.
    c. Water-soluble vitamins must be provided through daily intake.
    d. Hypervitaminosis of water-soluble vitamins does not occur.
17. What is the primary role of minerals in biochemical reactions?
18. Complete the table by describing the function of the

vitamin or mineral, three major food sources, and common manifestations of deficiency.

Nutrient	Function	Sources	Effects of Deficiency
Vitamins			
B₁ (thiamin)			
B₂ (riboflavin)			
Niacin			
B₆ (pyridoxine, pyridoxal, pyridoxamine)			
Folacin, folic acid, folate			
B₁₂ (cobalamin)			
Pantothenic acid			
Biotin			
C			
A			
D			
E			
K			
Minerals			
Calcium			
Magnesium			
Phosphorus			
Copper			
Fluoride			
Iodine			
Iron			
Zinc			

19. Match the food substance with the enzyme that aids its digestion.

Substance

   a. Protein _____
   b. Carbohydrate _____
   c. Fat _____

Enzyme
   1. Ptyalin
   2. Pepsin
   3. Lipase
   4. Polypeptidase
   5. Amylase
   6. Sucrase
   7. Maltase
   8. Lactase
   9. Trypsin
20. The major portion of digestion and absorption occurs in the:
    a. mouth.
    b. stomach.
    c. small intestine.
    d. large intestine.
21. The primary nutrient absorbed from the large intestine is:
    a. water.

b. vitamin E.

c. bile.

d. iron.

22. The metabolic process responsible for the breakdown of chemical substances into simpler substances is:
    a. anabolism.
    b. catabolism.
    c. emulsion.
    d. absorption.

23. Diagram and label the food guide pyramid developed by the U.S. Department of Agriculture (USDA).

24. What is the purpose of the food guide pyramid?

25. Define RDA.

26. What is the significance of the National Labeling and Education Act (NLEA) of 1990?

27. List five of the dietary guidelines for Americans issued by the USDA and the Department of Health and Human Services.

    a.

    b.

    c.

    d.

    e.

28. Match the category of vegetarianism with the characteristic diet.

Category

    a. Lactovegetarian _____

    b. Ovolactovegetarian _____

    c. Vegans _____

Diet

    1. Consume only plant foods
    2. Consume plant foods and milk but avoid eggs
    3. Consume plant foods, eggs, and milk

29. The birth weight of the typical infant characteristically doubles at:
    a. 2 to 3 months.
    b. 4 to 5 months.
    c. 6 to 8 months.
    d. 1 year.

30. Neonates are unable to digest:
    a. simple carbohydrates.
    b. complex carbohydrates.
    c. emulsified fats.
    d. simple proteins.

31. The recommended nutritional source for infants during the first 4 to 6 months is:
    a. breast milk.
    b. prepared formula.
    c. whole milk.
    d. enriched rice cereal.

32. List four nutrients that must be supplemented in the breast-fed infant.

    a.

b.

c.

d.

33. At what age are solid foods best introduced into the infant's diet?

34. Describe at least four indications of infant readiness to begin solid foods.

    a.

    b.

    c.

    d.

35. Mrs. Carson asks the nurse the kind of milk to purchase for her 12-month-old daughter. The nurse should advise Mrs. Carson to buy:
    a. the most economical milk available.
    b. skim or low-fat (1%) milk.
    c. 2% fat milk.
    d. whole milk.

36. The nutritional needs of toddlers include:
    a. increased total kilocalories.
    b. decreased total protein intake.
    c. a minimum of 28 oz. of milk daily.
    d. half of all proteins of high biological value.

37. During adolescence, the best guide to nutritional needs is:
    a. desired body weight.
    b. chronological age.
    c. physiological age.
    d. body image and appearance.

38. Which statement about nutrition in pregnancy is inaccurate?
    a. Poor nutrition can cause low birth weight and decreased neonatal survival.
    b. Fetal nutritional needs are generally met at the expense of the mother.
    c. The nutritional status of the mother at the time of conception is of little importance.
    d. A maternal weight gain of 22 to 33 pounds is recommended.

39. Compared to the pregnant woman, the lactating mother requires an increased amount of:
    a. calcium and phosphorus.
    b. iron.
    c. protein.
    d. calories and water.

40. List four factors influencing nutritional status of the older adult; using an asterisk, identify one factor considered to be the most important.

    a.

    b.

    c.

    d.

41. List the four components of a nutritional assessment.

    a.

    b.

c.

d.

42. List seven factors influencing dietary patterns.

a.

b.

c.

d.

e.

f.

g.

43. Describe three ways that excessive alcohol ingestion may contribute to nutritional deficiencies.

a.

b.

c.

44. For each assessment area, list at least two signs of poor nutrition.
a. General appearance

(1)

(2)

b. General vitality

(1)

(2)

c. Weight

(1)

(2)

d. Hair

(1)

(2)

e. Skin

(1)

(2)

f. Mouth (lips, gums, teeth, and mucous membranes)

(1)

(2)

g. Eyes

(1)

(2)

h. Gastrointestinal function

(1)

(2)

i. Cardiovascular function

(1)

(2)

j. Neurological function

(1)

(2)

45. List five common anthropometric measurements.

a.

b.

c.

d.

e.

46. The laboratory data most useful in determining protein-calorie malnutrition are:
a. hemoglobin and hematocrit.
b. total lymphocyte count and red cell count.
c. serum albumin and transferrin.
d. blood urea nitrogen and urine creatinine.

47. Answer the following:
a. The eating disorder characterized by self-imposed starvation is _____ .
b. The eating disorder characterized by abnormal food craving, gorging, and induced vomiting is _____ .

48. List at least two common goals for any client presenting with nutritional problems.

a.

b.

49. List the five nutrients provided through total parenteral nutrition (TPN).

a.

b.

c.

d.

e.

50. List three nursing measures to foster an environment conducive to eating.

a.

b.

c.

51. The regular hospital diet contains approximately:
a. 1500 kilocalories.
b. 1800 kilocalories.
c. 2200 kilocalories.
d. 2500 kilocalories.

52. Fill in the name of each special diet described.
a. Transparent fluids, egg whites, and gelatin _____
b. Foods from the regular diet that are easily chewed and digested _____
c. Limits fibers, milk and milk products, cheese, fried foods, and fruits _____

d. Allows all food, but minimizes those that are difficult to digest or fried _____

e. Food is served warm or cool; eliminates any foods that are irritating, stimulating, or spicy _____

f. Foods that are liquid at room or body temperature _____

g. Increases amounts of raw fruits and vegetables _____

53. List the two major modes of enteral feeding.

a.

b.

54. Tube feedings are appropriate for all of the following situations except:
a. a client unable to digest or absorb nutrients.
b. a client unable to ingest nutrients.
c. a client unable to adequately chew foods.
d. a client unable to swallow foods.

55. Which tube type is preferred for enteral tube feedings?
a. Large-bore nasogastric tubes
b. Large-bore rubber or plastic feeding tubes
c. Small-bore flexible feedings tubes
d. Small-bore rigid feeding tubes

56. Describe the method for determining the appropriate tube length for feeding tubes placed in the
a. stomach.
b. duodenum or jejunum.

57. List two methods for nurses to use at the bedside to determine gastric tube placement.

58. Auscultation of air is a reliable indicator to verify placement of small-bore feeding tubes. (True or false?)

59. Define gastric residual.

60. How often should gastric residual be routinely checked in a client receiving continuous tube feedings?
a. Every 2 to 4 hours
b. Every 4 to 6 hours
c. Every 6 to 8 hours
d. Every 12 hours

61. Why is it important for the nurse to assess abdominal distention, nausea, and vomiting in a client receiving tube feedings through a small-bore tube?

62. The most reliable method for determining feeding tube placement is:
a. aspiration of gastric contents.
b. radiographic verification.
c. auscultation of air injection.
d. examination of the posterior oral pharynx.

63. In what position should the client be placed before the nurse administers a tube feeding?

64. Briefly describe the rationale for each action associated with initiation and maintenance of total parenteral nutrition.
a. Trendelenburg position
b. Valsalva maneuver

c. Chest x-ray examination
d. Sterile technique and dressings
e. Infusion pump and careful infusion regulation
f. Monitoring blood glucose at least every 4 hours (or as ordered by the physician)

65. A client receiving TPN displays the following signs and symptoms: headache, cold and clammy skin, dizziness, tachycardia, and circumoral tingling. The most likely reason for these manifestations is:
a. fluid overload.
b. hyperglycemia.
c. hypoglycemia.
d. air embolism.

66. If a TPN solution falls behind schedule, the nurse should attempt to catch up to ensure that the client receives the prescribed amount. (True or false?)

CRITICAL THINKING AND EXPERIENTIAL EXERCISES

1. Client education: food guide pyramid and dietary guidelines for health promotion
a. Select a specific developmental level (preschool, school age, adolescent, young and middle adult, or older adult).
b. Based on developmental characteristics and specific nutritional needs for the age group, develop a teaching plan that presents the food guide pyramid and the USDA dietary guidelines.
c. Present your teaching plan to a peer group and instructor for feedback.
d. If possible, using your instructor as a resource, arrange to present your teaching session to the identified population in your community.

2. Diet history
a. Using the tool provided in your text, elicit a diet history from a peer or an assigned client. Formulate a list of nursing diagnoses based on the data obtained.
b. Keep a dietary log of your own intake for 3 days, including a weekend. Analyze and describe your intake, and formulate recommendations in relation to:
  (1) the food guide pyramid.
  (2) RDAs.
  (3) USDA dietary guidelines.

3. Nutritional assessment
a. Perform a comprehensive nursing assessment of a selected client (and/or review the medical record of the client).
b. Identify data pertinent to the client's nutritional state including:
  (1) factors influencing dietary patterns.
  (2) anthropometric data.
  (3) clinical signs of nutritional status.
  (4) laboratory data.
c. Formulate actual and potential nursing diagnoses pertinent to the client's nutritional status.
d. Develop a plan of care to address the priority diagnosis.

4. Special therapeutic diets
   a. Review the nursing or dietary Kardex for clients in any health care setting.
   b. Identify the types of diets that are ordered for selected clients.
   c. Using the institution's diet manual or other appropriate resources, determine the characteristics of the special diets ordered.
   d. Determine the reason for the prescribed diet.
5. Community resources
   Independently, or in a small group, identify resources available in your community to assist clients in meeting their nutritional needs (at least two for each of the identified resource areas listed).
   a. Government programs
   b. Private agencies
   c. Volunteer agencies
6. Clinical situation: developmental and therapeutic nutritional variables
   Outline a nutritional plan for the following clients:
   a. A 2-year-old admitted to the hospital with chronic diarrhea
   b. A 12-year-old who has just had oral surgery
   c. A 17-year-old pregnant girl who has been seen in the prenatal clinic with a diagnosis of altered nutrition: less than body requirements related to lack of information
   d. An obese 40-year-old teacher, wife, and mother
   e. A 53-year-old man who has recently had a myocardial infarction
   f. A 60-year-old woman with cancer who is receiving radiation therapy
   g. An 82-year-old with complaints of chronic constipation
7. Clinical situation: nutrition and the nursing process
   Mrs. Kirk is a 72-year-old widow who lives alone on a limited income. Her apartment is about six blocks from the nearest grocery store. To reach a larger supermarket, Mrs. Kirk must catch two buses. Mrs. Kirk has arthritis, which makes walking or carrying large, heavy bags of groceries very difficult and painful.
   Mrs. Kirk has been admitted to the hospital because of iron-deficiency anemia and low blood pressure. She complains of feeling very tired and weak "all the time."
   When questioned about her normal dietary patterns, Mrs. Kirk states that she usually has a small bowl of soup with crackers for lunch and tea and a piece of toast at supper. She states, "It's no fun eating alone, and I don't have much money to spend on food because I won't be able to pay my bills."
   Mrs. Kirk weighs 45 kg (98 pounds), and she is 157.5 cm (63 inches) tall. She states, "I guess I've lost some weight lately because my clothes are much looser." At lunchtime, the nurse notes that Mrs. Kirk has eaten very little of the roast chicken and vegetables. When asked if she did not like the food, Mrs. Kirk replies, "Oh, no, it tasted all right; I'm just too tired to eat."

1. Develop a comprehensive care plan for Mrs. Kirk that addresses her short-term nutritional needs while in the hospital and her nutritional needs after she is discharged.

SKILL AND TECHNIQUE ACTIVITIES

1. Feeding techniques
   a. Visit a day-care center and observe the feeding techniques and methods of assisting children during meals. Compare the techniques and methods of assisting with the developmental levels of the children.
   b. Observe a nurse or family member feeding or assisting an adult at mealtime. What techniques seem effective or ineffective? What are the similarities and differences between the techniques you observed and those you studied?
   c. Eat a meal with a peer. Take turns feeding each other. Be sure to include different food forms (for example, liquids, solids, semisolids) and use a variety of utensils (spoon, fork, straw, cup). Share how you felt in the roles of the nurse and client. Based on your experiences, identify ways to make the client more comfortable during mealtime.
2. Enteral tube feeding techniques
   a. Examine your institution's policies and procedures regarding administration of tube feedings.
   b. In the nursing laboratory or on your clinical unit, examine the various types of gastric and enteral tubes and associated equipment.
   c. In the nursing laboratory or on your clinical unit, examine any available pumps used to administer continuous enteral tube feedings.
   d. Talk with your institution's dietitian or nutritionist to determine the types of tube feeding preparations most often ordered for clients.
   e. Observe clients receiving tube feedings in the clinical area. Compare the techniques that you observed in monitoring the client and administering the tube feeding to those described in your text. Share your observations with your instructor.
   f. In the nursing laboratory, using a demonstration mannequin with a feeding tube in place, have a peer observe and critique your performance as you:
      (1) practice the techniques of assessment specific to a client receiving tube feedings.
      (2) practice the techniques of checking for feeding tube placement.
      (3) practice the techniques of administering a tube feeding.
   g. Elicit an instructor's evaluation of your assessment of a client requiring a tube feeding and your technique for administering it.

ADDITIONAL READINGS

Bockus S: Troubleshooting your tube feedings, *Am J Nurs* 91(5):24, 1991.
   A continuing education program addressing techniques for tube feeding administration. Includes illustrations and multiple-choice examination.

Eisenberg PG: Pulmonary complications for enteral nutrition, *Crit Care Nurs Clin North Am* 3(4):641, 1991.

Reviews current literature addressing common pulmonary complications of enteral feedings. Details nursing measures to reduce the incidence of complications associated with improper tube placement, tube displacement and aspiration, metabolic complications, and medication and formula incompatibility.

Ferraro AR, Huddleston KC: Safe administration of small volume enteral feedings: an alternative to intravenous pumps, *J Pediatr Nurs* 6(5):352, 1991.

Presents practical tips for providing safe enteral feedings to pediatric clients.

Hoyt MJ, Staats JR: Wasting and malnutrition in patients with HIV/AIDS, *J Assoc Nurses Aids Care* 2(3):16, 1991.

Outlines nursing interventions for nutritional care to increase the quality and quantity of lives of clients with HIV or AIDS.

Palmer TA: Anorexia nervosa, bulimia nervosa, causal theories and treatment, *Nurs Pract* 15(4):12, 1990.

Overviews medical management, psychotherapy, behavioral management, food management, and nutritional counseling in the care of clients with eating disorders. Emphasizes the importance of a multidisciplinary approach for successful treatment.

Plehn KW: Anorexia nervosa and bulimia: incidence and diagnosis, *Nurs Pract* 15(4):22, 1990.

Discusses signs and symptoms of common eating disorders. Emphasizes the role of nurses in case finding for early intervention.

Testerman EJ: Current trends in pediatric total parenteral nutrition, *J Intravenous Nurs* 12(3):152, 1989.

Overviews the evolution of pediatric TPN, indications for therapy, components of solutions, potential complications, monitoring guidelines, and nursing care. Well referenced to guide additional reading.

White JH: Feminism, eating and mental health, *ANS* 13(3):68, 1991.

Discusses the cultural, political, and social phenomena affecting eating disorders. Parallels eating disorders with other mental illnesses of women. Suggests a new view of anorexia nervosa and bulimia through feminist-based research.

Williams SR: *Nutrition and diet therapy,* ed 6, St Louis, 1989, Mosby–Year Book.

Comprehensively addresses normal and therapeutic nutrition. Approaches nutritional needs from developmental, physical, psychological, and cultural perspectives.

Worthington PH, Wagner BA: Total parenteral nutrition, *Nurs Clin North Am* 24(2):355, 1989.

One in a series of articles addressing nutritional care. Emphasizes the importance of nursing management through competent technical skills and physical and psychosocial support.

Chapter 36
Sleep

PREREQUISITE READING
Chapter 36, pp. 1144 to 1173

OBJECTIVES

Mastery of content in this chapter will enable the student to:

- Define selected terms associated with sleep and sleep disorders.
- Compare the characteristics of sleep and rest.
- Explain the effect the 24-hour sleep-wake cycle has on biological function.
- Discuss mechanisms that regulate sleep.
- Describe the stages of a normal sleep cycle.
- Explain the functions of sleep.
- Compare and contrast the sleep requirements of persons in different age groups.
- Identify factors that normally promote and disrupt sleep.
- Discuss characteristics of common sleep disorders.
- Conduct a sleep history for a client.
- Identify nursing diagnoses appropriate for clients with sleep alterations.
- Identify nursing interventions designed to promote normal sleep cycles for clients of all ages.
- Describe ways to evaluate sleep therapies

REVIEW OF KEY CONCEPTS

1. Define rest.
2. Define sleep.
3. List three basic conditions required for proper rest.

    a.

    b.

    c.

4. Which biological rhythm would describe the rapid eye movement (REM) stage of sleep?
    a. Diurnal
    b. Infradian
    c. Ultradian
    d. Circadian
5. Karen Finnigan is a 24-year-old registered nurse working a day/night rotation on a general surgical nursing unit. When she switches from the day to the night shift, she has difficulty sleeping. An alteration in her biological sleep cycle:

a. will occur immediately if Karen is healthy.
b. often takes several weeks before her body will adjust.
c. has little influence on Karen's actual physiological function.
d. is unrelated to environmental temperature or light.

6. Complete the table comparing the cerebral mechanisms responsible for sleep regulation.

	Sleep Mechanisms	Arousal Mechanisms
Name		
Anatomical location		
Neurotransmitter		

7. Match the sleep stage with the characteristic description.

Stage

    a. Stage 1: NREM _____

    b. Stage 2: NREM _____

    c. Stage 3: NREM _____

    d. Stage 4: NREM _____

    e. REM _____

Description

1. Complete muscle relaxation
2. If awakened, feels as if daydreaming
3. Responsible for mental restoration
4. Sound sleep, progressive relaxation
5. Responsible for restoring and resting body

8. The physical benefits derived from sleep include:
    a. cardiac function preservation.
    b. growth hormone production.
    c. energy conservation.
    d. all of the above.
9. The amount of time spent in REM sleep is greatest for:
    a. infants.
    b. school-age children.

c. adolescents.

d. older adults.

10. Sleep pattern changes in an older person are primarily a result of psychological problems. (True or false?)

11. List and briefly described five factors affecting sleep.

a.

b.

c.

d.

e.

12. A protein found in milk, cheese, and meats that may help a person to sleep is _____ .

13. Identify the sleep disorder described in each of the following client situations.

Description

a. While engaged in an argument with a co-worker, Mr. Warren suddenly falls asleep at his desk. _____

b. Mrs. Lewis, who has been depressed for several weeks, awakens each day at 3 AM and is unable to get back to sleep. _____

c. Todd is awakened by his mother and is surprised to find himself standing in the middle of the family room. _____

d. Mr. Hoyle reports that he has had difficulty falling asleep for the past 6 months. _____

e. Mr. Glenn has recently gained 50 pounds. His wife reports that she is awakened by his increased snoring. She has observed episodes when there is no sound of breathing but accentuated breathing movements. _____

f. Jimmy, 7 years old, begins to experience nightly bedwetting. _____

g. Mr. Smyth reports that since his wife's recent stroke, he has often noted that she stops breathing for 15- to 20-second periods during the night. _____

h. Mrs. Webster reports that she has been awakening three to four times every night for the past several weeks. _____

Disorder

1. Initial insomnia
2. Intermittent insomnia
3. Terminal insomnia
4. Central sleep apnea
5. Obstructive sleep apnea
6. Narcolepsy
7. Somnambulism
8. Nocturnal enuresis

14. Define sleep deprivation.

15. List four physiological and four psychological manifestations of sleep deprivation.

Physiological Symptoms	Psychological Symptoms
a.	a.
b.	b.
c.	c.
d.	d.

16. The most effective treatment for sleep deprivation is:

a. use of CPAP.

b. administration of hypnotic sleeping medications.

c. provision of comfort measures to induce relaxation and sleep.

d. elimination of factors disrupting the normal sleep pattern.

17. List five areas to be assessed when obtaining a sleep history.

a.

b.

c.

d.

e.

18. List three goals appropriate for a client needing rest or sleep.

a.

b.

c.

19. List six areas to consider when promoting a client's normal sleep pattern.

a.

b.

c.

d.

e.

f.

20. Which intervention would be expected to promote safe, restful sleep in an infant?

a. Keep the room softly lit.

b. Provide a soft pillow and light blanket.

c. Maintain the room temperature at 78° F.

d. Position the crib near an open window for fresh air.

21. Which intervention(s) would be expected to promote safe, restful sleep in a confused adult?

a. Position the bed's side rails up.

b. Keep the room dimly lit.

c. Provide additional covers.

d. All of the above.

22. Bedtime rituals are particularly important for:
    a. neonates and infants.
    b. toddlers and preschoolers.
    c. school-age children.
    d. adolescents.
23. List five bedtime rituals appropriate for an adult.

    a.

    b.

    c.

    d.

    e.
24. List six comfort measures the nurse may initiate to promote a client's sleep.

    a.

    b.

    c.

    d.

    e.

    f.
25. A client with initial insomnia should be encouraged to stay in bed and concentrate on falling asleep. (True or false?)
26. Roberta Kimball, RN, is working on the night shift. While making rounds at 1 AM, she finds a client who is unable to fall asleep. The most appropriate action would be to:
    a. provide the client with a hypnotic medication.
    b. tell other staff members to avoid going into the client's room.
    c. talk with the client to determine factors contributing to the sleeplessness.
    d. encourage the client to stay in bed and read or watch television until he or she feels tired.
27. Brian, 5 years old, frequently awakens during the night. He tells his mother that he is afraid to stay in his room. The best approach to this problem would be to:
    a. allow Brian to get up and watch television until he feels sleepy.
    b. provide Brian with a snack of milk and cookies.
    c. let Brian come into his parents' bed until he falls asleep.
    d. talk with Brian about his fears and comfort him in his own bed.
28. Which of the following snacks would be appropriate for a client experiencing difficulty falling asleep.
    a. Hot tea and crackers
    b. Cocoa and bread with butter
    c. Wine and cheese
    d. Gelatin with fruit
29. Regular use of sleeping medication may result in:
    a. insomnia.
    b. drug tolerance.

    c. drug withdrawal.
    d. all of the above.

CRITICAL THINKING AND EXPERIENTIAL EXERCISES

1. Sleep history
   a. Develop a sleep history assessment tool based on the components described in your text on pp. 1158-1163.
   b. Examine the nursing assessment form used in your health care setting. Identify areas of the tool providing pertinent information about client rest and sleep patterns.
   c. Elicit a sleep history from a partner using the tool you developed or The Sleep Questionnaire provided in your text on p. 1159. Based on your assessment, identify actual or potential sleeping problems and formulate possible interventions to promote rest and sleep. Share your assessment and interventions with your instructor for feedback.
2. Effect of the health care environment on rest and sleep
   a. Negotiate with your instructor to observe clients on a general nursing unit and, if possible, in an intensive care unit. (Although nighttime observation would be preferred, daytime assessment will provide useful information for the exercise.)
   b. Based on your observations, identify factors in each setting that actually or potentially interfere with rest and sleep patterns.
   c. Describe any client behaviors you observed that could be associated with sleep deprivation.
   d. Discuss specific actions to control environmental factors interfering with clients' rest and sleep.
3. Client education: normal sleep requirements
   a. Develop a teaching tool (for example, chart, table, pamphlet, booklet) that could be used to teach parents about the sleep requirements of their children from infancy through adolescence. Include each of the following areas.
      (1) Each developmental age group (that is, infants, toddlers, preschoolers, school-age children, and adolescents)
      (2) Total amounts of sleep required
      (3) Frequency and duration of naps
      (4) Common factors that disrupt sleep patterns
      (5) Actions to minimize sleep pattern disruption
   b. Submit the tool to your instructor for feedback.
   c. If possible, using your instructor as a resource, arrange to use your tool as a basis for discussion with parents or child-care providers in a community setting. (Possible locations may be day-care centers, schools, churches, or parent support groups.)
4. Factors affecting sleep in the hospitalized client
   a. Review the medical record of a selected client, including diagnosis, prescribed medications, and treatments.

b. Analyze the data obtained to determine the influence of each of the following factors on the child's rest and sleep patterns.
   (1) Medical diagnosis
   (2) Medications
   (3) Routine hospital care
   (4) Treatments and procedures
c. Share your analysis with your instructor for feedback.

5. Clinical situation: factors affecting rest and sleep
Mr. Styles is a 39-year-old engineer for the city power company. He is married and has four children (2, 4, 5, and 8 years old). His wife does not work outside of the home. Lately, he has been increasingly irritable and fatigued. He states that regardless of the amount of time he spends sleeping, he still feels tired.

Mr. Styles rotates from a straight day to an evening shift every 4 weeks. When he comes home from work, he typically drinks three or four cans of beer. Mr. Styles has been a smoker for 15 years and is approximately 40 pounds over the recommended weight for a man his size. He does not engage in any regular exercise program but does participate in summer softball and winter bowling leagues.

a. What factors may contribute to Mr. Styles' complaints of fatigue and irritability. Describe how these factors influence normal rest and sleep patterns.
b. What modifications in lifestyle could be explored with Mr. Styles to promote rest and sleep?

6. Clinical situation: nursing process with clients experiencing sleep problems
Mrs. McLean is a 58-year-old woman who is seen in the medical clinic for the first time. The nursing history reveals that Mrs. McLean has had great difficulty falling asleep since her discharge from the hospital 4 months ago. She indicates that before her hospitalization she used to sleep 7 or 8 hours every night but now she just "tosses and turns." She states, "My husband gets so angry when I can't relax. During the day, I feel so tired and irritable."

Mrs. McLean has had chronic bronchitis for several years and continues to smoke 1 to 2 packs of cigarettes per day. She tells the nurse, "I get short of breath sometimes when I lie flat." Her current medications include aminophylline (a bronchodilator) and prednisone (a corticosteroid). Several years ago Mrs. McLean took sleeping pills, but the physician will not prescribe them because of her current respiratory condition.

a. Discuss additional assessment data you would need from Mrs. McLean to address her current rest/sleep status.
b. What factors may be contributing to Mrs. McLean's difficulty sleeping?
c. What effect would sleeping pills have on Mrs. McLean's respiratory condition?
d. Based on the information provided in the situation, formulate actual and potential nursing diagnoses related to Mrs. McLean's sleeping problems.
e. Identify at least two goals for Mrs. McLean's care related to her need for sleep.
f. For each goal, formulate at least one expected outcome and three individualized nursing interventions.

ADDITIONAL READINGS

Balsmeyer B: Sleep disturbances in the infant and toddler, *Pediatr Nurs* 16(5):447, 1990.
   Discusses in detail common infant and toddler sleep disturbances, including sleeplessness and arousal disorders. Presents information to minimize the effect of these problems on the family.
Biddle C, Oaster TRF: The nature of sleep, *AANA J* 58(1):36, 1990.
   Describes sleep physiology, including dynamics of non-REM and REM sleep. Explores common sleep disorders.
Boomer H, Deakin A: Getting children to sleep, *Nurs Times* 87(12):40, 1991.
   Describes common sleep disorders of infants and children. Includes discussions of treatment and supportive nursing care.
Denner DS, Reman MK, Roth T: Help for geriatric sleep problems, *Patient Care* 23(8):74, 1989.
   Discusses sleep disorders common to geriatric clients. Presents unique therapies for this selected population.
Emra KL, Herrera CO: When your patient tells you he can't sleep, *RN* 52(9):79, 1989.
   Presents practical tips for the support of the hospitalized client who is unable to sleep.
Hart LK, Freel MI, Milde FL: Fatigue, *Nurs Clin North Am* 25(4):967, 1990.
   Discusses assessment and interventions for clients with fatigue. Includes nursing actions to support rest and sleep and alternative therapies such as relaxation strategies, activity and exercise, nutrition, and natural healing techniques.
Weaver TE, Millman RP: Broken sleep, *Am J Nurs* 86:146, 1986.
   In-depth exploration of obstructive and central sleep apnea. Describes pathophysiological mechanisms, clinical features, and treatments.

Chapter 37
Comfort

PREREQUISITE READING

Chapter 37, pp. 1174 to 1215

OBJECTIVES

Mastery of content in this chapter will enable the student to:

- Define selected terms describing pain and therapies to increase comfort.
- Discuss common misconceptions about pain.
- Identify components of the pain experience.
- Discuss the three phases of behavioral responses to pain.
- Explain the relationship of the gate-control theory to selected nursing therapies for pain relief.
- Perform an assessment of a client experiencing pain.
- Describe guidelines for individualizing pain therapies.
- Identify the techniques and rationales for selecting pain therapies.
- Explain common causes for undertreatment of pain with analgesics.
- Discuss the purpose and services of a hospice program.
- Provide nursing therapies that prevent or reduce a client's pain.

REVIEW OF KEY CONCEPTS

1. Define pain as described by the International Association for the Study of Pain (IASP).
2. Pain is:
   a. easily measured and described.
   b. rarely influenced by psychosocial and cultural factors.
   c. a protective mechanism or warning of tissue damage.
   d. associated only with acute illness or disease states.
3. A nurse's response to client pain is often based on personal perceptions and value systems. (True or false?)
4. Which statement about pain is accurate?
   a. Psychogenic pain is just as real as pain associated with physiological disturbances.
   b. Clients with a history of drug or alcohol abuse tend to overreact to pain.
   c. Clients with minor illnesses have less pain than those with severe diseases.
   d. Administering analgesics regularly will lead to a client's drug dependence.
5. List and briefly describe the three components of the pain experience.
   a.
   b.
   c.
6. Define pain threshold.
7. Compare the two types of peripheral nerve fibers responsible for conducting painful stimuli by completing the table.

Type	A Fibers	C Fibers
Fiber type		
Myelination status		
Transmission speed		
Nature of pain message		

8. Match the neuroregulator with the neurophysiological function.

Neuroregulator

   a. Substance P _____
   b. Serotonin _____
   c. Prostaglandins _____
   d. Endorphins _____
   e. Bradykinin _____

Function

1. Generated by breakdown of phospholipids in cell membranes
2. Body's natural supply of morphinelike substances activated by stress and pain
3. Required for pain impulse transmission from the periphery to higher brain centers
4. Released from plasma leaking from blood vessels at the site of tissue injury and binds to peripheral receptors increasing pain stimuli

5. Released from the brainstem and dorsal horn to inhibit pain transmission

9. Neuromodulators altering neuron activity by increasing or decreasing the effects of particular neurotransmitters include:
  a. bradykinin.
  b. substance P.
  c. serotonin.
  d. prostaglandins.

10. List the three interactional systems of pain perception described by Meinhart and McCaffery.
  a.
  b.
  c.

11. Pain that is severe or unrelenting stimulates the sympathetic nervous system. (True or false?)

12. Place the letter "S" for sympathetic or "P" for parasympathetic to describe the physiological response to pain.
  a. Increased pulse rate _____
  b. Nausea and vomiting _____
  c. Rapid, irregular breathing _____
  d. Dilated pupils _____
  e. Diaphoresis _____
  f. Decreased blood pressure _____

13. List and briefly describe the three phases of the pain experience.
  a.
  b.
  c.

14. Define pain tolerance.

15. Describe the basic concept underlying the gate-control theory of pain.

16. The use of client distraction in pain control is based on the principle that:
  a. small C fibers transmit impulses via the spinothalamic tract.
  b. the reticular formation can send inhibitory signals to gating mechanisms.
  c. large A fibers compete with pain impulses to close gates to painful stimuli.
  d. transmission of pain impulses from the spinal cord to the cerebral cortex can be inhibited.

17. List four characteristics of acute pain.
  a.
  b.
  c.
  d.

18. Pain that has periods of remissions and exacerbations would most appropriately be described as:
  a. acute.
  b. intractable.
  c. chronic.
  d. psychosomatic.

19. List four symptoms associated with chronic pain.
  a.
  b.
  c.
  d.

20. The nurse's primary goal in caring for the client with chronic pain is to:
  a. foster feelings of hope for a cure.
  b. reduce the client's perception of pain.
  c. eliminate the source of the pain.
  d. alter the client's reaction to pain.

21. List seven factors influencing pain perception.
  a.
  b.
  c.
  d.
  e.
  f.
  g.

22. When Mr. Owns bends over, the pain in his back seems to travel down his right leg. This is an example of:
  a. phantom limb pain.
  b. deep visceral pain.
  c. radiating pain.
  d. cutaneous pain.

23. Which assessment statement is most likely to yield accurate information about the quality of the client's pain?
  a. "Tell me how you would rate your pain on a scale of 1 to 10."
  b. "Would you describe your pain as pricking, burning, or aching?"
  c. "What events seemed to cause your pain?"
  d. "Tell me what your pain feels like."

24. Whatever a client uses safely and effectively to relieve pain should also be tried by the nurse. (True or false?)

25. Define concomitant symptom.

26. Identify the four major behavioral indicators of the effects of pain and cite at least two examples for each indicator.
  a.
    (1)
    (2)

b.

(1)

(2)

c.

(1)

(2)

d.

(1)

(2)

27. When the client presents with severe, acute pain, the nurse gives priority to:
   a. emotional support.
   b. analgesic administration.
   c. relaxation techniques.
   d. positioning and body alignment.
28. List three goals appropriate for the client experiencing pain.

   a.

   b.

   c.
29. Teaching a child about painful procedures is best achieved by:
   a. early warnings of the anticipated pain.
   b. story telling about the upcoming procedure.
   c. relevant play directed toward procedure activities.
   d. avoiding explanations until the pain is experienced.
30. List eight general guidelines for individualizing approaches to a client's pain relief.

   a.

   b.

   c.

   d.

   e.

   f.

   g.

   h.
31. When implementing pain relief measures, the least invasive or safest therapy should be tried first. (True or false?)
32. Match the nursing measure with the principle for promoting client comfort.

Nursing measure

   a. Teaching guided imagery _____

   b. Application of heat or cold _____
   c. Turning a client alternately from the back to
      sides _____

   d. Using distraction _____
   e. Encouraging fluids and fiber to avoid constipation _____
   f. Giving a massage _____
   g. Using progressive relaxation techniques _____

Principle

1. Preventing pain reception
2. Lessening pain perception
3. Modifying pain reaction

33. What is TENS and how is it believed to reduce pain?
34. Which type of pain is most likely to respond to the use of distraction?
   a. Intractable cancer pain
   b. Chronic pain of moderate intensity
   c. Acute, intense pain of short duration
   d. Chronic visceral pain
35. Which action is appropriate when using music to control pain?
   a. Encourage the client to concentrate on the music's rhythm.
   b. When pain is acute, reduce the volume.
   c. When the client's mood is low, select music that is upbeat.
   d. Avoid selecting music based on client age and background.
36. Under certain circumstances, it is appropriate for the nurse to obtain a physician's order for relaxation therapy. (True or false?)
37. The nurse has just taught a relaxation technique to a client with chronic tension headaches. The client subsequently develops a tension headache and finds that the technique is ineffective in reducing pain. The best action by the nurse would be to:
   a. tell the client that the technique was probably done incorrectly.
   b. teach the client a new technique because this one is ineffective.
   c. inform the client that relaxation techniques are inappropriate for tension headaches.
   d. assure the client that the technique may need to be practiced repeatedly to be effective.
38. List five areas to include when providing a client with anticipatory guidance about pain.

   a.

   b.

   c.

   d.

   e.
39. List six characteristics of an ideal analgesic.

   a.

   b.

   c.

   d.

e.

f.

40. Describe four major principles for analgesic administration.

a.

b.

c.

d.

41. Which statement about analgesic administration is correct?
   a. Narcotic injections provide longer, more sustained relief for clients with chronic pain.
   b. The same dose of a drug, when administered by a different route, will produce the same level of analgesia.
   c. The best time to administer analgesics is after the client has been active.
   d. More severe pain requires a greater amount of analgesic for relief.

42. What is PCA?

43. Describe three benefits of PCA.

a.

b.

c.

44. Nursing care for clients receiving a local anesthetic includes:
   a. warning the client that loss of motor function occurs before loss of senstion.
   b. protecting the client from injury.
   c. explaining that the initial injection will be painless.
   d. encouraging the client to use the anesthetized body part.

45. List four goals and one action for each goal related to care of clients with intraspinal infusions.

a.

b.

c.

d.

46. Define placebo.

47. The nurse may administer a placebo without the physician's order. (True or false?)

48. Which action would be inappropriate when administering a placebo.
   a. Promoting a relaxing environment before administration
   b. Explaining that the purpose of the placebo is to relieve pain
   c. Assessing the client's pain and evaluating the effect of the placebo
   d. Using the placebo as a way to determine the presence of genuine pain

49. The administration of a local anesthetic in the lumbosacral region of the spinal cord is:
   a. an epidural nerve block.
   b. an infiltration.
   c. a peripheral nerve block.
   d. a spinal nerve block.

50. The surgical procedure cutting the dorsal roots of a spinal nerve to control pain is a

_____ .

51. With current technology, intractable pain may be permanently relieved. (True or false?)

52. Treatment of severe, acute pain and cancer-related pain are the same. (True or false?)

53. Diagram and label the three-step approach to cancer pain management recommended by the World Health Organization (WHO, 1986).

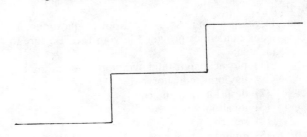

54. When providing analgesics to clients with intractable cancer pain, it is important to know that:
   a. medication addiction is high among these clients.
   b. the goal of treatment is to anticipate and minimize pain.
   c. administration of analgesics is best provided on a prn basis.
   d. the overall goal of treatment is to cure the pain.

55. List four guidelines for safe administration of morphine sulfate via ambulatory infusion pumps.

a.

b.

c.

d.

56. The best resource for evaluating the effectiveness of pain-relief measures is the:
   a. client.
   b. nurse.
   c. family member.
   d. physician.

CRITICAL THINKING AND EXPERIENTIAL EXERCISES

1. Personal pain perspectives
   a. Identify a personal experience in which you or someone you know experienced physiological pain.
   b. Describe the etiology of the pain and the individual's response to the painful stimuli.

c. Discuss how other people (family, friends, and health care providers) responded to the individual experiencing pain.

d. Analyze how this experience has influenced your personal perspectives about pain and the pain experience.

e. Explore how your personal perspective may influence the care you provide to clients experiencing pain.

f. Share your analysis with your instructor for feedback.

2. Pain reception, perception, and reaction
   a. Using the example of stepping on a nail, trace the transmission of the pain impulse from reception through perception and reaction. (Be sure to identify the specific neurological components involved.)

3. Pain
   a. Develop a pain assessment tool or questionnaire using guidelines provided in your text. Be sure to include:
      (1) physical signs and symptoms, including behavioral indicators.
      (2) descriptive pain scales.
      (3) location.
      (4) severity.
      (5) quality.
      (6) time and duration.
      (7) precipitating and aggravating factors.
      (8) relieving factors.
      (9) concomitant symptoms.
      (10) past experiences.
      (11) effects on activities of daily living.
      (12) available coping resources.
   b. Identify the essential data (from the information listed previously) that you would attempt to elicit if a client has acute, severe pain in an emergency room (before pain relief or reduction).
   c. Use the tool or questionnaire to assess a peer's or assigned client's pain.
   d. Based on the assessed data, formulate nursing diagnoses pertinent to the peer's or client's pain.

4. Analgesics
   a. Care for a client requiring analgesics for pain control (or review the medical records of a client experiencing pain who is receiving analgesics).
   b. Review the medical and nursing diagnoses to determine the source of the pain and variables influencing the client's reception, perception, and response.
   c. Review the medication record or Kardex to identify ordered analgesics. Prepare medication cards or papers that indicate the:
      (1) medication classification.
      (2) indications for use.
      (3) usual dose and frequency of administration.
      (4) actions.
      (5) side and toxic effects.
      (6) the antidote.
      (7) nursing implications.

5. Client teaching: anticipatory guidance for pain management
   Develop a teaching plan for each client requiring a venipuncture to obtain a blood specimen. Include the components of anticipatory guidance described in your text to design a developmentally appropriate plan for a:
   a. 3-year-old toddler.
   b. 9-year-old school child.
   c. 22-year-old college student.
   d. 82-year-old man with impaired hearing.

6. Clinical situation: pain assessment
   Mr. Williams is a carpenter experiencing acute neck pain for 2 weeks. He describes it as "a sharp knife cutting into the muscle behind my head."
   a. State the questions you would ask Mr. WIlliams to more thoroughly asess his pain. (If possible, consider role playing this situation with a peer and audiotaping it for review and self-evaluation.)

7. Clinical situation: nursing process for pain management
   Maria Lombardo, a 32-year-old woman of Italian descent, is recovering from a cholecystectomy. She has a large dressing on an upper abdominal incision.

   Her physician has ordered the choice of a narcotic analgesic meperidine (Demerol) to be given intramuscularly every 3 to 4 hours for severe pain or acetaminophen with codeine (Tylenol 3) to be given every 3 to 4 hours for mild to moderate pain. Mrs. Lombardo is to be assisted with ambulation and requires deep breathing and coughing exercises every 2 hours.

   Mrs. Lombardo is anxious "to get better," but she is also very tense and rigid when she gets up to walk. She is also reluctant to do her exercises because "it hurts too much." Her pain is described as "sharp and burning," and she also complains of a backache.
   a. What assessment criteria will you use to determine whether Mrs. Lombardo receives meperidine or acetaminophen with codiene?
   b. Develop a list of actual and potential nursing diagnoses for Mrs. Lombardo related to her current pain problem.
   c. Identify the priority nursing diagnosis associated with her pain problem and formulate two short-term goals for care.
   d. For each goal statement, describe at least three individualized nursing interventions and the rationale for their selection.
   e. For each goal formulated, describe at least one outcome criterion to be used in evaluating the success of the plan of care.

SKILL AND TECHNIQUE ACTIVITIES

1. Massage techniques
   a. Practice the procedure for massage of a body part with a partner. Ask your partner to critique your performance and report subjective feelings during and after the massage.
   b. Elicit an instructor's evaluation of your massage technique.

2. Pain-control techniques

    a. Observe client care in a clinic or a nursing unit where clients experiencing chronic or intractable pain receive care.

    b. Identify pain-control modalities being used for the client (for example, TENS, continuous morphine infusions, guided imagery, and relaxation techniques).

    c. Identify the role of the nurse in applying or monitoring pain-control equipment or modalities.

    d. Talk to the client about the pain experience, its effect on lifestyle, and the effectiveness of pain-relief measures.

    e. Discuss your observations with your instructor.

ADDITONAL READINGS

Baily LM: Music's soothing charms, *Am J Nurs* 85:1280, 1985.
Briefly discusses music's effect on anxiety and fear associated with pain. Overviews responsibilities associated with the use of music as a pain-control measure. Selects references that cite experimental studies in which music was an effective technique for pain control.

DiMotto JW: Relaxation, *Am J Nurs* 84:754, 1984.
Summarizes characteristics of relaxation methods and their effects on physical, cognitive, and behavioral functioning. Describes six specific relaxation methods. Useful for client care and the nurse's personal health-promotion activities.

Heath AH: Imagery: helping ICU patients control pain and anxiety, *DCCN* 11(1):57, 1992.
Presents relaxation and imagery strategies to help clients cope with symptoms, treatments and the critical care environment.

Harrison A: Assessing patients' pain: identifying reasons for error, *J Adv Nurs* 16:1018, 1991.
Emphasizes the importance of careful pain assessment in effective pain management. Provides guidance for nursing assessment of pain.

Holm K et al: Effect of personal pain experience on pain assessment, *Image J Nurs Sch* 21(2):72, 1989.
Discusses the effect of a nurse's personal pain experiences on client assessment and subsequent pain-control interventions. Emphasizes the significance of personal attitude and values in client care.

McCaffrey M: Would you administer placebos for pain? These facts can help you decide, *Nurs 82* 12(2):80, 1982.
Describes common myths and misconceptions about administration of placebos. Presents circumstances in which placebos could be used and describes when and how they should be administered. Explores the legal and ethical issues surrounding placebo administration.

Moore DE, Blacker HM: How effective is TENS for chronic pain? *Am J Nurs* 83:1175, 1983.
Discusses history and theoretical concepts underlying the use of TENS. Discusses a study involving the use of TENS by clients with chronic pain.

Ryder E: All about patient-controlled analgesia, *J Intravenous Nurs* 14(6):372, 1991.
Describes the technology associated with patient-controlled analgesia (PCA), indications for administration, and monitoring parameters in the hospital and home.

Walding MF: Pain, anxiety, and powerlessness, *J Adv Nurs* 16(4):388, 1991.
Explores physiological mechanisms of postoperative pain and factors influencing client perception of pain. Correlates the interaction of pain, anxiety, and powerlessness with adequate pain control. Emphasizes the need for detailed assessment and intervention in all three areas to promote client comfort.

Chapter Chapter 38
Oxygenation

PREREQUISITE READING
Chapter 38, pp. 1216 to 1273

OBJECTIVES

Mastery of content in this chapter will enable the student to:
- Define selected terms associated with respiratory function and oxygenation.
- Describe the gross structure and function of the cardiopulmonary system.
- Identify physiological processes in maintaining cardiac output, myocardial blood flow, and coronary artery circulation.
- Describe the electrical conduction system of the heart.
- Describe how cardiac output can be altered by preload, afterload, contractility, and heart rate.
- Identify physiological processes involved in ventilation, perfusion, and exchange of respiratory gases.
- Describe neural and chemical regulation of respiration.
- Explain the ways a client's level of health, age, lifestyle, and environment can affect tissue oxygenation.
- Identify causes and effects of disturbances in conduction, altered cardiac output, impaired valvular function, myocardial ischemia, and impaired tissue perfusion.
- Identify causes and effects of hyperventilation, hypoventilation, and hypoxemia.
- Perform a nursing assessment of the cardiopulmonary system.
- Develop nursing diagnoses for altered oxygenation.
- Describe nursing interventions to increase activity tolerance, maintain or promote lung expansion, promote mobilization of pulmonary secretions, maintain a patent airway, promote oxygenation, and restore cardiopulmonary function.
- Develop evaluation criteria for the nursing care plan for the client with altered oxygenation.

REVIEW OF KEY CONCEPTS

1. Describe the Frank-Starling law of the heart.
2. Which statement about myocardial blood flow is accurate?
   a. During ventricular diastole, the atrioventricular valves close.
   b. Blood flows from the higher pressure atria into the relaxed ventricles during systole.
   c. The systolic phase begins after ventricular filling.
   d. The semilunar valves prevent backflow of blood into the atria.
3. The myocardium derives oxygen and nutrient requirements from blood flow through the atria and ventricles. (True or false?)
4. Match the term with the most accurate description.

Term
   a. Cardiac output _____
   b. Stroke volume _____
   c. Preload _____
   d. Afterload _____
   e. Myocardial contractility _____

Description
   1. Force of cardiac contraction
   2. Amount of blood ejected from the left ventricle with each contraction
   3. Resistance to left ventricular ejection
   4. Stroke volume multiplied by heart rate
   5. End diastolic volume
5. Diagram and label the electrical conduction system of the heart.
6. Draw and label the components of the ECG waveform for normal sinus rhythm (NSR).
7. Define ventilation.
8. The major inspiratory muscle is innervated by the _____ .
9. Spinal cord disruption impairing diaphragmatic function would be characterized by damage at which spinal cord level?
   a. First thoracic level
   b. Fourth cervical level
   c. Second thoracolumbar level
   d. Seventh cervical level
10. Match the following activities involved in the work of breathing with the most accurate description.

Description
   a. Pressure difference between the mouth and alveoli _____

b. Use of muscle groups to contract the lungs
_____

c. Ability of the lungs and thorax to expand
_____

d. Sternocleidomastoid group _____

Activities

1. Compliance
2. Airway resistance
3. Active expiration
4. Accessory muscles

11. An instrument used to measure the volume of air entering or leaving the lungs is a _____.

12. Define perfusion.

13. The exchange of gases in pulmonary circulation occurs in the:
   a. pulmonary artery.
   b. pulmonary vein.
   c. pulmonary capillary bed
   d. pulmonary venules.

14. Define diffusion.

15. List four factors required for oxygen transport and delivery.

   a.

   b.

   c.

   d.

16. List and briefly describe two regulatory mechanisms of respiration.

   a.

   b.

17. Match the physical condition or disease with the mechanism affecting oxygenation.

Condition or disease

   a. Fever _____

   b. Heart failure _____

   c. Anemia _____

   d. Stroke _____

   e. Rib fracture _____

   f. Hypovolemia _____

   g. Pregnancy _____

   h. Muscular dystrophy _____

   i. Cigarette smoking _____

Mechanism

   1. Decreased oxygen-carrying capacity of the blood
   2. Decreased cardiac output
   3. Hypovolemia

4. Increased metabolic rate
5. Conditions affecting chest wall movement
6. Altered central nervous system function

18. List the three basic mechanisms contributing to anemia.

   a.

   b.

   c.

19. Anemia is characterized by:
   a. pallor and fatigue.
   b. decreased exercise tolerance.
   c. increased heart and respiratory rate.
   d. all of the above.

20. List at least one physiological factor influencing tissue oxygenation for each developmental level listed.
   a. Premature infant
   b. Infant and toddler
   c. School-age child and adolescent
   d. Young adult
   e. Older adult

21. List and briefly describe the five behavioral (lifestyle) factors influencing respiratory function.

   a.

   b.

   c.

   d.

   e.

22. An abnormal cardiac rhythm resulting from a disturbance in conduction is a _____.

23. Match the term with the correct definition.

Term

   a. Bradycardia _____

   b. Tachycardia _____

   c. Supraventricular dysrhythmia _____

   d. Junctional dysrhythmia _____

   e. Ventricular dysrhythmia _____

Definition

   1. Abnormal rhythm originating above the ventricles
   2. Abnormal rhythm originating in the ventricles
   3. Abnormal rhythm originating above or below the AV node
   4. Heart rate of greater than 100 beats/min
   5. Heart rate of less than 60 beats/min

24. Tachycardias can reduce cardiac output by:
   a. decreasing diastolic filling time.
   b. decreasing systolic filling time.
   c. decreasing the heart rate.
   d. increasing stroke volume.

25. Left-sided cardiac failure is characterized by:
    a. weight gain.
    b. peripheral edema.
    c. dyspnea.
    d. all of the above.
26. A decrease in coronary blood flow or an increase in myocardial oxygen demand without adequate coronary perfusion is known as:
    a. angina pectoris.
    b. myocardial infarction.
    c. ventricular hypertrophy.
    d. aortic stenosis.
27. Briefly compare the pain experienced with angina pectoris and the pain of myocardial infarction in relation to pain onset, precipitating factors, relieving factors, characteristics, and duration.
28. Define hyperventilation.
29. Hyperventilation refers to an increased respiratory rate. (True or false?)
30. List six signs and symptoms of alveolar hyperventilation.

    a.

    b.

    c.

    d.

    e.

    f.
31. Hypoventilation is best described as a state in which:
    a. the respiratory rate decreases.
    b. thoracic excursion decreases.
    c. carbon dioxide increases.
    d. inspired oxygen decreases.
32. List two causes of hypoventilation.

    a.

    b.
33. Briefly discuss why clients with chronic obstructive pulmonary disease (COPD) should not receive high concentrations of oxygen.
34. List five signs and symptoms of alveolar hypoventilation.

    a.

    b.

    c.

    d.

    e.
35. Define hypoxia.
36. List four major physiological conditions that can cause hypoxia.

    a.

    b.

    c.

    d.
37. List seven signs and symptoms of hypoxia.

    a.

    b.

    c.

    d.

    e.

    f.

    g.
38. Which statement about cyanosis is accurate?
    a. Cyanosis is an early sign of hypoxia.
    b. Cyanosis from hypoxemia is best observed in the fingernail beds.
    c. An absence of cyanosis indicates adequate oxygenation.
    d. Cyanosis is a result of desaturation of hemoglobin.
39. Define dyspnea.
40. List eight areas to include in a nursing history for oxygenation.

    a.

    b.

    c.

    d.

    e.

    f.

    g.

    h.
41. List the five major characteristics to be included in a description of sputum.

    a.

    b.

    c.

    d.

    e.
42. A term for blood-tinged sputum is:
    a. hematemesis.
    b. hematuria.
    c. hemothorax.
    d. hemoptysis.
43. An abnormal condition in which the person must stand, sit, or use multiple pillows to breathe when lying down is _____.
44. Define wheezing.
45. Identify the possible cause for each of the following cardiopulmonary assessment findings.
    a. Peripheral cyanosis

b. Dependent edema
c. Neck vein distention
d. Intercostal retractions
e. Pale conjunctivae
f. Corneal arcus
g. Cyanotic mucous membranes
h. Nail-bed clubbing
i. Xanthelasma

46. Match the following breathing pattern with the most accurate description provided.

Description

a. Abnormally slow respiratory rate _____
b. Alternating periods of apnea and deep, rapid breathing _____
c. Abnormally rapid, shallow breathing _____
d. Absence of coordinated rate or depth of respirations _____
e. Abnormally deep, rapid, sighing type of respiration _____
f. Normal respiratory rate _____

Pattern

1. Eupnea
2. Tachypnea
3. Bradypnea
4. Kussmaul
5. Ataxic
6. Cheyne-Stokes

47. Describe what is meant by paradoxical breathing.
48. The sound produced by percussion over normal adult lung tissue during inspiration would be:
a. resonance.
b. hyperresonance.
c. dullness.
d. tympany.

49. Which of the following cardiovascular assessment findings would be considered normal?
a. Presence of S_1 and S_2
b. Presence of S_3 and S_4
c. Carotid bruits
d. Murmurs and rubs

50. The continuous measurement of capillary oxygen saturation through a cutaneous sensor is _____.

51. What information about oxygenation is obtained through arterial blood gas studies?
52. In relation to safety, what is the most important information to present to a client before thoracentesis?
53. List four possible classifications of nursing diagnoses for a client with altered oxygenation.

a.

b.

c.

d.

54. List five goals appropriate for clients with actual or potential oxygenation needs.

a.

b.

c.

d.

e.

55. Describe selected nursing interventions used to promote and maintain adequate oxygenation by completing the following table. Include the purpose of the intervention.

Nursing intervention	Purpose
Positioning the client	
Pursed-lip breathing	
Diaphragmatic breathing	
Using flow-oriented incentive spirometer	
Maintaining hydration	
Inserting an oral airway	

56. An acceptable postoperative inspiratory capacity for a client must equal:
a. the preoperative inspiratory volume.
b. one-half to three-fourths the preoperative volume.
c. one-fourth to one-half the preoperative volume.
d. one-eighth to one-fourth the preoperative volume.

57. A collection of air or other gas in the pleural space is a _____.

58. The absence of fluctuation of the water level in the water-seal chamber of a chest tube may indicate that:
a. the client is lying on the tubing.
b. the tubing has been occluded by a clot.
c. the lung is reexpanded.
d. all of the above.

59. A client had a chest tube inserted for a pneumothorax 3 days ago. On entering the room, the nurse finds that there is continuous bubbling in the water-seal chamber. Which action should be taken immediately?
a. No action is required because this is an expected finding.
b. Check for any air leaks in the system.
c. Call for a chest x-ray film.
d. Clamp the tube until the physician can evaluate it.

60. Humidification is necessary for clients receiving oxygen therapy. (True or false?)
61. List and briefly describe the three activities involved in chest physiotherapy (CPT).

a.

b.

c.

62. Chest percussion would be contraindicated in all of the following except:
   a. a client with a bleeding disorder.
   b. a client with osteoporosis.
   c. a client with a rib fracture.
   d. infants and children.

63. Vibration is contraindicated in chest physiotherapy for which age group?
   a. Infants and toddlers
   b. School-age children
   c. Adolescents
   d. Older adults

64. Vibration is performed during:
   a. inhalation.
   b. exhalation.
   c. either inhalation or exhalation.

65. Liquification of pulmonary secretions can be achieved by all of the following except:
   a. increased fluid intake.
   b. inhaling humidified air.
   c. chest physiotherapy.
   d. nebulization.

66. In most situations, the client should be positioned so that the lung segment requiring postural drainage is:
   a. dependent.
   b. elevated.

67. List the three interventions used to maintain a patent airway.

   a.

   b.

   c.

68. Describe the characteristics of coughing techniques by completing the table below.

Cough	Technique	Action/benefits
Controlled cough		
Cascade cough		
Huff cough		
Quad cough		

69. List two criteria to use in evaluating the effectiveness of coughing.

   a.

   b.

70. Which principle governing suctioning techniques is correct?
   a. Nasopharyngeal suctioning is indicated for clients unable to cough effectively.
   b. Suction should be applied intermittently during catheter insertion.
   c. Tracheal suctioning should always precede oropharyngeal suctioning.

   d. The suctioning procedure should take 20 to 30 seconds.

71. The nurse auscultates rhonchi over an area of the left lung. To optimally suction from the left bronchus, the nurse positions the client's head:
   a. to the left.
   b. to the right.
   c. in a neutral position.
   d. forward, with chin touching the chest.

72. Describe the "five rights" of medication administration as they pertain to oxygen administration.

   a.

   b.

   c.

   d.

   e.

73. List three safety measures to be instituted when a client requires oxygen administration.

   a.

   b.

   c.

74. List the three signs of cardiac arrest.

   a.

   b.

   c.

75. List the three goals of cardiopulmonary resuscitation (CPR).

   a.

   b.

   c.

CRITICAL THINKING AND EXPERIENTIAL EXERCISES

1. Assessment of cardiopulmonary function and oxygenation
   a. Structure an assessment tool to be used specifically for clients with altered cardiopulmonary function or oxygenation (or identify the elements in the comprehensive assessment tool used by your institution that address cardiopulmonary function).
   b. Using an appropriate tool (self-developed or modified), assess a client or partner for evidence of cardiopulmonary dysfunction or diminished oxygenation levels.
   c. Request that an instructor or other experienced staff nurse confirm your cardiopulmonary assessment findings.
   d. Based on the data obtained, identify physiological, developmental stage, lifestyle, and environmental factors that are influencing the client's respiratory state (positively or negatively).

e. Based on the data obtained, identify actual or potential diagnoses that relate to the individual's respiratory status.
2. Diagnostic tests
   a. Review a client's medical record for the presence of any laboratory or diagnostic tests associated with oxygenation and cardiopulmonary function.
   b. Determine whether the findings are normal or abnormal. Identify factors that may be contributing to any abnormal findings (for example, disease process, physiological factors, developmental stage, lifestyle, or environment). Describe how these findings may influence delivery of nursing care.
   c. Describe nursing responsibilities associated with at least two of the diagnostic tests.
3. Clinical situation: cardiopulmonary reconditioning — client education
   Mrs. Theiss is a 34-year-old homemaker who has been experiencing increased fatigue and shortness of breath with exertion. She states that she is tired all the time and seems anxious during her clinic visit. She reports no formal health maintenance behaviors. She has three children under 5 years of age. Her husband has recently been working two jobs to "make ends meet."
   The physician informs Mrs. Theiss, after examination and diagnostic testing, that there are no major physical problems contributing to her condition. The physician recommends cardiopulmonary reconditioning to assist in improving her activity tolerance.
   a. Structure a client teaching program for Mrs. Theiss that may assist in improving her activity tolerance. Be sure to include the major activities included in cardiopulmonary reconditioning that may be adapted to her home environment and financial situation.
4. Clinical situation: interpretation of physical findings
   a. Explain why cyanosis in an anemic client would reflect a more critical oxygenation problem than cyanosis in a client with polycythemia.
5. Water-seal systems
   Draw a picture of each of the water-seal systems listed below. Be sure to include the water-seal straws and water level. Label the tubes to client, to suction, or to air.
   a. One-bottle system
   b. Two-bottle system
   c. Suction—three bottle system
6. Chest physiotherapy
   Prepare a chart that illustrates the positions for postural drainage in the adult or pediatric client. Include in the chart the lung segment being treated with the appropriate client position.
7. Clinical situation: nursing process in clients with altered oxygenation
   Mr. Mathews is a 56-year-old bank manager admitted to the hospital. He states that he is having trouble "catching his breath" when he walks short distances.

Occasionally he coughs and expectorates small amounts of tenacious greenish sputum. He smokes one and one-half packs of cigarettes per day.
His thorax has bilateral chest wall movement. Vital signs are as follows: pulse, 112 beats/min, regular, bounding; blood pressure, 168/102 mm Hg; temperature 37.2° C (99° F); and respirations 28, labored, shallow, and wheezy. His skin is warm and moist to the touch. He is 5 feet 10 inches tall (170 cm) and he weighs 190 pounds (86 kg).
During the admission interview, Mr. Mathews readily attempts to answer all questions, but he has difficulty breathing when he speaks. He is unable to lie in a supine position. He indicates he has less difficulty breathing if he is sitting upright.
   a. Based on the data presented, state three nursing diagnoses related to Mr. Mathews' current respiratory state. Identify the data supporting each diagnosis.
   b. Write two goal statements for each nursing diagnosis. Identify expected outcomes that could be used to measure goal achievement.
   c. Describe nursing actions and rationale for two interventions addressing each goal.

SKILLS AND TECHNIQUE ACTIVITIES
1. Cardiopulmonary assessment
   a. Practice cardiopulmonary assessment with a partner. Validate your findings with your instructor or nursing laboratory supervisor.
   b. Record your assessment findings using correct medical terminology, and submit them to your instructor for evaluation.
   c. In any client care setting, identify individuals with normal and abnormal cardiopulmonary conditions and, with their permission, perform cardiopulmonary assessment. Confirm your findings with your instructor or other experienced staff members. Record your findings on a separate piece of paper and compare them with assessment findings reported in the client's medical record.
2. Breathing and coughing exercises
   a. Independently, or with a partner, practice the techniques of deep breathing, pursed-lip breathing, and abdominal-diaphragmatic breathing.
   b. Independently, or with a partner, practice the coughing techniques for controlled cough, cascade cough, and huff cough.
3. Incentive spirometry and blow bottles
   a. Examine the types of incentive spirometers and blow bottles used in your institution.
   b. Practice setting up incentive spirometers and blow bottles with the assistance of your instructor or laboratory supervisor.
   c. Practice using the incentive spirometers and blow bottles.
4. Care of chest tubes
   a. Examine your institution's policies for care of clients with chest tubes.

   b. In a clinical laboratory or hospital setting, examine equipment and supplies required by clients with chest tubes. Compare the parts of the water-seal bottle system to the Pleuravac system.

   c. With the assistance of an instructor or laboratory supervisor, practice setting up a water-seal drainage system.

   d. In the clinical setting, observe chest tube drainage systems being used by clients. Observe other staff as they monitor and provide care unique to the client with chest tubes.

5. Chest physiotherapy

   a. Observe a respiratory therapist, physical therapist, or experienced nurse administering chest physiotherapy.

   b. In the laboratory setting, practice the techniques of chest physiotherapy (percussion, vibration, and postural drainage) with a partner. For the practice situation, position your partner to promote drainage from each of the following lung segments:

     (1) Left upper lobe

     (2) Right middle lobe

     (3) Posterior lower lobes

6. Artificial airways and suctioning technique

   a. Examine your institution's policies for airway management and suctioning techniques.

   b. Examine a variety of artificial airways (for example, endotracheal tubes, nasotracheal tubes, tracheal tubes, oral airways, and nasal airways) provided by your instructor or available in your clinical setting.

   c. Formulate a list of all of the equipment and supplies required for client airway suctioning.

   d. In the laboratory setting, practice the following techniques on a simulation mannequin:

     (1) Placement of an oral airway

     (2) Placement of a nasal airway

     (3) Oropharyngeal and nasopharyngeal suctioning

     (4) Nasotracheal suctioning

     (5) Tracheal tube suctioning

7. Oxygen administration

   a. Examine your institution's policies for oxygen administration.

   b. Request a respiratory therapist, experienced respiratory care nurse, or your instructor to show you various oxygen delivery equipment and methods for setting up and changing systems.

   c. Practice setting up or changing the oxygen administration system in the laboratory setting.

   d. Observe other nursing staff as they care for clients receiving oxygen therapy. Identify actions taken that reflect the "five rights" and safety considerations associated with oxygen administration. Discuss your observations with your instructor.

8. CPR

Reading about CPR technique or limited independent practice in a laboratory setting is not adequate preparation for this life-saving skill. It is of utmost im-portance that you enroll in a CPR course that provides repetition and reinforcement of the necessary psychomotor skills. This course may be offered through your nursing program, National Safety Council, American Red Cross, or American Heart Association. You should be recertified in these skills on an annual basis.

ADDITIONAL READINGS

Andreoli KG, Zipes DP, Wallace AG, Kinney MR, Fowkes VK: *Comprehensive cardiac care,* ed 6, St Louis, 1987, Mosby–Year Book.

   Well-referenced resource in care of clients with cardiac disease. Clearly presents an overview of anatomy and physiology, diagnosis, and treatment of cardiac diseases. Includes nursing care for a variety of cardiac conditions.

Dennison R: Cardiopulmonary assessment: how to do it better in 15 easy steps, *Nurs 86* 16(4):34, 1986.

   Presents clear, concise approach for cardiopulmonary assessment. Useful for clinical practice.

Dettenmeier PA: *Pulmonary nursing care,* St Louis, 1990, Mosby–Year Book.

   Comprehensively presents basic concepts of anatomy, physiology, diagnosis, and treatment of clients with pulmonary disease. Details nursing interventions for a variety of respiratory disease states.

Duncan CR, Erickson RS, Weigel RM: Effect of chest tube management on drainage after cardiac surgery, *Heart Lung* 16(1):1, 1987.

   Compares three methods of chest tube management on mediastinal drainage volume in postoperative cardiac surgery clients. Compares the efficacy of suction, intermittent stripping, single, and sump catheters.

Farley J: About chest tubes, *Nurs 88* 18(6):16, 1988.

   Describes chest tube management and related client care. Includes illustrations to clarify major points.

Gift AD: Dyspnea, *Nurs Clin North Am* 25(4):955, 1990.

   Details the nature and clinical manifestations of dyspnea. Examines physiological and psychological factors affecting dyspnea experienced by clients.

Gift AG, Bolbiano CS, Cunningham J: Sensations during chest tube removal, *Heart Lung* 20(2):131, 1991.

   Describes client sensory experiences during chest tube removal, which can be incorporated into client teaching to minimize anxiety and discomfort during chest tube removal.

Hoffman L, Wesmiller S: Home Oxygen: transtracheal and other options, *Am J Nurs* 88(4):464, 1988.

   Describes alternative home oxygen delivery systems. Places emphasis on the transtracheal approach. Provides guidelines for nursing care of the client using transtracheal oxygen. Compares efficacy, advantages, and disadvantages of frequently used home systems.

Sonnesso G: Are you ready to use pulse oximetry? *Nurs 91* 21(8):60, 1991.

   Presents techniques for effective use of pulse oximetry through concise explanation and helpful illustrations.

Weaver TE: New life for lungs . . . through incentive spirometers, *Nurs 81* 11(2):53, 1981.

   Discusses types of incentive spirometers and mechanisms of function. Provides guide to the 10 common brands and their characteristics. Can guide selection of the most appropriate spirometer for the client and assist in client education about spirometer use.

Chapter 39
Fluid, Electrolyte, and Acid-Base Balances

PREREQUISITE READING
Chapter 39, pp. 1274 to 1331

OBJECTIVES
Mastery of content in this chapter will enable the student to:
- Define selected terms associated with fluid, electrolyte, and acid-base balances.
- Describe the regulation and imbalances of sodium, potassium, calcium, magnesium, chloride, bicarbonate, phosphate, and acid-base.
- Describe the isotonic fluid imbalances of fluid volume excess and fluid volume deficit.
- Describe the alterations in serum osmolality caused by water excess and deficit.
- Describe third-space syndrome.
- Discuss the variables affecting fluid, electrolyte, and acid-base balances.
- Compile a nursing history and complete a physical examination for fluid, electrolyte, and acid-base balances.
- Describe laboratory studies associated with fluid, electrolyte, and acid-base imbalances.
- Develop a nursing care plan for clients with fluid, electrolyte, and acid-base disturbance.
- Discuss the purpose of intravenous (IV) therapy.
- Distinguish between peripheral and central venous lines.
- Describe the procedures for initiating and maintaining an intravenous line and calculating intravenous flow rate.
- Demonstrate how to change intravenous solutions, tubing, and dressings and how to discontinue an infusion.
- Discuss the complications of IV therapy.
- Discuss the procedure for administering a blood transfusion and nursing actions for a transfusion reaction.

REVIEW OF KEY CONCEPTS
1. The portion of body fluids comprising the interstitial fluid and blood plasma are:
   a. intracellular.
   b. extracellular.
   c. hypotonic.
   d. hypertonic.

2. Define electrolyte.
3. List and briefly describe the four factors responsible for movement of body fluids.

   a.

   b.

   c.

   d.
4. The movement of body fluids and electrolytes that requires metabolic function and energy expenditure is:
   a. diffusion.
   b. osmosis.
   c. active transport.
   d. fluid pressure.
5. The pressure exerted by blood as it enters the capillaries is:
   a. hydrostatic pressure.
   b. osmotic pressure.
   c. diffusion gradient.
   d. active transport.
6. Answer the following:
   a. A solution with the same osmotic pressure or osmolality as blood plasma is _____ .
   b. A solution with a lower osmotic pressure or osmolality than blood plasma is _____ .
   c. A solution with a higher osmotic pressure or osmolality than blood plasma is _____ .
7. Briefly describe the physiological stimuli triggering the thirst mechanisms.
8. List the four organs contributing to body fluid loss.

   a.

   b.

   c.

   d.
9. Approximately what hourly urine output would be expected from a client weighing 55 kg?

10. Define insensible water loss.

11. For each hormone, identify the stimuli for its release and its influence on fluid and electrolyte balance.

Hormone	Stimuli	Action
ADH		
Aldosterone		
Glucocorticoids		

12. The primary intracellular cation is:
   a. calcium.
   b. magnesium.
   c. potassium.
   d. sodium.

13. Give normal values, function, and regulatory mechanisms for the following major body electrolytes:
   a. Sodium
   b. Potassium
   c. Calcium
   d. Magnesium
   e. Chloride
   f. Bicarbonate
   g. Phosphate

14. An increased acid component of the blood would be reflected by:
   a. an increased pH and a rising hydrogen ion concentration.
   b. a decreased pH and a falling hydrogen ion concentration.
   c. an increased pH and a falling hydrogen ion concentration.
   d. a decreased pH and a rising hydrogen ion concentration.

15. What is the normal value for an arterial blood pH?

16. Identify and describe the acid-base regulatory mechanisms for each of the following buffering systems.
   a. Chemical regulation
   b. Biological regulation
   c. Physiological regulation

17. Body pH is most rapidly regulated by:
   a. the lungs.
   b. the kidneys.
   c. biological buffering.
   d. carbonic acid–bicarbonate buffering.

18. List three ways in which the kidneys can regulate hydrogen ion concentration.

   a.

   b.

   c.

19. Define and briefly describe the two major classifications of fluid imbalance.

   a.

   b.

20. Match the following fluid imbalances with the most accurate description or definition.

Description

   a. Occurs with excess intake of water or excess ADH; results in dilution of extracellular fluid volume with shift of water into cells _____
   b. Loss of extracellular fluid into a body space, where it becomes trapped; results in fluid volume deficit _____
   c. Loss of water without a proportionate loss of electrolytes, or a gain in osmotically active substances; results in intracellular dehydration _____
   d. Occurs when water and sodium are retained in isotonic proportions; results in hypervolemia _____
   e. Occurs when water and electrolytes are lost in isotonic proportions; results in hypovolemia _____

Imbalance
   1. Third space syndrome
   2. Fluid volume excess
   3. Fluid volume deficit
   4. Hyperosmolar imbalance
   5. Hypoosmolar imbalance

21. List six signs of isotonic fluid volume deficit.

   a.

   b.

   c.

   d.

   e.

   f.

22. List five signs of isotonic fluid volume excess.

   a.

   b.

   c.

   d.

   e.

23. For each electrolyte disturbance, identify the diagnostic laboratory finding and list at least four characteristic signs and symptoms.

Imbalance	Lab Finding	Signs and Symptoms
Hyponatremia		
Hypernatremia		
Hypokalemia		
Hyperkalemia		
Hypocalcemia		
Hypercalcemia		
Hypmagnesemia		
Hypermagnesemia		

24. Mr. Lusk, 65 years old, complains of stomach pains and ingests sodium bicarbonate eight times a day. For which acid-base imbalance is Mr. Lusk at risk?
  a. Respiratory acidosis
  b. Respiratory alkalosis
  c. Metabolic acidosis
  d. Metabolic alkalosis

25. Mary Ellen Wharton, 17 years old, is admitted to the hospital. Her respirations are very deep and rapid (32 breaths/min). She is disoriented. Her pH is 7.34, and her PCO_2 is 38 mm Hg. These findings probably indicate:
  a. Respiratory acidosis
  b. Respiratory alkalosis
  c. Metabolic acidosis
  d. Metabolic alkalosis

26. Mr. Donaldson enters the emergency room complaining of light-headedness and numbness and tingling of his extremities. Vital signs are blood pressure, 126/82 mm Hg; temperature 37° C (98.6° F); pulse, 100 beats/min; and respirations, 36 breaths/min. He states that he is "nervous and jumpy." He appears very uncomfortable and anxious. Based on the assessment data presented, which acid-base disturbance would Mr. Donaldson most likely be experiencing?
  a. Respiratory acidosis
  b. Respiratory alkalosis
  c. Metabolic acidosis
  d. Metabolic alkalosis

27. List the five major factors that can affect fluid and electrolyte status.
  a.
  b.
  c.
  d.
  e.

28. Briefly describe the influence of each lifestyle habit on fluid and electrolyte balance.
  a. Diet
  b. Stress
  c. Exercise

29. Briefly discuss the fluid and electrolyte imbalances commonly experienced by clients with each of the following conditions.
  a. Surgical trauma
  b. Burns
  c. Cardiovascular disorders
  d. Renal disorders
  e. Cancer

30. List six major categories of risk factors for fluid, electrolyte, and acid-base imbalances.
  a.
  b.
  c.

  d.
  e.
  f.

31. Indicate the possible fluid, electrolyte, or acid-base imbalance associated with each assessment finding.
  a. Weight loss of 6% to 9% _____
  b. Irritability _____
  c. Lethargy _____
  d. Bulging fontanels (infant) _____
  e. Periorbital edema _____
  f. Sticky, dry mucous membranes _____
  g. Chvostek's signs _____
  h. Distended neck veins _____
  i. Dysrhythmias _____
  j. Weak pulse _____
  k. Low blood pressure _____
  l. Third heart sound _____
  m. Increased respiratory rate _____
  n. Crackles _____
  o. Anorexia _____
  p. Abdominal cramps _____
  q. Poor skin turgor _____
  r. Oliguria or anuria _____
  s. Increased specific gravity _____
  t. Muscle cramps, tetany _____
  u. Hypertonicity of muscles on palpation

  _____
  v. Decreased or absent deep tendon reflexes

  _____
  w. Increased temperature _____
  x. Distended abdomen _____
  y. Skin cold, clammy _____
  z. 2+ edema _____

32. Which of the following should be recorded as fluid intake?
  a. A bowl of gelatin
  b. A liquid antacid given through a feeding tube
  c. Intravenous fluids
  d. All of the above

33. The nurse requires a physician's order to place a client on intake and output. (True or false?)

34. Complete the table comparing the laboratory findings for each acid-base imbalance.

Lab Value	Metabolic Alkalois	Metabolic Acidosis	Respiratory Alkalosis	Respiratory Acidosis
pH				
$PaCO_2$				
HCO_3				
K^+				

35. The laboratory test most useful in measuring kidney function is:
 a. urine specific gravity.
 b. blood creatinine.
 c. CBC.
 d. serum electrolytes.

36. What is the normal value for urine specific gravity?

37. List two goals appropriate for the client with altered fluid, electrolyte, or acid-base imbalance.

 a.

 b.

38. Calculate the fluid intake in metric measurements for the following meal:

 a. 4 oz. tomato juice _____

 b. 2 poached eggs _____

 c. 2 slices bacon _____

 d. one-half pint milk _____

 e. 1 cup coffee _____

 f. 1 tablespoon cream _____

 g. Total _____

39. Up to 10 pounds of fluid is retained before edema appears. (True or false?)

40. The preferred route for fluid replacement in most clients is:
 a. oral.
 b. nasogastric feeding tubes.
 c. jejunostomy feedings.
 d. parenteral.

41. When a client is placed on fluid restriction, which food form would be considered a fluid?
 a. Ice cream
 b. Ice chips
 c. Liquid medication
 d. All of the above

42. According to the recommendation described in the text, allocate a 1000-ml fluid restriction over 24 hours.
 a. 0800 to 1600
 b. 1600 to 2400
 c. 2400 to 0800

43. State the primary goal of IV fluid administration.

44. The fluids generally used for extracellular volume replacement are:
 a. hypertonic.
 b. hypotonic.
 c. isotonic.

45. Which IV fluid additive would be expected when a client with normal kidney function is NPO:
 a. Sodium
 b. Potassium
 c. Multivitamins
 d. Calcium

46. List three groups of clients in whom venipuncture may be difficult.

 a.

 b.

 c.

47. Briefly describe the differences between peripheral and central venous lines in relation to location, catheter size, and purpose.

48. Complete the following calculations.
 a. 1000 ml D5W to run 12 hours: how many milliliters per hour?
 b. 1000 NS to run over 8 hours (drop factor = 10 gtts/ml): how many drops per minute?
 c. 500 ml Ringer's lactate to run over 6 hours (drop factor = 15 gtts/ml): how many drops per minute?
 d. 50 ml D5W with 500 mg ampicillin to run over 30 minutes (drop factor = 60 gtts/ml): how many drops per minute?
 e. 1000 ml D5W with 20 mEq KCl to run over 12 hours (drop factor = 10 gtts/ml): how many drops per minute?

49. List four factors that may affect IV flow rates.

 a.

 b.

 c.

 d.

50. Identify two major purposes of infusion pumps.

 a.

 b.

51. When using volume control devices, such as Volutrol or buret, how much fluid is routinely added to the device?
 a. The total buret capacity (approximately 150 ml)
 b. The total amount of solution ordered for the shift
 c. Two hours worth of solution
 d. One hours worth of solution

52. How often should a nurse routinely check an IV infusion?
 a. Every hour
 b. Every 2 hours
 c. Every 4 hours
 d. Once per shift

53. Indicate the sequence to be followed when changing a gown of a client with an IV line.
 a. Place the IV bottle or bag and tubing through the sleeve of the clean gown. _____

b. Remove the sleeve of the gown from the uninvolved arm. _____

c. Place the uninvolved arm through the gown sleeve. _____

d. Remove the IV bottle or bag from its stand and pass it and the tubing through the sleeve. _____

e. Place the involved arm through the gown sleeve. _____

f. Remove the sleeve of the gown from the involved arm.

54. Describe the instructions to be given to a client with a peripheral IV line who is able to ambulate independently.

55. What is the average infusion flow to keep the vein open (KVO)?
  a. 5 ml/hr
  b. 10 to 15 ml/hr
  c. 25 to 50 ml/hr
  d. 100 ml/hr

56. Complete the table describing complications of IV therapy.

Complication	Assessment Finding	Nursing Action
Infiltration		
Phlebitis		
Fluid overload		
Bleeding		

57. List four interventions that can reduce the risk of infusion-related infections.
  a.
  b.
  c.
  d.

58. The nurse should wear disposable gloves when discontinuing IV infusions. (True or false?)

59. How long should pressure be applied to an IV site when an infusion has been discontinued?

60. List the three objectives for blood transfusion.
  a.
  b.
  c.

61. Complete the table describing the major blood groups.

	Blood Type			
	A	B	O	AB
Antigens present				
Antibodies produced				

62. a. The blood group of the universal donor is _____ .

  b. The blood group of the universal recipient is _____ .

63. Define autotransfusion.

64. In an emergency situation it is acceptable for the nurse to hang blood without double checking the information about the blood product and client with another registered nurse. (True or false?)

65. Describe the rationale for each of the following nursing actions associated with blood transfusions.
  a. Confirm placement of an 18- or 19-gauge angiocath.
  b. Prime the tubing only with 0.9% normal saline.
  c. Ask the client if he or she has ever experienced a transfusion reaction.
  d. Obtain baseline vital signs.
  e. Begin the infusion slowly (2 ml/min) for the first 15 minutes and remain with the client.

66. The most common type of adverse reaction to blood transfusion is:
  a. febrile and nonhemolytic.
  b. allergic urticarial.
  c. hemolytic.
  d. anaphylactic.

67. List five signs and symptoms most commonly associated with transfusion reaction.
  a.
  b.
  c.
  d.
  e.

68. When a transfusion reaction is suspected in a client receiving blood, the nurse should:
  a. close the roller clamp to the blood and open the roller clamp to the 0.9% normal saline.
  b. slow the blood transfusion until the physician is notified.
  c. stop the transfusion and "piggyback" 0.9% normal saline into the IV line.
  d. continue the blood transfusion until symptoms clearly indicate a transfusion reaction.

69. How long should pressure be applied over an arterial puncture site?

CRITICAL THINKING AND EXPERIENTIAL EXERCISES

1. Monitoring fluid, electrolyte, and acid-base balance
  a. Perform a comprehensive assessment of an assigned client, or obtain assessment data from the medical record, using a standard or self-developed form. (If it is not feasible to do this on a client, select a peer, friend, or family member as your "client.")
  b. Identify variables that influence the client's fluid, electrolyte, and acid-base balance.

c. Identify factors in the health history that indicate that the client may be at risk for fluid, electrolyte, or acid-base disturbance. Describe why these place the client at risk.

d. Identify signs and symptoms from your assessment that indicate that there is an acutual or potential fluid, electrolyte, or acid-base disturbance.

e. Review the medical records to identify pertinent laboratory data reflecting the client's current fluid, electrolyte, and acid-base status. Analyze whether these data are normal. If they are abnormal, attempt to determine the factors contributing to these findings.

f. From the information obtained, describe specific nursing interventions for the client that relate to fluid, electrolyte, or acid-base status.

2. Clinical situation: blood transfustion
Mrs. Smith is receiving her second unit of whole blood when she demonstrates signs of an acute hemolytic transfusion reaction.

a. List at least seven signs and symptoms that Mrs. Smith may demonstrate.

b. List, in priority order, the actions you would take as Mrs. Smith's nurse.

3. Clinical situation: acid-base imbalance
Ms. English, 22 years old, was admitted to the hospital because of repeated episodes of fainting while at work. While completing her nursing history, Ms. English tells the nurse she has been trying to lose weight. Her diet consists mostly of black coffee, diet cola, and some vegetables. She admits to taking a "water pill" the past two mornings and evenings.

a. What is the most likely acid-base disturbance described in this situation?

b. List the assessment criteria that support your conclusion.

c. What additional data would you wish to obtain to better care for Ms. English?

d. Identify at least three interventions specific to the acid-base disturbance identified.

4. Clinical situation: nursing process for clients with fluid and electrolyte imbalance
Ms. Wanda Marconi, 16 years old, is admitted to the hospital after experiencing severe vomiting and diarrhea for the past 3 days. The onset of these symptoms was sudden. During the initial nursing assessment, Wanda states that she has had "a couple of glasses of ginger ale in the past few days but neither of them stayed down." She states she has been having loose green liquid stools every 2 or 3 hours accompanied by cramps.

On admission, Wanda was able to void 75 ml of concentrated dark amber urine for a urinalysis; the specific gravity was 1.030. Her skin turgor is poor. Her lips are dry and cracked. Her tongue is covered with a white-gray coating. She says she is thirsty but is afraid to drink anything. Vital signs are as follows: temperature 37.2° C (99° F); pulse, 116; respirations, 28 and shallow; blood pressure, 104/62 supine and 90/50 sitting.

a. What fluid, electrolyte, and acid-base disturbances are present or potentially exist in the client? Support your answer with the assessment data provided.

b. Identify laboratory data that you would review to gain a clearer understanding of the client's condition.

c. Formulate nursing diagnoses that relate to the client's fluid, electrolyte, or acid-base status.

d. For the primary diagnoses, identify three nursing goals.

e. For each goal, describe at least two interventions.

SKILL AND TECHNIQUE ACTIVITIES

1. Intake and output
a. Obtain copies of the intake and output records used in your institution (or review the samples provided on pp. 180 and 181).
b. Complete the records using the information from a simulated 8-hour shift provided below.
0730—voided 250 ml
0800—50 ml D5W with 500 mg Keflin IVPB
0815—1 cup coffee, 4 oz. juice
0830—½ cup water
0900—voided 300 ml
1000—1 cup water
1200—½ pint milk, 4 oz. juice, 1 cup iced tea
1330—350 ml diarrhea
1400—¾ cup water
    Voided 200 ml
    Hemovac drainage: 150 ml
The infusion pump is set to deliver 100 ml/hr, and the 1400 reading indicates that 800 ml has infused since previous readings were cleared at 0600.
c. Submit your completed I & O forms to your instructor for feedback.

2. IV calculation problems
Complete the following calculation problems and submit them to your instructor for validation of the correct answer.
a. 250 ml of packed cells to infuse over 2 hours (drip factor: 12 gtts/ml)
b. 100 ml D5W with 40 mg gentamicin to infuse over 40 minutes (drip factor: 60 gtts/ml)
c. 2500 ml D5W to infuse over 24 hours (drip factor: 10 gtts/ml)
d. 2000 ml TPN solution to infuse over 24 hours through an infusion pump. Infusion pump requires nurse to dial in number of milliliters per hour. What is the correct setting?
e. 450 ml of whole blood to infuse over 3 hours (drip factor: 15 gtts/ml)

3. Parenteral solution administration
a. Review your institution's policies for IV fluid administration.
b. In the nursing laboratory, or on the clinical unit, examine the various types of fluids, vascular access devices, delivery systems, and equipment used for IV fluid administration.

c. Write a list of all the equipment needed to:
 (1) start an IV.
 (2) change IV tubing.
 (3) change an IV dressing.
 (4) discontinue an IV.
d. In the nursing laboratory practice each of the following skills using available equipment and, if possible, a simulation mannequin. Have another student critique your performance and provide feedback on your technique.
 (1) Changing the gown with an IV placed in the hand or forearm (If a mannequin is not available for this, tape the IV tubing to a partner's arm and attach the tubing to an IV bag or bottle.)
 (2) Changing the IV bag or bottle but continuing to use the current tubing
 (3) Changing the tubing but continuing to use the current IV fluid bottle or bag
 (4) Changing the tubing and IV fluid bottle or bag at the IV catheter
 (5) Changing the IV dressing
e. When you feel comfortable with the preceding skills, elicit an instructor's evaluation of your technique.
f. Observe an experienced nurse providing care to a client receiving parenteral fluids. Identify techniques that are specific to needs associated with parenteral fluid administration. Share your observations with your instructor.
g. In the nursing laboratory setting, practice the following infusion pump techniques with a partner:
 (1) Setting up the pump
 (2) Changing a client gown when the pump is in use
 (3) Changing the IV tubing when the pump is in use
 (4) Changing the flow rate on the pump
 (5) Obtaining the total intake computed by the pump (if it has the capacity) and clearing the totals
 (6) Responding to the various alarm modes
h. In the nursing laboratory setting, with the assistance of an instructor or laboratory supervisor, practice venipuncture techniques on an appropriate mannequin. When you have become proficient in your practice, request an opportunity to practice on a peer with the close supervision of an instructor.
4. Arterial puncture
 a. Review your institution's policies on arterial punctures or "sticks" with particular attention to the nursing role in this procedure.
 b. List the equipment required when assisting with an arterial puncture.
 c. Observe a qualified staff member obtaining an arterial blood sample. Be sure to interact with, and provide support to, the client. Share your observations with your instructor.
5. Blood transfusions
 a. Review your institution's policies on blood transfusions. Pay particular attention to the responsibilities of the nurse and compare them to the information presented in your text.
 b. In the laboratory setting, or on the clinical division, examine the equipment and supplies needed to transfuse a client.
 c. Observe or assist an experienced nurse caring for a client being transfused. Share your observations with your instructor.

Barnes Hospital
DAILY INTAKE AND OUTPUT RECORD
B-8

17-4 Rev. 2/83

FROM 0700   /   /   TO 0700   /   /   Addressograph Plate

INTAKE		OUTPUT	

Coffee mug - 180cc
Ice tea container to clear line (without ice) - 250cc
Ice cream container (melted) - 30cc
Sherbet container (melted) - 50cc
Juice container - 120cc
Milk carton - 240cc
Paper cup (1/4 from brim) - 240cc
Soup bowl (broth) - 180cc
Gelatin container (melted) - 100cc

ORDERS: (CIRCLE)
NPO
WATER
CLEAR FLUIDS
FULL FLUIDS
AMT. DESIRED   CC

SOURCE KEY:
V = VOIDED
C = CATHETER
INC = INCONTINENT

SOURCE KEY:
VOM. = VOMITUS
LIQ. S. = LIQUID STOOL
HV. = HEMOVAC
L.T. = LEVIN TUBE
T.T. = T. TUBE
OTHER

RATE   GTTS/MIN.   CC/HR.

TIME	SOLUTION IN BOTTLE KIND / AMT.(CC)	AMT.(CC) ABSORBED	ORAL KIND	AMT.(CC)	URINE SOURCE	AMT.(CC)	OTHER SOURCE	AMT.(CC)
0700 0800								
0800 0900								
0900 1000								
1000 1100								
1100 1200								
1200 1300								
1300 1400								
1400 1500								
8 HR. TOT.			8 HR. TOT.		8 HR. TOT.		8 HR. TOT.	
1500 1600								
1600 1700								
1700 1800								
1800 1900								
1900 2000								
2000 2100								
2100 2200								
2200 2300								
8 HR. TOT.			8 HR. TOT.		8 HR. TOT.		8 HR. TOT.	
2300 2400								
2400 0100								
0100 0200								
0200 0300								
0300 0400								
0400 0500								
0500 0600								
0600 0700								
8 HR. TOT.			8 HR. TOT.		8 HR. TOT.		8 HR. TOT.	
24 HR. TOT.			24HR. TOT.		24 HR. TOT.		24 HR. TOT.	

B-17

BARNES HOSPITAL
24 HOUR
INTAKE AND OUTPUT SUMMARY
(Retain in Patient's Record)

STAMP ADDRESSOGRAPH PLATE HERE

		INTAKE			OUTPUT		
DATE	SHIFT	ORAL and/or TUBE FEEDING	IV (Incl. Blood and Plasma)		URINE	GASTRIC	OTHER (specify)
	07000 1500						
	1500 2300						
	2300 0700						
	TOTAL						
	07000 1500						
	1500 2300						
	2300 0700						
	TOTAL						
	07000 1500						
	1500 2300						
	2300 0700						
	TOTAL						
	07000 1500						
	1500 2300						
	2300 0700						
	TOTAL						
	07000 1500						
	1500 2300						
	2300 0700						
	TOTAL						
	07000 1500						
	1500 2300						
	2300 0700						
	TOTAL						
	07000 1500						
	1500 2300						
	2300 0700						
	TOTAL						

ADDITIONAL READINGS

Chenevey B: Overview of fluid and electrolytes, *Nurs Cl North Am* 22(4):749, 1987.

The first in a series of articles addressing the complex topic of fluid and electrolyte balance. Other articles in this edition of the journal explore specific disease states associated with fluid and electrolyte imbalance and provide guidelines for nursing care.

Hahn, K: Monitoring blood transfusion, *Nurs 89* 19:20, 1989

Describes guidelines for safe blood administration. Includes information about nursing assessment and intervention during a transfusion reaction.

Hazinski MF: Understanding fluid balance in the seriously ill child, *Pediatr Nurs* 14(3):231, 1988.

A concise review of fluid balance with a pediatric focus.

Lancaster LE: Renal and endocrine regulation of water and electrolyte balance, *Nurs Cl North Am* 22(4):761, 1987.

A detailed review of the anatomy and physiology of water and electrolyte regulation.

Messner RL, Gorse GJ: Nursing management of peripheral intravenous sites, *Focus Crit Care* 14(2):25, 1987.

Analyzes research related to peripheral IV infection. Describes common factors predisposing clients to peripheral IV infection, characteristic manifestations, and preventive care techniques. Tables summarize essential steps in infection prevention and the related rationale.

Metheny NM, editor: *Overview of fluid and electrolyte balance: nursing considerations*, ed 2, Philadelphia, 1992, Lippincott.

An excellent, clear presentation of a complex and often confusing clinical topic. A comprehensive reference describing the normal regulation of fluids and electrolytes and balance disturbances. Includes nursing assessment and care from a developmental perspective. Describes specific nursing care unique to each fluid or electrolyte disturbance. Discusses many special topics related to maintenance of fluid and electrolyte balance, including parenteral therapy and nutritional support. Also addresses fluid and electrolyte imbalances associated with disease states and treatment modalities.

Chapter 40
Urinary Elimination

PREREQUISITE READING

Chapter 40, pp. 1332 to 1385

OBJECTIVES

Mastery of content in this chapter will enable the student to:

- Define selected terms associated with urinary elimination.
- Explain the function of each organ in the urinary system.
- Describe the process of urination.
- Identify factors that commonly influence urinary elimination.
- Compare and contrast common alterations in urinary elimination.
- Obtain a nursing history for a client with urinary elimination problems.
- Identify nursing diagnoses appropriate for clients with alterations in urinary elimination.
- Obtain urine specimens.
- Describe characteristics of normal and abnormal urine.
- Describe the nursing implications of common diagnostic tests of the urinary system.
- Discuss nursing measures to promote normal micturition and reduce episodes of incontinence.
- Insert a urinary catheter.
- Discuss nursing measures to reduce urinary tract infection.
- Irrigate a urinary catheter.
- Identify two modalities of renal replacement therapy.
- Discuss organ system alterations in urinary system failure.
- Understand basic principles in selecting urinary catheters.

REVIEW OF KEY CONCEPTS

1. List and summarize the function of each organ in the urinary system.

   a.

   b.

   c.

   d.

2. The functional unit of the kidney responsible for the formation of urine is the _____ .
3. All of the following substances are normally filtrated through the glomeruli except:
   a. protein.
   b. glucose.
   c. creatine.
   d. electrolytes.
4. All of the substances filtered through the glomeruli are excreted as urine. (True or false?)
5. Which urinary output measurement would be associated with altered renal function?
   a. 1500 ml in 24 hours
   b. 1800 ml in 24 hours
   c. 60 ml per hour
   d. 25 ml per hour

6. Excessive urination at night is _____ .
7. The process by which urine is expelled from the urinary bladder is called:
   a. urination.
   b. micturition.
   c. voiding.
   d. all of the above.
8. Number the steps describing the normal act of micturition in sequential order.
   a. Parasympathetic impules from micturition center cause detrusor muscle to begin contracting. _____

   b. External bladder sphincter relaxes. _____
   c. Impulses travel to cerebral cortex, making the person conscious of the need to void. _____

   d. Detrusor muscle contracts. _____
   e. Internal urethral sphincter relaxes, allowing urine to enter urethra. _____

   f. Urine passes through urethral meatus. _____
   g. Volume of urine stretches bladder walls, sending impulses to spinal cord. _____

9. Full control of micturition generally occurs at age:
   a. 12 to 16 months.
   b. 18 to 24 months.
   c. 2 to 3 years.
   d. 4 to 5 years.
10. The process of aging causes all of the following changes in urination except:
   a. increased concentration of urine.
   b. loss of bladder tone.
   c. increased frequency.
   d. urinary retention.
11. Briefly explain how each of the following factors can influence urinary elimination.
   a. Anxiety
   b. Childbirth
   c. Long-term use of indwelling catheter
   d. Increased fluid intake
   e. Diabetes mellitus
   f. Narcotic analgesics
12. The accumulation of urine in the bladder with the inability of the bladder to empty fully is _____ .
13. What are the mechanisms associated with "retention with overflow"?
14. List three factors that may cause urinary retention.
   a.
   b.
   c.
15. The most common cause of infection in the urinary tract is:
   a. poor perineal hygiene.
   b. bladder distention.
   c. instrumentation.
   d. sexual intercourse.
16. Blood-tinged urine is described as _____ .
17. List six signs or symptoms of urinary tract infections.
   a.
   b.
   c.
   d.
   e.
   f.
18. The loss of control over micturition is _____ .
19. Define enuresis.
20. Match the following types of urinary incontinence with the most accurate definition or description.

Description

   a. Involuntary passage of urine after a strong urge to void _____
   b. Involuntary passage of urine when a specific bladder volume is reached _____

   c. Strong urge to void, causing loss of urine before reaching appropriate facilities _____
   d. Constant flow of urine at unpredictable times, unawareness of bladder filling or emptying ___
   e. Dribbling of urine with coughing, laughing, vomiting, or lifting _____

Incontinence type
   1. Total
   2. Functional
   3. Stress
   4. Urge
   5. Reflex
21. What is a urinary diversion?
22. The urinary diversion in which the end of one or both ureters is brought to the abdominal surface is:
   a. an ileal loop.
   b. an ileal conduit.
   c. urethral fistula.
   d. ureterostomy.
23. List the three major factors to be explored during a nursing history concerning urinary elimination.
   a.
   b.
   c.
24. Match the following common symptoms of urinary alterations with the correct description.

Decription
   a. Voiding at frequent intervals _____
   b. Leakage of urine despite voluntary control of urination _____
   c. Difficulty initiating urination _____
   d. Diminished urinary output _____
   e. Painful or difficult urination _____
   f. Feeling of the need to void immediately _____
   g. Voiding a large amount of urine _____

Symptoms
   1. Urgency
   2. Dysuria
   3. Frequency
   4. Hesitancy
   5. Polyuria
   6. Oliguria
   7. Dribbling
25. Which of the following is the best description of the normal bladder?
   a. Normally nonpalpable; when distended feels smooth and rounded
   b. Normally palpable just below symphysis pubis; feels smooth and rounded

c. Normally nonpalpable; palpation may cause urge to urinate; when distended feels smooth and rounded

d. Normally palpable; palpation causes urge to urinate

26. What physical examination technique may be used to assess the presence of kidney infection or inflammation?

27. A congenitally formed opening of the urethra on the undersurface of the penis is _____ .

28. The scale on the outside of a urinary drainage bag may be used for accurate volume measurement. (True or false?)

29. When urine is red, it is appropriate to assume that the client has hematuria. (True or false)

30. A sterile urine specimen may be collected from a urinary drainage bag. (True or false?)

31. Which of the following assessment findings would be characteristic of normal urine?
    a. Clear, straw colored, and aromatic
    b. Pink tinged, clear, and aromatic
    c. Dark amber, clear, and smelling of ammonia
    d. Cloudy, thick, and smelling of ammonia

32. When a clean voided specimen is collected, the nurse follows all of the following steps except:
    a. sends the specimen to the laboratory within 15 minutes or refrigerates it.
    b. collects a midstream specimen.
    c. discards the first specimen and obtains a second specimen in 30 to 45 minutes.
    d. washes the urethral meatus of the female from above urethral orifice toward the anus.

33. Which technique would be appropriate for obtaining a sterile specimen from an indwelling retention catheter?
    a. Clamp the tubing just above the site chosen for withdrawal
    b. Cleanse the catheter with soap and water before obtaining the specimen.
    c. Insert the needle at a 90-degree angle.
    d. use a small-gauge (no. 23 or 25) needle on a sterile syringe.

34. Briefly describe the method of obtaining a timed urine collection.

35. Which measurement would be considered a normal value in a routine urinalysis?
    a. pH of 5.6
    b. Specific gravity of 1.035
    c. Protein of 10 mg/100 ml
    d. Glucose of 2^+

36. An accurate measurement of urinary glucose and ketones always requires a double-voided specimen. (True or false?)

37. Which of the following diagnostic tests allows direct visualization of the urinary structures?
    a. Intravenous pyelogram (IVP)
    b. Renal scan
    c. Cystoscopy
    d. All of the above

38. List four nursing interventions appropriate for the client following cystoscopy.
    a.
    b.
    c.
    d.

39. List four goals appropriate for promoting a client's normal urinary elimination.
    a.
    b.
    c.
    d.

40. List five techniques that may be used to stimulate the micturition reflex.
    a.
    b.
    c.
    d.
    e.

41. Describe two pelvic floor (Kegel) exercises.
    a.
    b.

42. A client with urge incontinence is likely to benefit most from:
    a. catheterization.
    b. diuretics.
    c. anticholinergic medications.
    d. cholinergic medications.

43. The physician has ordered bethanechol (Urecholine) for a client with retention and overflow incontinence. Nursing actions to enhance the effectiveness of the first dose include:
    a. administration immediately after voiding.
    b. administration immediately before micturition.
    c. administration 3 or 4 hours after voiding.
    d. restriction of oral fluids.

44. State the goal of bladder retraining.

45. Match the client situation with the most appropriate type of catheterization.

Situation

a. Mr. Powers received 10 mg of morphine every 4 hours for the past 12 hours. His bladder is palpable, but he cannot void. _____

b. Ms. Spencer lives in a nursing home. She cannot sense the need to void. She has severe excoriation of her perineum. _____

c. Ms. Pine enters the clinic with a high fever. Her doctor suspects urinary infection and orders a specimen. Ms. Pine is unable to void. _____

d. Mr. Ahrens is admitted to the hospital with severe congestive heart failure. To treat his fluid volume overload, the physician requests that the nurses monitor his intake and output hourly. _____

Catheterization type

1. Intermittent
2. Indwelling

46. Indicate the catheter size appropriate for:
    a. Children
    b. Women
    c. Men

47. To ensure easy insertion of a urinary catheter into a male client, the best technique would include:
    a. lowering the penis and introducing the catheter as the client bears down to void.
    b. lifting the penis perpendicular to the body and asking the client to breathe deeply.
    c. lifting the penis perpendicular to the body, applying light traction, and asking the client to bear down.
    d. holding the penis at a 45-degree angle to the body and applying light traction.

48. When urine flows out of the end of a retention catheter during insertion, how much further should it be advanced?
    a. 2.5 cm
    b. 5 cm
    c. 7.5 cm
    d. 10 cm

49. The nurse should never raise a drainage bag and tubing above the level of the client's bladder. (True or false?)

50. All of the following would be routine methods for maintaining the patency of the urinary drainage system except:
    a. irrigating the tubing using sterile saline.
    b. checking for kinks or bends in the tubing.
    c. avoiding positioning the client on the drainage tubing.
    d. observing for clots or sediment that may occlude the collecting tubing.

51. List two important principles to follow when removing an indwelling catheter.

    a.

    b.

52. It is normal for the client to experience dysuria immediately after removal of an indwelling catheter. (True or false?)

53. Describe a suprapubic catheter.

54. List two precautions that should be taken to ensure client safety and comfort when using a condom catheter.

    a.

    b.

55. List three general measures to prevent urinary tract infection in clients without indwelling urinary catheters.

    a.

    b.

    c.

56. Describe six ways to minimize the risk of urinary tract infection in catheterized clients.

    a.

    b.

    c.

    d.

    e.

    f.

57. All of the following would be appropriate foods for acidifying the urine to inhibit growth of microorganisms except:
    a. orange or grapefruit juice.
    b. meats and eggs.
    c. whole grain breads.
    d. cranberries and plums.

58. A physician's order is required for catheter irrigations. (True or false?)

59. Describe renal replacement therapy.

60. What is the best way to remove urine from the skin?

61. A comfort measure for the client with dysuria could include all of the following except:
    a. warm sitz baths.
    b. administration of urinary analgesics.
    c. fluid restriction to reduce frequency.
    d. encouraging fluid intake.

CRITICAL THINKING AND EXPERIENTIAL EXERCISES

1. Urinary system anatomy and physiology
    a. Trace the formation and flow of urine from the glomerulus to the urethra.

2. Client teaching: pelvic floor exercises
    a. Develop a teaching tool (chart, table, paper, pamphlet, or booklet) to assist clients in learning pelvic floor (Kegel) exercises.
    b. Practice these exercises yourself, following the directions in the teaching tool.
    c. Practice explaining or teaching these exercises to a partner (or audio-tape for practice and self-evaluation).
    d. Submit your teaching tool to your instructor for feedback before using in an actual client education situation.

3. Clinical situation: urinary tract infection
    Ms. Giles is a 58-year-old woman with a lower uri-

nary tract infection. She is alert and reports no other acute or chronic health problems.

  a. Describe normal physiological mechanisms that prevent urinary tract infections.
  b. Describe the criteria to be used in collecting a nursing history on Ms. Giles.
  c. Identify the signs and symptoms that would be expected for a lower urinary tract infection.
  d. What laboratory examinations would you expect to be ordered for Ms. Giles? What results would indicate a urinary tract infection?
  e. Formulate a discharge teaching plan for Ms. Giles that is directed toward prevention of future urinary tract infections.

4. Clinical situation: diagnostic examinations
  Mr. Kent is a 58-year-old business executive with a long history of pipe smoking and recent onset of lower abdominal discomfort and hematuria. He has entered the hospital for diagnostic studies to determine the source of his symptoms.

  a. The physician has ordered lower GI studies, including a barium enema and an IVP. Which test should be scheduled first? Why?
  b. What is the purpose of an IVP?
  c. Describe at least five nursing responsibilities before the procedure.
  d. What responsibilities does the nurse have during the IVP? (Name at least two.)
  e. What specific nursing interventions are appropriate when Mr. Kent returns from the IVP?

5. Clinical situation: bladder retraining
  Mrs. Sharp is a 37-year-old woman who sustained a bladder injury during a traumatic childbirth 3 months ago. Since that time she has experienced problems initating voiding and urge incontinence. Formulate a bladder retraining program for this client.

6. Clinical situation: nursing process for clients with altered urinary elimination
  Mrs. Pender is a 63-year-old woman with urinary retention. Her problem developed 1 year ago after having surgery for a vaginal tumor. Mrs. Pender is a highly anxious person and becomes embarrassed when outflow of urine accidentally occurs. She states that this problem has caused her to curtail all social activities and prevents her from attending church services. She also suffers from degenerative arthritis and has pain in her knees with joint motion.

  a. List actual and potential nursing diagnoses associated with Mrs. Pender's elimination problem.
  b. Identify one goal for each of the top two priority nursing diagnoses.
  c. For each goal, describe at least three interventions. (State the rationale for the interventions selected.)

SKILL AND TECHNIQUE ACTIVITIES

1. Obtaining urine specimens
  a. Review your institution's procedures for obtaining routine urinalysis, clean voided specimens, timed (24-hour) collections, and specimens for glucose and acetone. Locate the needed equipment for collection and laboratory requisitions (or computer menu) on your clinical unit.
  b. Obtain a sample of your own urine and practice each of these skills in the laboratory setting: specific gravity, Keto-Diastix, and Multistix. Have an instructor or laboratory supervisor validate your findings.
  c. In the laboratory setting, using indwelling catheter demonstration equipment, practice the technique for obtaining a sterile specimen from a catheter. Have another student observe and critique your performance. Elicit an instructor's evaluation of your technique.

2. Use of bedpans and urinals
  a. In the nursing laboratory, or on the clinical unit, examine the various types of bedpans and urinals available in your institution. Review institutional procedures regarding distribution and cleaning of these items.
  b. In the nursing laboratory, practice assisting a partner on and off a regular and orthopedic (fracture) bedpan.

3. Urinary catheterization
  a. Review your institution's procedure for intermittent and indwelling catheterization.
  b. Examine equipment used for catheterization insertion, drainage, and maintenance in your nursing laboratory or on the clinical unit.
  c. In the nursing laboratory, using demonstration mannequins or models (male or female), practice the techniques of intermittent catheterization and indwelling catherization. Have another student observe and critique your performance. Elicit an instructor's evaluation of your technique.
  d. In the nursing laboratory, using a demonstration mannequin or model, practice removing an indwelling catheter. Have another student observe and critique your performance. Elicit an instructor's evaluation of your technique.
  e. In the nursing laboratory, using a demonstration mannequin or model, practice the technique of perineal care and catheter care.
  f. In the nursing laboratory, tape a urinary catheter to the leg of a partner and attach the catheter to a urinary drainage bag. Practice each of the following techniques: turning and positioning in bed, dangling, moving from bed to wheelchair, and ambulation. Be sure to monitor the level of the drainage bag, tube patency, and the tension on the tubing during these maneuvers.

g. In the nursing laboratory, using a demonstration mannequin or model, practice application of a condom catheter.

ADDITIONAL READINGS

Burgener S: Justification of closed intermittent urinary catheter irrigation/instillation: a review of current literature and practice, *J Adv Nurs* 12:229, 1987.

Reviews current literature on the pathogenesis of urinary tract infection, catheter irrigation techniques, and specific outcomes. Based on findings cited, recommends use of closed-system technique in catheter irrigations and instillations.

Erickson PJ: Ostomies: the art of pouching, *Nurs Clin North Am* 22:311, 1987.

Describes practical approaches for pouching a stoma. Useful for students and experienced nurses. May be easily incorporated into a client teaching plan.

Kaltrieder DL et al: Can reminders curb incontinence? *Geriatr Nurs* 11(1):17, 1990.

Presents the position that contextual reminders reduce the frequency of incontinence in the older client.

Petillo MH, editor: Enterostomal therapy, *Nurs Clin North Am* 22(2):253, 1987.

Addresses, in a series of articles, urinary and intestinal ostomy therapy. Includes specific information about management of urinary and intestinal ostomies. Discusses special topics applicable to ostomy clients, including developmental implications, psychosocial considerations, sexuality, and skin care.

Petillo MH: The patient with a urinary stoma, *Nurs Clin North Am* 22:261, 1987.

Discusses in detail specific nursing care measures appropriate for clients with urinary stomas.

Wilde MH: Living with a Foley, *Am J Nurs* 86:1212, 1986.

Describes variations in technique required when a client has a long-term indwelling urinary catheter. Makes specific recommendations for procedure modification appropriate to the home.

Chapter 41
Bowel Elimination

PREREQUISITE READING

Chapter 41, pp. 1386 to 1427

OBJECTIVES

Mastery of content in this chapter will enable the student to:
- Define selected terms associated with gastrointestinal (GI) function.
- Discuss the role of gastrointestinal organs in digestion and elimination.
- Describe four functions of the large intestine.
- Explain the physiological aspects of normal defecation.
- Discuss psychological and physiological factors that influence the elimination process.
- Describe common physiological alterations in elimination.
- Assess a client's elimination pattern.
- Perform a guaiac test for occult blood.
- List nursing diagnoses related to alterations in elimination.
- Describe nursing implications for common diagnostic examinations of the gastrointestinal tract.
- Administer an enema.
- List nursing measures that promote normal elimination.
- Discuss the relationship between the structure and function of bowel diversions and nursing care required.

REVIEW OF KEY CONCEPTS

1. List the three major purposes of the gastrointestinal tract.

   a.

   b.

   c.

2. Mechanical and chemical digestion begins in the:
   a. mouth.
   b. stomach.
   c. small intestine.
   d. large intestine.

3. Most nutrients and electrolytes are absorbed in the:
   a. large intestine.
   b. small intestine.
   c. cecum.
   d. stomach.

4. List and briefly describe the four functions of the colon.

   a.

   b.

   c.

   d.

5. The medical term for intestinal gas is

   _____.

6. Waste products reaching the sigmoid portion of the colon are _____.

7. Permanent dilations of the rectal veins are

   _____.

8. Indicate the correct sequence of mechanisms involved in normal defecation.
   a. Increased intraabdominal pressure or the Valsalva maneuver occurs. _____
   b. The external sphincter relaxes. _____
   c. The internal sphincter relaxes, and awareness of the need to defecate occurs. _____
   d. The levator ani muscles relax. _____
   e. Sensory nerves are stimulated via rectal distention. _____

9. Describe the Valsalva maneuver.

10. List six changes occurring in the GI system of the older adult that impair normal digestion and elimination.

    a.

    b.

    c.

    d.

    e.

    f.

11. What mechanisms causes high-fiber diets to promote elimination?

12. List four types of foods considered high in fiber.

    a.

    b.

    c.

    d.

13. Inability to digest milk and milk products, resulting in diarrhea, gaseous distention and cramping, is

    _____.

14. Bowel elimination is facilitated by all of the following except:
    a. increasing fluid intake to 1400 to 2000 ml daily.
    b. drinking hot beverages.
    c. drinking fruit juices.
    d. drinking milk.

15. General anesthesia and surgery tend to stimulate peristalsis. (True or false?)

16. Describe the effect of each medication on elimination.
    a. Mineral oil
    b. Dicyclomine hydrochloride (Bentyl)
    c. Narcotics
    d. Anticholinergics (atropine and glycopyrrolate)
    e. Antibiotics

17. Chronic use of cathartics can make the large intestine less responsive to laxatives. (True or false?)

18. What treatment would be anticipated in a client who has had a barium examination procedure?

19. All of the following describe constipation except:
    a. it is a symptom.
    b. it is a decrease in the frequency of bowel movements.
    c. it is the passage of hard, dry stools.
    d. it is the inability to have a daily bowel movement.

20. List and briefly describe four causes of constipation.

    a.

    b.

    c.

    d.

21. List three groups of clients in whom constipation could pose a significant health hazard.

    a.

    b.

    c.

22. How can the Valsalva maneuver be avoided?

23. Define fecal impaction.

24. List four signs and symptoms of fecal impaction.

    a.

    b.

    c.

    d.

25. Define diarrhea.

26. List the two major complications associated with diarrhea.

    a.

    b.

27. Mr. Wilms had an appendectomy 2 days ago. He currently complains of abdominal pain and shortness of breath. The nurse observes abdominal distention. The most likely cause of Mr. Wilms' current condition is:
    a. increased peristalsis.
    b. flatulence.
    c. constipation.
    d. slowed esophageal emptying.

28. An artificial opening in the abdominal wall is a(n)

    _____.

29. A surgical opening formed from the ileum to the

    abdominal wall is an _____.

30. A surgical opening formed from the colon to the

    abdominal wall is a _____.

31. Feces with the most normal consistency and appearance would be expected from:
    a. an ileostomy.
    b. a sigmoid colostomy.
    c. a transverse colostomy.
    d. an ascending colostomy.

32. List eight factors to be included in a nursing history for clients with altered elimination status.

    a.

    b.

    c.

    d.

    e.

    f.

    g.

    h.

33. The nurse auscultates the abdomen for bowel sounds before performing palpation because:
    a. the action minimizes the client's anxiety.
    b. it is less intrusive than palpation.
    c. palpation may change the frequency of bowel sounds.
    d. palpation may alter the location of bowel sounds.

34. Identify the possible cause for each of the following abdominal assessment findings.
    a. Increased pitch or "tinkling" bowel sounds
    b. Hypoactive or absent bowel sounds
    c. Hyperactive bowel sounds
    d. Percussion of tympanic sounds
    e. Percussion of dull sounds

35. To increase client comfort by relaxing the anal sphincter during rectal examination, the nurse instructs the client to:
    a. bear down.
    b. deep breathe.
    c. pant.
    d. hold breath.
36. For each of the fecal characteristics below, indicate the possible cause.
    a. white or clay colored
    b. Black or tarry
    c. Melena
    d. Liquid consistency
    e. Narrow, pencil shaped
37. Nurses should wear disposable gloves when handling specimens. (True or false?)
38. Mr. Rogers has been receiving an anticoagulant (Coumadin) for a clotting disorder. The nurse notes that Mr. Rogers' stools appear darker. The test most likely to be ordered for Mr. Rodgers would be a:
    a. sigmoidoscopy.
    b. stool for guaiac.
    c. proctoscopy.
    d. stool for culture.
39. Answer the following:
    a. State three risk factors for colon cancer.

    (1)

    (2)

    (3)
    b. Identify two warning signs of colon cancer.

    (1)

    (2)
40. Which diagnostic examination requires that the client remain NPO before the test?
    a. Sigmoidoscopy
    b. Guaiac
    c. Gastroscopy
    d. Proctoscopy
41. List four nursing interventions appropriate for clients following gastroscopy.

    a.

    b.

    c.

    d.
42. List five goals appropriate for clients with elimination problems.

    a.

    b.

    c.

    d.

    e.

43. List three ways to promote regular bowel habits in the hospitalized client.

    a.

    b.

    c.
44. The proper technique for positioning a client on a bedpan is to:
    a. place client high in bed, raise head 30 degrees, and assist client in bending knees and lifting hips upward.
    b. place client high in bed, position head of bed flat, and instruct client to bend knees and raise hips.
    c. place client low in bed, elevate head 30 degrees, and instruct client to extend back and raise hips.
    d. raise head of bed 30 degrees, roll client to side, place pan over buttocks, and roll client to supine position.
45. When is the best time to administer cathartic suppositories?
46. Match the laxative classification to its primary action.

Action

    a. Intestinal mucosa is irritated to increase motility.

    _____
    b. Osmotic effect increases pressure in bowel to

    stimulate peristalsis. _____
    c. High fiber content absorbs water and increases

    intestinal bulk. _____
    d. Fecal contents are coated, allowing for easier

    passage. _____
    e. Detergents lower surface tension of feces, allow-

    ing penetration of water and fat. _____

Classification

    1. Bulk forming
    2. Emollient (wetting)
    3. Saline
    4. Stimulant cathartics
    5. Lubricants
47. The safest solution to use for repeated enemas would be:
    a. tap water.
    b. saline.
    c. soapsuds.
    d. sterile water.
48. Which enema would be ordered to provide relief from gaseous distention?
    a. Carminative (MGW)
    b. Medicated (Kayexalate)
    c. Oil retention
    d. Soapsuds

49. What height would be appropriate for elevation of the enema bag or bottle for a cleansing enema?
    a. Less than 12 inches above the hips
    b. 12 to 18 inches above the hips
    c. 18 to 24 inches above the hips
    d. Slightly below the hips
50. What is the meaning of the order "enemas 'til clear"?
51. It is acceptable to give an enema while the client is seated on the toilet. (True or false?)
52. The most appropriate action to take when a client complains of abdominal cramping during an enema would be to:
    a. remove the rectal tube.
    b. encourage the client to change positions.
    c. temporarily lower the container or clamp the tubing.
    d. take no action (this is expected).
53. A physician's order is necessary for the nurse to remove a fecal impaction. (True or false?)
54. Why is it necessary to assess a client's heart rate when digitally removing stool?
55. List five factors to consider when selecting a pouching system for an ostomate.

    a.

    b.

    c.

    d.

    e.

56. A nurse with special education in the care of clients with an ostomy is an _____.
57. List six contraindications to colostomy irrigation.

    a.

    b.

    c.

    d.

    e.

    f.

58. Describe two exercises for prevention of constipation in the bedridden client.

    a.

    b.

59. The most effective means of local heat application for painful hemorrhoids would be:
    a. warm soaks.
    b. sitz baths.
    c. a heating pad.
    d. a heat lamp.
60. A client is experiencing discomfort from postoperative flatulence. Which actions will assist in decreasing flatus or promoting its escape?
    a. Drinking soda
    b. Sucking on hard candy
    c. Maintaining a right, side-lying position
    d. Ambulation
61. Baby powder or cornstarch offers effective skin protection for debilitated, incontinent clients. (True or false?)
62. List and describe four interventions that may assist in restoring self-concept in a client with bowel elimination problems.

    a.

    b.

    c.

    d.

63. Mr. Clancy has an ascending colostomy. What information would be appropriate to include in his individualized teaching plan?
    a. Techniques for colostomy irrigation
    b. Daily use of stool softeners
    c. Skin care and pouching techniques
    d. Activity and exercise restrictions

CRITICAL THINKING AND EXPERIENTIAL EXERCISES

1. GI tract anatomy and physiology
    a. Trace the pathway of ingested foods through the GI tract. Include the anatomical structures and primary functions of each section of the tract and the functions of accessory organs (liver, gallbladder, and pancreas).
2. Assessment of bowel elimination
    a. Formulate an assessment tool to evaluate a client's bowel elimination status (or examine the assessment tool used in your health care setting and identify those components that are pertinent to the assessment of bowel elimination).
    b. Use the formulated or modified form to evaluate bowel elimination of an assigned client or partner.
    c. From the information obtained, identify factors promoting or impairing effective elimination and any other actual or potential abnormalities in GI function.
    d. Formulate pertinent nursing diagnoses based on your findings.
3. Medications and GI function
    After a client care experience or after reviewing a selected client's medication records, identify each of the following:
    a. The effect of prescribed medications on GI function
    b. Medications that are laxatives or cathartics
    c. In the case of laxatives or cathartics, identify the particular classification, action, side effects, and nursing implications for safe administration
4. Clinical situation: care of the client with chronic constipation
    Mr. Truscott, a 58-year-old business executive, has

come to the clinic for his annual employment physical. During the assessment interview, Mr. Truscott tells the nurse that he travels extensively and most of his mornings are rushed by trying to catch early-morning flights to his next business destination. He reports that he frequently ignores the urge to defecate. Most of his meals are in restaurants or at fast food outlets. His fluid intake is limited to mealtimes, which are often rushed. His "normal" bowel elimination pattern varies. It is not uncommon for Mr. Truscott to have only one bowel movement every 5 to 7 days. His stool is hard and dry. He frequently requires a lot of straining to pass the stool. He often experiences pain, and occasionally bleeding, with bowel movements. When he is not traveling, he takes laxatives to relieve his constipation.

a. What factors are currently influencing Mr. Truscott's elimination status?

b. Develop a teaching plan for Mr. Truscott that promotes regular bowel habits. Be sure to individualize the plan to his lifestyle and developmental level.

5. Clinical situation: care of the client with diarrhea
Jamie Rose is a 9-month-old with gastroenteritis. Jamie's mother reports that he has had 10 or more greenish watery stools each day for the past 2 days.

a. Describe at least three major nursing diagnoses appropriate for Jamie at this time.

b. State at least one goal for each nursing diagnosis formulated.

c. Identify three nursing interventions for each goal.

6. Clinical situation: client teaching, ileostomy care
Ms. Bowen is a single, 35-year-old executive secretary with a prestigious law firm. One week ago Ms. Bowen had an ileostomy for treatment of inflammatory bowel disease.

a. Outline a discharge teaching plan for Ms. Bowen that reflects her developmental level and the nature of her bowel diversion. Include good health practices (foods, fluids, exercise, and comfort), self-concept, sexuality, and specifics about care of the ostomy.

7. Clinical situation: bowel training
James Hamet is a 48-year-old college professor with multiple sclerosis. Recently Dr. Hamet has had an exacerbation of his symptoms, including problems with bowel control. He has responded well to treatment and continues to have the ability to ambulate with the assistance of a walker. He is alert and oriented and hopes to return to work after his hospitalization. He is, however, extremely concerned about regaining bowel control. He reports that his office is near a bathroom, but that his classrooms are not always accessible to toilet facilities.

a. Describe and appropriately modify the components of a successful bowel training program based on Dr. Hamet's age, disease state, work environment, and developmental level.

SKILL AND TECHNIQUE ACTIVITIES

1. Obtaining stool specimens
a. Review your institution's procedures for obtaining the following stool specimens: guaiac stools, stools for ova and parasites, and fecal fat.
b. Obtain a Hemocult slide testing kit from your nursing laboratory and practice a guaiac test on your own stool sample.
2. Positioning for bowel elimination
a. In the nursing laboratory, practice the following maneuvers with a partner:
(1) Positioning on a regular bedpan using a hip-lift approach
(2) Positioning on a regular bedpan using a rolling technique
3. Enema administration
a. Review your institution's procedure for giving enemas.
b. In the nursing laboratory, or on the clinical unit, locate and examine the equipment needed to administer the following enemas: soapsuds, saline, and MGW.
c. In the nursing laboratory, using an appropriate mannequin or simulation model, practice administering a tap water enema. Have another student observe and critique your performance. Elicit an instructor's evaluation of your technique.
4. Ostomy care
a. Review your institution's procedure for ostomy care.
b. In the nursing laboratory, or on the clinical unit, locate and examine the equipment available for care of the client with an ostomy.
c. In the nursing laboratory, using an appropriate mannequin or simulation model, practice the following skills with a partner and have your instructor evaluate your performance:
(1) Skin and stoma care
(2) Pouching the ostomy
(3) Changing the ostomy pouch
(4) Irrigating the colostomy
d. Identify clinicians or experienced nurses in your health care setting with expertise in the care of the client with an ostomy. Determine the mechanisms for client and staff referral.

ADDITIONAL READINGS

Alterescu V: The ostomy, what do you teach the patient? *Am J Nurs* 85:1250, 1985.
Discusses client education for the preoperative and postoperative ostomate. Presents information to include in a discharge plan, including common "do's and don'ts" and sample instruction sheets.
Bellan A: Coloplast-update on the conseal plug, *Ostomy Internat* 11(2):15, 1990.
Describes the use of the new disposable colostomy plug for achievement of stomal continence.

Brown MK, Everett I: Gentler bowel fitness with fiber, *Geriatr Nurs* 11(1):26, 1990.

Discusses the problem of bowel elimination associated with the aging process. Describes the role of fiber in minimizing the use of laxatives and cathartics.

Erickson PJ: Ostomies: the art of pouching, *Nurs Clin North Am* 22:311, 1987.

Describes practical approaches for the technique of pouching a stoma. Useful for students and experienced nurses. May be easily incorporated into discharge teaching plans.

Petillo MH, editor: Enterostomal therapy, *Nurs Clin North Am* 22(2):253, 1987.

Addresses, in a series of articles, urinary and intestinal ostomy therapy. Includes specific information about the management of urinary and intestinal ostomies. Discusses special topics applicable to ostomy clients, including developmental implication, psychosocial considerations, sexuality, and skin care.

Smith DB: The ostomy: how is it managed? *Am J Nurs* 85:1246, 1985.

Describes nursing interventions for ostomy management. May be readily applied to client education.

Watt R: The ostomy: why is it created? *Am J Nurs* 85:1242, 1985.

Describes conditions requiring an ostomy. Includes actual photographs and compares these with drawings depicting the specific surgical diversions created. Useful illustrations for client education.

Chapter 42
Safety

PREREQUISITE READING

Chapter 42, pp. 1430 to 1459

OBJECTIVES

Mastery of content in this chapter will enable the student to:

- Define selected terms associated with client safety.
- Describe how unmet basic physiological needs of oxygen, fluids, nutrition, and temperature can threaten a client's safety.
- Discuss methods to reduce physical hazards.
- Describe current methods to reduce the transmission of pathogens and parasites.
- Describe present methods of pollution control.
- Discuss the specific risks to safety related to developmental age.
- Describe the four categories of risks in a health care agency.
- State nursing diagnoses associated with risks to safety.
- Develop a care plan for clients whose safety is threatened.
- Describe nursing interventions specific to the client's age for reducing risks of falls, fires, poisonings, and electrical hazards.
- Describe methods to evaluate interventions designed to maintain or promote safety.

REVIEW OF KEY CONCEPTS

1. List five characteristics of a safe environment.

   a.

   b.

   c.

   d.

   e.

2. An individual's safety would be threatened by:
   a. lack of an adequate water supply.
   b. unrefrigerated fresh vegetables.
   c. atmospheric carbon dioxide.
   d. atmospheric humidity of 70%.

3. List three general measures to decrease physical hazards in the home.

   a.

   b.

   c.

4. Define pathogen.
5. Define parasite.
6. The process by which resistance to infectious disease is produced or augmented is _____ .
7. Which of the following would be considered a source of environmental pollution?
   a. Vehicle exhaust
   b. Flooding
   c. Rock concert
   d. All of the above
8. List four potential problems associated with sensory overload.

   a.

   b.

   c.

   d.

9. List five factors that influence a client's safety in the community.

   a.

   b.

   c.

   d.

   e.

10. The greatest risk of death from home accidents occurs in children:
    a. less than 5 years old.
    b. between 5 and 8 years old.
    c. between 9 and 12 years old.
    d. between 12 and 16 years old.

11. Accidents involving children are largely preventable through parental education. (True or false?)

12. The majority of childhood fatalities are associated with:
    a. accidental poisoning.
    b. accidents.
    c. congenital diseases.
    d. infectious diseases.

13. Information about safer sexual practices and birth control is appropriate to provide to the adolescent client. (True or false?)

14. Threats to an adult client's safety are frequently related to lifestyle habits. (True or false?)

15. Describe eight physiological changes that increase the risk of falls in the older client.

    a.

    b.

    c.

    d.

    e.

    f.

    g.

    h.

16. List the four major risks to client safety in the health care environment.

    a.

    b.

    c.

    d.

17. When an accident involving a client occurs, the nurse should do all of the following except:
    a. notify the attending physician.
    b. complete an incident report.
    c. document the incident and its effect on the client in the medical record.
    d. document in the medical record that an incident report was completed.

18. Incorrect administration of a medication to a client is an example of:
    a. a client-inherent accident.
    b. a procedure-related accident.
    c. an equipment-related accident.

19. List six electrical hazards that increase the risk of injury or fire.

    a.

    b.

    c.

    d.

    e.

    f.

20. The nurse experiences a small shock when unplugging a suction machine from a wall outlet. The nurse should:
    a. plug the machine back into the same outlet and unplug it again to determine whether the shock can be replicated.
    b. plug the machine into a different outlet to determine whether the shock was caused by a defective outlet.
    c. ignore the incident because the client no longer requires the suction machine.
    d. label the machine as defective and report the incident.

21. List four signs that could indicate potential depression in the school-age child.

    a.

    b.

    c.

    d.

22. Select the nursing intervention that best promotes safety in a hospitalized toddler.
    a. Provide child-size knife, fork, and spoon at mealtime.
    b. Allow unattended bathtub play in less than 3 inches of water.
    c. Provide minature (matchbox) cars for group play.
    d. Cover electrical outlets with protective covers.

23. Describe five measures to reduce the risk of accidents in adolescents.

    a.

    b.

    c.

    d.

    e.

24. List the three most common injuries in the older adult.

    a.

    b.

    c.

25. List eight measures to prevent falls in the health care setting.

    a.

    b.

    c.

    d.

    e.

    f.

    g.

    h.

26. Mr. Brimford, an active 72-year-old, is admitted to the hospital for prostate surgery. He tells you he usually gets up to the bathroom at least twice each night. As a safety precaution the nurse should:
    a. apply a restraint jacket so he cannot get up at night.
    b. leave a night light on so he can see where he is going.
    c. insist that he use the urinal in bed instead of getting up.
    d. put the side rails up on his bed so he won't fall out.

27. List the four purposes for restraints.

    a.

    b.

    c.

    d.

28. Any restraint applied to a bedridden client should be secured to the:
    a. side rail.
    b. head board.
    c. bed frame.
    d. most easily accessible spot.

29. Restraints should be removed at least:
    a. every 30 minutes.
    b. every 60 minutes.
    c. every 2 hours.
    d. every 4 hours.

30. Mr. George is confused and frequently pulls out his peripheral IV. The restraint method most appropriate for this problem would be:
    a. jacket restraint.
    b. bilateral wrist restraint.
    c. mitten restraints.
    d. mummy restraint.

31. Short-term restraint of a small infant or child for treatments involving the head or neck is best accomplished by:
    a. jacket restraint.
    b. mummy restraint.
    c. mitten restraints.
    d. clove-hitch restraints.

32. Although Mr. Norton is confused at times, he enjoys sitting in a chair and watching the activity around him. To prevent Mr. Norton from falling out of his chair, the nurse can apply a(n):
    a. elbow or arm restraint.
    b. close-hitch restraint.
    c. mitten restraint.
    d. jacket restraint.

33. What is the best method for preventing falls in a confused client confined to bed?

34. Describe six fire containment guidelines.

    a.

    b.

    c.

    d.

    e.

    f.

35. List three nursing priorities when a fire occurs in a health care agency. Using an asterisk, identify which of the three should always take highest priority.

    a.

    b.

    c.

36. The electrical cord on a heating lamp has started to smoke. Which fire extinguisher would be most appropriate for controlling this type of fire?
    a. Soda and acid
    b. Water pump
    c. Antifreeze
    d. Dry chemical

37. Identify priorities in a fire using the acronym *RACE*.

38. When vomiting is indicated after accidental poisoning, the substance of choice for inducing vomiting is _____ .

39. The best initial action after accidental poisoning is to:
    a. induce vomiting.
    b. call the poison control center.
    c. administer serum of Ipecac.
    d. call 911.

40. If a client receives an electric shock, the nurse's first action should be to:
    a. assess the client's pulse.
    b. assess the client for thermal injury.
    c. notify the physician.
    d. notify the maintenance department.

CRITICAL THINKING AND EXPERIENTIAL EXERCISES

1. Accident prevention in children
   Complete the following table to identify methods to protect children from hazards located in their home and environment. For each injury, identify at least one safety precaution specific to each age group.

Injury	Age Group	Safety Precautions
Burns	Infant	
	Toddlers	
	Preschooler	
Falls	Infant	
	Toddlers	
	Preschooler	
Poisons	Infant	
	Toddlers	
	Preschooler	
Asphyxiation	Infant	
	Toddlers	
	Preschooler	
Motor vehicle accidents	Infant	
	Toddlers	
	Preschooler	
	School-age child	
Play	Infant	
	Toddlers	
	Preschooler	
	School-age child	

2. Clients at risk for hospital falls
   a. Using the risk for fall assessment tool in your text, complete an assessment on a selected client.

b. From the information gathered, indicate whether the individual is at high risk for falls. Discuss the factors that contribute to the identified risk.

c. Formulate nursing interventions that will prevent or minimize the client's risk of experiencing a fall.

3. Environmental safety assessment

   a. Perform an assessment of your home or residence to identify environmental hazards. Summarize your findings of safety hazards and potential solutions for each of the following areas:
      (1) Falls
      (2) Electrical safety
      (3) Fire
      (4) Toxic substances (poisoning)

   b. Perform an environmental assessment of your home and identify modifications that would be required if your environment included:
      (1) a 5-month-old infant.
      (2) an 18-month-old toddler.
      (3) a 4-year-old preschooler.
      (4) an 8-year-old school-age child.
      (5) an 88-year-old person who needs a walker for ambulating.

   c. Survey any health care setting to identify:
      (1) safety promotion activities being implemented.
      (2) actual or potential safety hazards.

   d. Share your observations with your instructor, and be sure to bring any hazards to the immediate attention of your instructor or supervisor.

4. Adolescent safety

   a. Formulate a teaching session to present measures for adolescent accident prevention.

   b. Incorporate teaching strategies appropriate to the adolescent development level.

   c. Present the teaching session to a peer group (or audio tape or videotape it) for evaluation.

   d. With your instructor as a resource, present this session to a selected group (for example, teenagers, parents of teenagers, or teachers).

5. Accident prevention for the older adult

   a. Select one of the three accidents responsible for the majority of injuries in the older adult population: falls, automobile accidents, or burns.

   b. Develop a teaching tool (paper, chart, pamphlet, or booklet) focusing on one of these three areas.

   c. Submit your teaching tool to your instructor for feedback.

   d. Use your tool in presenting a safety session to a population of older adult clients in the community (or families or health care providers who work with the older adult population in the community).

6. Clinical situation: application of restraints
   Mrs. Ferris is a 70-year-old woman who recently sustained a fractured femur. After surgery to repair the fracture, Mrs. Ferris is restless, confused, and picking at her IV site.

   a. What factors must be considered before applying any type of restraint on Mrs. Ferris?

   b. If a decision is made to restrain Mrs. Ferris, what guidelines must be followed? (Include the rationale for the nursing actions taken.)

   c. What type of restraint might be appropriate for Mrs. Ferris? Why?

   d. If the situation is presenting a hazard to Mrs. Ferris' safety and the nurse is unable to immediately obtain a physician's order before applying restraints, what actions must be taken?

7. Clinical situation: fire containment
   Ms. Varga is a paraplegic. After entering her room, you smell smoke. Upon investigation, you realize that Ms. Varga has fallen asleep while smoking and that her mattress is smoldering.

   a. Describe the sequence of actions you would take. Include the rationale for each action.

   b. What type of fire extinguisher could be used to put out this fire?

8. Clinical situation: hospital falls
   During the night, Mr. Jackson, 74 years old, gets up to go to the bathroom. While in the bathroom, he slips and falls.

   a. List and describe four possible factors that could have contributed to this accident.

   b. State a nursing diagnosis (related to safety) that the nurse could include on Mr. Jackson's nursing care plan.

   c. List five nursing interventions and their rationale that may have prevented this accident.

SKILL AND TECHNIQUE ACTIVITIES

1. Application of restraints

   a. Review your institution's policies regarding the use of restraints.

   b. In the nursing laboratory, practice applying each of the following types of restraints to a partner (as client) in bed or in a chair:
      (1) Jacket restraint
      (2) Belt restraint
      (3) Extremity restraint (commercially prepared or clove hitch)
      (4) Mitten restraint

   c. In the nursing laboratory, practice applying each of the following types of restraints to an infant mannequin:
      (1) Mummy restraint
      (2) Elbow restraint

2. Fire containment

   a. Review your institution's fire containment policies.

   b. Identify your institution's methods for reporting a fire.

   c. Request an opportunity to have your institution's safety, security, or maintenance department review the use of fire extinguishers and fire hoses found in client care areas.

   d. Visit a client care area and locate each of the following:
      (1) Fire escape routes

(2) Oxygen and electrical outlet shutoff valves
(3) Fire alarm boxes
(4) Fire extinguishers or hoses

ADDITIONAL READINGS

Brower HT: The alternative to restraints, *J Gerontol Nurs* 17(2):18, 1991.

  Provides practical approaches for maintaining safety of the older adult. Useful for working with clients at home or in health care settings.

Cooper KL: Electrical safety: the electrically sensitive ICU patient, *Focus Crit Care* 10:17, 1983.

  Identifies electrical hazards present in the ICU. Emphasizes the physiological alterations present in ICU clients, placing them at even higher risk for injury.

Hernandez M, Miller J: How to reduce falls, *Geriatr Nurs* 2:97, 1986.

  Describes a program developed to decrease falls in geropsychiatric settings. Identifies common risk factors. Presents an assessment of a protocol for "fall precautions."

  Makes specific recommendations for nursing care to minimize risk of falls.

Hoffman Y: Surviving a child's suicide, *Am J Nurs* 87:955, 1987.

  Provides personal reflections on the loss of a child from suicide. Provides insights that may enhance care of families experiencing loss.

Jankin JK, Reynolds BA, Swiech K: Patient falls in the acute care setting: identifying the risk factors, *Nurs Res* 35:214, 1986.

  Describes retrospective chart review on hospitalized older adults to determine factors increasing the risk of client injury. Assists in determining clients at risk and modifying care to prevent client injury in the acute care setting.

Jones MK: Fire *Am J Nurs* 84:1368, 1984.

  Graphically describes the disaster inherent when fires occur in the health care setting. From data based on interviews with survivors, makes specific recommendations about appropriate nursing actions in this crisis.

Chapter 43
Mobility and Immobility

PREREQUISITE READING
Chapter 43, pp. 1460 to 1521

OBJECTIVES

Mastery of content in this chapter will enable the student to:
- Define terms associated with mobility and body alignment.
- Describe the roles of the skeleton, skeletal muscles, and nervous system in regulation of movement.
- Discuss physiological and pathological influences on body alignment and joint mobility.
- Identify changes in physiological and psychosocial function associated with mobility.
- Assess for impaired body alignment and mobility.
- State correct nursing diagnoses for impaired body alignment and mobility.
- Write nursing care plans for impaired body alignment and mobility.
- Describe the procedures for assisting a client to move up in bed, repositioning a helpless client, assisting a client to a sitting position, and transferring a client from a bed to a chair or a bed to a stretcher.
- Describe complete range of motion (ROM) exercises.
- Describe crutch safety.
- Evaluate the nursing plan for maintaining body alignment and mobility.

REVIEW OF KEY CONCEPTS

1. Define body mechanics.
2. The positioning of the joints, tendons, ligaments, and muscles while in a lying, sitting, or standing position is:
   a. body alignment.
   b. body balance.
   c. center of gravity.
   d. passive motion.
3. Define friction.
4. List two techniques that maximize body balance.

   a.

   b.
5. List the three systems responsible for coordinated body movements.

   a.

   b.

   c.
6. List four functions of the skeletal system.

   a.

   b.

   c.

   d.
7. Fractures associated with weight-bearing activities in clients with osteoporosis are _____.
8. Match the following terms with the most accurate description or definition.

Description

   a. Tissues connecting muscles to bone _____
   b. Connection between ribs and sternum _____
   c. Hip _____
   d. Nonvascular supporting connective tissue _____
   e. Tissue binding joints _____
   f. Connection between tibia and fibula _____
   g. Sacrum _____

Term

   1. Synostatic joint
   2. Ligament
   3. Cartilaginous joint
   4. Tendons
   5. Fibrous joint
   6. Cartilage
   7. Synovial joint
9. Muscle contraction that occurs when increased muscle tension results in shortening of the muscle is _____.
10. Muscle contraction that causes an increase in muscle tension without shortening the muscle is _____.
11. Posture and movement can be reflections of personality and mood. (True or false?)

200

12. The normal state of balanced muscle tension is:
    a. posture.
    b. muscle movement.
    c. muscle tone.
    d. balance.
13. Muscles that permit an individual to maintain a sitting posture are:
    a. antagonistic muscles.
    b. antigravity muscles.
    c. synergistic muscles.
    d. complementary muscles.
14. Awareness of the body's spatial position and muscular activity is _____.
15. Maintenance of balance is primarily achieved by the:
    a. cerebral cortex.
    b. proprioceptors.
    c. motor strip and spinal cord.
    d. cerebellum and inner ear.
16. Proper body mechanics is as important to the nurse's health as it is to the client's. (True or false?)
17. Which statement about the principles of body mechanics is correct?
    a. Equilibrium is maintained with least effort when the base of support is narrow.
    b. Lifting requires less force than pushing, pulling, or sliding an object.
    c. Stooping with hips and knees flexed and trunk in alignment helps to prevent back strain.
    d. The higher the center of gravity, the greater the stability of the nurse.
18. Match the following postural abnormality with the description provided.

Description

    a. Dorsiflexion, inability to invert foot because of peroneal nerve damage _____
    b. Hip instability with limited abduction of hips _____
    c. Increased convexity in curvature of the thoracic spine _____
    d. Medial deviation and plantar flexion of the foot _____
    e. Exaggeration of the anterior, convex curve of the lumbar spine _____
    f. Lateral curvature of the spine, unequal heights of hips and shoulders _____
    g. Inclining of head to one side in association with contraction of sternocleidomastoid muscle _____

Abnormality

    1. Lordosis
    2. Kyphosis
    3. Scoliosis
    4. Clubfoot
    5. Congenital hip dysplasia
    6. Foot-drop
    7. Torticollis

19. Mr. Moore has had a cerebrovascular accident (stroke) in the right cerebral hemisphere. The nurse would anticipate the Mr. Moore would have motor weakness or paralysis:
    a. on the left side of his body.
    b. on the right side of his body.
    c. bilaterally in the lower extremities.
    d. bilaterally in the upper extremities.
20. Disruption of bone tissue continuity is a _____.
21. List four conditions that may result in immobility.
    a.
    b.
    c.
    d.
22. List three objectives of therapeutic bedrest.
    a.
    b.
    c.
23. Young clients develop pronounced effects of immobility more quickly than older clients. (True or false?)
24. Immobility disrupts normal metabolism, as evidenced by:
    a. increased metabolic rate.
    b. increased anabolic processes.
    c. increased nitrogen excretion.
    d. decreased catabolic processes.
25. List at least two hazards of immobility for each area listed.
    a. Metabolic
    b. Respiratory
    c. Cardiovascular
    d. Muscular
    e. Skeletal
    f. Integumentary
    g. Elimination
26. Immobilization can lead to:
    a. emotional changes.
    b. intellectual changes.
    c. sensory changes.
    d. all of the above.
27. Match the following developmental stage with the most descriptive characteristics of body alignment and mobility.

Characteristic

    a. Tremendous but frequently uneven growth spurt _____
    b. Shift of gravity toward anterior and complaints of back pain _____

c. Decreased ROM and muscle mass _____

d. Spinal flexion and complete ROM _____

e. Swaybacked, broad-based gait with feet everted _____

f. Improved balance, coordination and fine motor movement _____

Stage

1. Infant
2. Toddler
3. School-age child
4. Adolescent
5. Pregnant woman
6. Older adult

28. List and briefly describe four major areas for assessment of client mobility.

a.

b.

c.

d.

29. For the nurse to accurately assess body alignment, the client must be standing. (True or false?)

30. Describe five objectives to be achieved during assessment of body alignment.

a.

b.

c.

d.

e.

31. List 10 goals appropriate for clients with actual or potential positioning and mobility needs.

a.

b.

c.

d.

e.

f.

g.

h.

i.

j.

32. List four criteria to be assessed before lifting a client or object.

a.

b.

c.

d.

33. How would you determine the maximum weight that is safe for you to carry?

34. Which of the following violates the principles of body mechanics and therefore could cause injury to the nurse when moving a client?

a. Standing with the feet together
b. Standing with the feet apart
c. Bending at the knees
d. Using body weight to assist with movement

35. In the following table, indicate the correct use for each positioning device listed.

Device	Uses
Pillow	
Footboard	
Trochanter roll	
Sandbag	
Hand-wrist splint	
Trapeze bar	
Side rail	
Bed board	

36. In an emergency, it would be acceptable to tie restraints to a side rail. (True or false?)

37. List three general guidelines to apply when positioning clients.

a.

b.

c.

38. Identify the unprotected pressure points associated with each position.

a. Fowler's
b. Supine (dorsal recumbent)
c. Prone
d. Side-lying
e. Sims'

39. Describe five general guidelines to apply in any transfer procedure.

a.

b.

c.

d.

e.

40. When a client experiences pain, it is best to provide analgesic medications:

a. before moving, positioning, or transferring.
b. after moving, positioning, or transferring.

41. List four areas for the nurse to consider to determine whether assistance is required when moving a client in bed.

a.

b.

c.

d.

42. Exercise in which the nurse moves each of the client's joints through its ROM are:
   a. active.
   b. passive.
43. In most situations, ROM exercises should be as active as the client's health and mobility allow. (True or false?)
44. Which principle about ROM exercise is correct?
   a. Passive ROM should begin 48 hours after the ability to move an extremity or joint is lost.
   b. Each movement should be performed twice during the exercise.
   c. Nurses should gently force a joint slightly beyond its capacity.
   d. Nurses should support the joint and extremity being exercised.
45. To maintain the functional position of the hand means that:
   a. the thumb is slightly adducted and the fingers are extended.
   b. the thumb is abducted and the fingers are extended.
   c. the thumb is slightly adducted and the fingers are slightly flexed.
   d. the thumb is abducted and the fingers are flexed.
46. Describe five steps to be taken by the nurse in preparing to assist the client to walk

   a.

   b.

   c.

   d.

   e.

47. When ambulating a client with hemiplegia or hemiparesis, the nurse should:
   a. stand on the unaffected side, holding the client's arm.
   b. stand on the affected side, holding the client's arm.
   c. stand on the unaffected side, with one arm around the client's waist and the other around the inferior aspect of the client's upper arm.
   d. stand on the affected side, with one arm around the client's waist and the other around the inferior aspect of the client's upper arm.
48. Mr. Taylor has left leg paralysis after a stroke. Which assistive walking device would be appropriate?
   a. Straight-legged cane
   b. Quad cane
   c. Lofstrand (forearm) crutch
   d. Axillary (wooden) crutch
49. Which guideline for ambulation with a single, straight-legged cane is correct?

   a. The cane should be kept on the weaker side of the body.
   b. The cane should be placed forward about 6 to 10 inches before moving the legs.
   c. The stronger leg should be moved forward first.
   d. The stronger leg should never be advanced past the cane.
50. Describe the appropriate measurements for axillary crutches.
51. List four crutch safety guidelines to be taught to clients before they are allowed to walk independently.

   a.

   b.

   c.

   d.

52. Match the crutch stance or gait with the most accurate description.

Description

   a. Weight is placed on the supported legs; the client places the crutches one stride in front and then swings to or through the crutches. The sequence is repeated.
   b. Weight is borne on the uninvolved leg and then on both crutches; the sequence is repeated.
   c. The crutches are placed 6 inches (15 cm) in front of and to the side of each foot.
   d. Each leg is moved alternately with each crutch so that three points of support are on the floor at all times.
   e. Each crutch is moved at the same time as the opposing leg, so crutch movements are similar to arm motion during normal walking.

Stance or gait

   1. Swing-through
   2. Two-point gait
   3. Three-point gait
   4. Four-point gait
   5. Tripod position

53. List the sequence of movement for ascending the stairs on crutches.
   a. Weight shifts from the crutches to the unaffected leg. _____
   b. The unaffected leg is advanced between crutches to the stairs. _____
   c. The client aligns both crutches on the stairs. _____
   d. Body weight is transferred to the crutches. _____
54. When descending the stairs while on crutches, the client moves the unaffected leg to the lower step before the crutches. (True or false?)

55. When preparing to sit in a chair while using crutches, the client:
    a. places the posterior aspect of the legs against the seat of the chair.
    b. holds both crutches in the hand on the same side as the affected leg.
    c. supports the body weight on the affected leg and crutches.
    d. all of the above.
56. Identify one to two nursing interventions to meet each of the following goals for the immobilized client.
    a. Maintain optimal nutritional (metabolic) state.
    b. Promote lung expansion.
    c. Prevent stasis of pulmonary secretions.
    d. Maintain patent airway.
    e. Minimize orthostatic hypotension.
    f. Decrease cardiac workload.
    g. Prevent thrombus formation.
    h. Maintain muscle strength and joint mobility.
    i. Maintain normal elimination patterns.
    j. Maintain usual psychosocial state.
57. Which statement regarding developmental changes and immobility is accurate?
    a. Immobility rarely influences normal development.
    b. Immobilized children should be placed with children of the same age who are also immobilized.
    c. Environmental stimuli should be minimized for older, inactive clients.
    d. Care plans for older clients may require more frequent ROM and position changes.

58. Orthostatic hypotension occurs when the client's blood pressure:
    a. increases by 15 mm Hg.
    b. decreases by 15 mm Hg.
    c. increases by 35 mm Hg.
    d. decreases by 25 mm Hg.
59. Immobilization can retard a child's intellectual development. (True or false?)
60. Elastic stockings should be removed at least twice per day. (True or false?)

CRITICAL THINKING AND EXPERIENTIAL EXERCISES

1. Principles of body mechanics
   From the following list, explain why each principle is important and identify clinical situations in which it may be regularly applied.
   a. Moving an object by pulling increases friction.
   b. A wide base of support increases stability.
   c. A lower center of gravity increases stability.
   d. The center of gravity passes through the base of support.
   e. A person should face in the direction of motion.
   f. A person should use more than one muscle group if possible.
2. Body alignment and mobility
   a. Using the guidelines provided in your text, perform an assessment of an assigned client or partner that includes the following:
      (1) Body alignment while standing
      (2) Body alignment while sitting
      (3) Body alignment while lying

Physiological effects	Client manifestations	Nursing interventions
Metabolic		
Fluid and electrolyte changes		
Bone demineralization		
Altered exchange of nutrients		
Altered exchange of gases		
Altered GI function		
Respiratory		
Decreased lung expansion		
Pooling of secretions		
Cardiovascular		
Orthostatic hypotension		
Increased cardiac work load		
Thrombus formation		
Musculoskeletal		
Decreased endurance		
Decreased muscle mass		
Atrophy		
Decreased stability		
Contracture formation		
Osteoporosis		
Skin		
Decubitus ulcer formation		

Physiological effects	Client manifestations	Nursing interventions
Elimination		
Renal calculi		
Stasis of urine		
Kidney infection		
Fecal constipation		
Fecal impaction		
Psychosocial		
Depression		
Behavioral changes		
Changes in sleep-wake cycles		
Decreased coping abilities		
Decreased problem-solving abilities		
Decreased interest in surroundings		
Increased isolation		
Sensory deprivation		
Developmental		
Increased rate of dependence		
Increased rate of loss of system functions		

(4) ROM
(5) Gait
(6) Exercise tolerance
  b. Summarize your findings.
  c. Formulate actual or potential nursing diagnoses based on your findings.
3. Therapeutic benefits of bed rest
  a. Discuss the physiological and psychological benefits (rationale for) therapeutic bed rest.
  b. Review the nursing Kardex from a selected client area. Identify clients on bed rest.
  c. Analyze information in the Kardex and medical record to determine the specific reason or reasons that bed rest was ordered for a particular client.
  d. Discuss the physiological and psychological benefits of bed rest expected for the identified client.
4. Multisystem effects of immobility
  a. Care for, assess, or review the medical records of a client for whom bed rest has been ordered.
  b. Using the table at left, identify the specific effects of immobility that the client is experiencing and formulate at least two interventions to control or correct the identified complication.
5. ROM
  a. Observe a client, family member, or friend performing ADLs.
  b. Formulate a two-column table, with one column reflecting the activity observed and the second identifying the ROM that is part of that activity (see the following example).

ADL	ROM
Nodding head "yes"	Neck flexion and extension

6. Clinical situation: nursing process for clients with altered mobility

Mr. Cobb is a 68-year-old retired train engineer. He has been hospitalized for total hip replacement. He has a history of degenerative arthritis that has resulted in limited ROM in his arms, hands, and both legs.

Mr. Cobb likes to be independent, but because of his limited mobility, he often finds this very difficult. His wife had been assisting him with his ADLs before his hospitalization.

Mr. Cobb's physician informed him that he will be confined to bed for at least 5 or 6 days after surgery. He will be able to be turned from his back to his unoperative side as long as a splint, designed to keep his leg in an abducted position, is in place.

Mr. Cobb is within normal weight limits for his age and height. He states that he would feel much better if he could be more independent. He is hoping that the surgery will enable him to be more mobile.
  a. Identify areas that will need to be considered to determine the number of persons required to safely move Mr. Cobb in bed.
  b. State three nursing diagnoses that would be related to Mr. Cobb's mobility.

  c. Formulate one goal for each nursing diagnosis.
  d. Formulate at least two nursing interventions and the rationale for each.
7. Clinical situation: nursing process for immobilized clients

Mr. Concord, a 62-year-old businessman, has been hospitalized because of a cerebrovascular accident (stroke). The stroke has resulted in right-sided hemiplegia and dysarthria (difficulty with clearly articulating words). The physician has ordered complete bed rest, a soft diet, stool softeners, and a physical therapy consultation.

Mr. Concord is very quiet and withdrawn. His wife visits him daily. She is very anxious for her husband to "get better" and is very attentive to his needs. You notice that Mrs. Concord frequently leaves her husband's bedside to go to the lounge to cry.
  a. Develop a list of nursing diagnoses related to Mr. Concord's immobility.
  b. Develop a nursing care plan based on the priority nursing diagnosis. (Include at least two goals and four interventions.)
  c. Describe at least two outcome criteria for evaluation of the care plan.

SKILL AND TECHNIQUE ACTIVITIES

1. Positioning in bed.
  a. In the nursing laboratory, practice positioning a partner in each of the following positions:
    (1) Fowler's
    (2) Supine
    (3) Prone
    (4) Lateral side-lying
    (5) Sims'
  b. After positioning your partner, evaluate the partner's body alignment, pressure points, and comfort level.
  c. When you have practiced these positions, elicit an instructor's evaluation of your partner's body alignment.
  d. In the nursing laboratory or on the clinical unit, identify positioning devices available in your institution. Practice using these devices when positioning your partner.
2. Assisting with ambulation
  a. In the nursing laboratory, practice each of the following with a partner as the client:
    (1) Preparation for walking
    (2) Ambulation
    (3) Lowering a fainting client to the floor
  b. In the nursing laboratory, with the assistance or supervision of an instructor, practice ambulation with each of the following assistive devices:
    (1) Walker
    (2) Single-legged cane
    (3) Quad cane
    (4) Crutches (tripod position, two-point gait, three-point gait, four-point gait, swing-to-swing-through)

    c. After you have practiced walking with an assistive device, teach another student to safely use the assistive device in the laboratory. If possible, spend part of a day ambulating with the device. Share your experiences and perceptions with other students and your instructor.

3. Assisting with exercise

    a. In the nursing laboratory, practice performing passive ROM on a partner. Attempt to put each joint on one side of the body through ROM. Switch places and have your partner perform passive ROM on you. Elicit an instructor's evaluation of your technique.

    b. Observe nurses caring for client in any health care setting. Identify active ROM that the nurse performs while caring for clients.

4. Lifting and moving

    a. In the nursing laboratory, incorporate good body mechanics as you practice each of the following techniques with one or more partners:

      (1) Pulling a client up in bed

      (2) Using a three-person carry

      (3) Moving a bed

      (4) Lifting a box

    b. Elicit an instructor's evaluation of your technique.

5. Transfer techniques

    a. In the nursing laboratory, practice each of the following techniques with a partner:

      (1) Assisting a client to a sitting position in bed

      (2) Assisting a client to a sitting position on the side of the bed

      (3) Assisting a client to transfer from the bed to a chair

      (4) Assisting a client to transfer from a chair to a bed

    b. Elicit an instructor's evaluation of your technique.

6. Application of elastic stockings

    a. In the nursing laboratory, measure a partner to determine the correct size of elastic hose to apply.

    b. Practice applying and removing an elastic hose without active assistance or cooperation of your partner (client). Keep in mind that often the client who requires elastic hose will be unable to assist in their application.

    c. Using the steps presented in your text, evaluate your own performance.

ADDITIONAL READINGS

Gordon M: Assessing activity tolerance, *Am J Nurs* 76:72, 1976.

    Provides guidelines for assessment before and during client activities. Analyzes the various parameters and their interpretation in relation to client activity tolerance.

Olson EV, editor: The hazards of immobility, *Am J Nurs* 67:799, 1967.

    A classic series of articles. Addresses the effects of immobility on each major body system. Includes the effect of immobility on metabolism and psychosocial equilibrium.

Rubin M: How bedrest changes perception, *Am J Nurs* 88:55, 1988.

    Describes alterations in sensory stimuli associated with bed rest. Discusses perceptual changes that commonly occur in clients on bed rest and suggests approaches to minimize altered perceptions.

Rubin M: The physiology of bedrest, *Am J Nurs* 88:50, 1988.

    Explores normal physiological respone to bed rest and its potential complications. Well referenced for additional reading.

Winslow EH, Weger TM: Progressive exercises to combat hazards of bedrest, *Am J Nurs* 80:440, 1980.

    Describes a progressive exercise program based on the needs of clients with cardiac disease. Presents normal, expected exercise responses and the signs and symptoms of more serious problems that indicate the need to stop or slow down exercise progression.

Chapter 44
Skin Integrity

PREREQUISITE READING
Chapter 44, pp. 1522 to 1551

OBJECTIVES
Mastery of content in this chapter will enable the student to:
- Define selected terms related to skin integrity.
- Describe the economic consequences of pressure ulcers.
- Describe four risk factors for pressure ulcer development.
- Discuss 10 contributing factors to pressure ulcer formation.
- Discuss the pathogenesis of pressure ulcers.
- List the four stages of pressure ulcer development.
- Complete an assessment for a client with impaired skin integrity.
- List nursing diagnoses associated with impaired skin integrity.
- Develop a nursing care plan for a client with impaired skin integrity.
- List appropriate nursing interventions for a client with impaired skin integrity.
- State evaluation criteria for a client with impaired skin integrity.

REVIEW OF KEY CONCEPTS
1. Define pressure ulcer.
2. Preventive measures for pressure ulcers need only be targeted to high-risk clients. (True or false?)
3. Name one of the tools for prediction of pressure ulcers and list its major assessment areas.
4. Define tissue ischemia.
5. A compensatory response to ischemia in which the tissues become reddened because of increased blood

   flow is _____ .
6. An area of localized edema associated with reactive

   hyperemia is _____ .
7. Abnormal reactive hyperemia may last up to 2 weeks after the removal of pressure. (True or false?)
8. List four risk factors for pressure ulcer development.

   a.

   b.

   c.

   d.

9. Describe why each mechanism contributes to pressure ulcer formation in the "at-risk" client.
   a. Shearing force
   b. Moisture
   c. Poor nutrition
   d. Anemia
   e. Fever
   f. Infection
   g. Impaired circulation
   h. Obesity
   i. Cachexia
   j. Age
10. Indicate the stages of pressure ulcer formation from the descriptions provided.
    a. Full-thickness skin loss with extensive destruction, tissue necrosis, or damage to muscle,

       bone, or supporting structures _____
    b. Loss of epidermis and/or dermis; similar to blister or abrasion; possible reddened surrounding

       area with or without serous drainage _____
    c. Nonblanchable erythema of intact skin _____
    d. Damage or necrosis of subcutaneous tissues that

       may extend to the fascia _____
11. Stage II pressure ulcers are potentially reversible. (True or false?)
12. List two areas of nutritional assessment integral to clients at risk for impaired skin integrity.

    a.

    b.
13. List four possible goals for the client at risk for pressure ulcers.

    a.

    b.

    c.

    d.
14. List at least 2 nursing interventions to minimize the pressure ulcer risk factors listed.
    a. Immobility
    b. Inactivity
    c. Incontinence
    d. Malnutrition

e. Diminished sensation, decreased mental status
f. Impaired skin integrity
15. Donut-shaped cushions help to reduce ischemia in clients sitting in a chair. (True or false?)
16. Hyperemic skin areas should be massaged to maximize blood flow and minimize tissue necrosis. (True or false?)
17. Which cleansing agent would be appropriate for pressure ulcer care when no necrotic tissue is present?
   a. Antiseptic agents
   b. Oxidizing agents
   c. Enzymes
   d. Dextranomer beads
18. The removal of necrotic tissue to allow healthy tissue to regenerate is:
   a. escharotomy.
   b. sloughing.
   c. debridement.
19. List three outcomes of care for clients with impaired skin integrity.

   a.

   b.

   c.

CRITICAL THINKING AND EXPERIENTIAL EXERCISES

1. Assessment for clients with impaired skin integrity
During a client care experience:
   a. Review the medical record of a hospitalized client. Identify risk factors and contributing factors for pressure ulcer formation.
   b. Conduct a physical assessment of the client. Using the Norton scale or the Braden scale, predict the client's risk for pressure ulcer development.
   c. Formulate nursing diagnoses appropriate for prevention or treatment of skin breakdown (pressure ulcers).
   d. Summarize your assessment and diagnoses and submit these to your instructor for feedback.
2. Care of clients with pressure ulcer
   a. During a client care experience, identify individuals who have pressure ulcers.
   b. In a discussion with your instructor and peers, compare the risk factors and contributing factors in each of these individuals. What factors are similar? What factors are different?
   c. Identify the pressure ulcer treatments being used for these clients. How are they similar? How are they different? What are the rationale underlying the treatment plans?
3. Nursing process for clients with pressure ulcers
Millie Boyken is 52 years old. She has had multiple sclerosis more than 30 years and is now totally disabled. She has contractures of the lower extremities and minimal range of motion in the upper extremities.

She requires assistance in all the activities of daily living (ADLs). She is frequently incontinent. She weighs 89 pounds and is 64 inches tall. On admission she had a 4-cm stage I pressure ulcer over her right scapula, a 2-cm by 4-cm stage III pressure ulcer over her left ilium, and a 5-cm by 7-cm stage IV sacral pressure ulcer.
   a. Identify nursing diagnoses related to skin integrity for this client.
   b. For each diagnosis, identify at least one outcome and four interventions directed toward improved skin integrity.
   c. How will you determine the type of treatment required for the ulcers? What care is appropriate for each ulcer?
   d. What type of mattress surface/therapeutic bed would you consider for this client? Why?

SKILL AND TECHNIQUE ACTIVITIES

1. Use of mechanical devices to prevent skin breakdown
   a. In the nursing laboratory or in the client care setting, identify the devices available in your institution to minimize the complications of immobility.
   b. In the nursing laboratory, examine and practice application or use of different mattress surfaces/therapeutic beds such as the egg-crate mattress, flotation pad, low-air-loss bed, oscillating support surface, air-fluidized bed, static air mattress, alternating air mattress, and water mattress. If possible, experience the mattress surfaces yourself.
   c. If possible, visit a clinical unit where you can observe special beds in use. Identify nursing responsibilities related to safe operation of these devices.

ADDITIONAL READINGS

Barnes SH: Patient/family education for the patient with a pressure necrosis, Nurs Clin North Am 22:463, 1987.
   Presents a plan for client and family teaching related to pressure ulcers.
Bergstrom N et al: The Braden scale for predicting pressure sore risk, Nurs Res 36:205, 1987.
   Provides criteria to evaluate clients at risk for pressure ulcer formation. Supports the reliability and validity of the tool, which permits early intervention to prevent or minimize the risk of pressure ulcers.
Jones PL, Lillman A: A three-part system to combat pressure sores, Geriatr Nurs 2:78, 1986.
   Describes a study at a large metropolitan hospital that included the development of an assessment tool for the identification of pressure ulcer risk. Discusses the protocol developed for treatment based on the identified stage of the pressure ulcer.
Mondous LA, editor: Pressure ulcers, Nurs Clin North Am 22(2):359, 1987.
   Through a series of articles, comprehensively addresses topics related to pressure ulcers, including etiology and prevention, nutritional support needs, assessment, treatment strategies, and supportive measures, client and family education, and current research.

Stonberg C, Petcock N, Myton D: Pressure sores in the home-bound: one solution, *Am J Nurs* 86:426, 1986.

Describes a study in which various home care techniques for pressure ulcer prevention were examined. Based on data obtained, makes specific recommendations for skin care and prevention of pressure ulcers in the homebound client.

Willey T: High-tech beds and mattress overlays: a decision guide, *Am J Nurs* 89:1142, 1989.

Provides practical, concise guidelines for determining the most appropriate therapeutic bed or mattress surface to promote comfort and prevent skin breakdown.

Chapter 45
Sensory Alterations

PREREQUISITE READING
Chapter 45, pp. 1552 to 1571

OBJECTIVES
Mastery of content in this chapter will enable the student to:
- Define selected terms associated with normal and altered sensory function.
- Differentiate among the processes of reception, perception, and reaction to sensory stimuli.
- Discuss common causes and effects of sensory alterations.
- Discuss common sensory changes that normally occur with aging.
- Identify factors to assess in determining sensory status.
- Describe behaviors indicating sensory alterations.
- Identify nursing diagnoses relevant to clients with sensory alterations.
- Develop a plan of care for clients with visual, auditory, tactile, speech, and olfactory deficits.
- Describe how a client's sensory alteration influences the nursing care approaches selected to improve sensory function.
- List interventions for preventing sensory deprivation and controlling sensory overload.
- Describe conditions in the health care agency or client's home that can be adjusted to promote meaningful sensory stimulation.
- Discuss ways to maintain a safe environment for clients with sensory deficits.

REVIEW OF KEY CONCEPTS
1. List the three functional components necessary for any sensory experience.

   a.

   b.

   c.

2. All sensory impulses that enter the nervous system:
   a. are received.
   b. are perceived.
   c. elicit a response.
   d. all of the above.

3. List seven factors that may influence sensory function.

   a.

   b.

   c.

   d.

   e.

   f.

   g.

4. Define sensory deficit.

5. A condition in which inadequate quality or quantity of stimulation impairs an individual's perception is known as _____.

6. List the three major types of sensory deprivation.

   a.

   b.

   c.

7. A condition in which there is a reception of multiple sensory stimuli that cannot be perceptually disregarded or selectively ignored is known as _____.

8. For each type of alteration associated with sensory deprivation, describe at least two associated symptoms experienced by the client.
   a. Cognitive
   b. Affective
   c. Perceptual

9. List three client groups at high risk for sensory alterations during hospitalization.

   a.

   b.

   c.

10. Complete the table by describing at least one assessment technique for the identified sensory func-

tion and one adult behavior that could indicate a sensory deficit.

Sense	Assessment technique	Deficit behavior
Vision		
Hearing		
Touch		
Smell		
Taste		
Position sense		

11. The adult with deafness:
    a. becomes more flexible in daily routines.
    b. shows greater independence than hearing adults.
    c. shows poor social judgment.
    d. prefers interaction with hearing adults.

12. The inability to understand or produce language is called _____.

13. A client who is unable to name common objects or express simple ideas in words or writing suffers from:
    a. expressive aphasia.
    b. receptive aphasia.
    c. global aphasia.
    d. mental retardation.

14. List five goals appropriate for clients with sensory alterations.

    a.

    b.

    c.

    d.

    e.

15. List four general measures to promote visual function.

    a.

    b.

    c.

    d.

16. List four ways to maximize residual hearing in an older adult.

    a.

    b.

    c.

    d.

17. All of the following interventions will enhance taste perception except:
    a. good oral hygiene.
    b. seasoning foods.
    c. chewing food thoroughly.
    d. blending or mixing foods.

18. Which nursing intervention would be appropriate for clients with hyperesthesia?
    a. Minimal use of direct touch
    b. Firm pressure when touching body parts
    c. Frequent back rubs
    d. Vigorous hair brushing

19. When ambulating a client with visual impairment, the nurse should:
    a. stand on the client's dominant side and grasp the client's arm.
    b. stand on the client's nondominant side, approximately one step behind the client, grasping the client's arm.
    c. stand slightly in front of the client, on the client's nondominant side, allowing the client to grasp the nurse's arm.
    d. stand on the client's dominant side slightly in front of the client, allowing the client to grasp the nurse's arm.

20. Painting the edge of a step with a bright color to prevent falls would be most helpful for clients with:
    a. reduced peripheral vision.
    b. color blindness.
    c. night blindness.
    d. altered depth perception.

21. All of the following communication methods would be appropriate for the client with aphasia except:
    a. allowing time for the client to respond.
    b. using short, simple sentences.
    c. speaking loudly and articulating clearly.
    d. using nonverbal clues.

22. Describe six communication methods appropriate for clients with hearing impairment.

    a.

    b.

    c.

    d.

    e.

    f.

23. An aphasic client should be considered intellectually impaired. (True or false?)

CRITICAL THINKING AND EXPERIENTIAL EXERCISES

1. Sensory deprivation
    a. Spend a limited time (for example, 1 hour) during which you experience a simulated sensory deficit. Select only one of the following sensory modifications for your experience:
       (1) Touch: wearing disposable latex gloves
       (2) Hearing: wearing earmuffs or plugging ears with cotton
       (3) Vision: wearing sunglasses covered with petroleum jelly or with a portion of the lenses covered with black construction paper

b. Be sure to have a partner who is not sensory impaired act as your monitor and ensure your safety.

c. After an hour (or sooner if you find this experience problematic) switch roles with your partner.

d. Summarize your perceptions of the experience and share them in a small-group discussion with peers or your instructor.

2. Assessment of sensory function

During a client care or observational experience, determine ways to evaluate the client's sensory function through your own observational skills. The goal is to determine how much information you are able to gather in the normal course of client care, without formal physical examination. Attempt to identify at least two observations for each of the sensory functions listed below.

a. Vision

b. Hearing

c. Touch

d. Smell

e. Taste

f. Position sense

3. Maintaining meaningful stimuli

a. During a client care or observational experience, identify at least three specific examples of environmental stimuli for each of the following areas:

(1) Meaningful stimuli present

(2) Stimuli to introduce

(3) Excessive stimuli present

(4) Methods to control excessive stimuli

b. Sit in any hospital area for 15 minutes. Avoid any interactions; you are there merely to experience the sensory stimuli present. If possible, close your eyes a moment to hear, more clearly, the activity around you. Share the nature of the stimuli, your perceptions, and the effect of the experience with a small group or your instructor. Identify how the activity may modify care you provide to clients.

4. Clinical situations: promoting sensory function

In each of the following situations, discuss nursing interventions that are needed to promote functioning of existing senses.

a. Mr. Abrams is reading his magazine by the light of a small bedside table. When the nurse says something to him about needing more light to read, he says he "can see just fine."

b. A 12-year-old girl is seen with a radio headset on. When the nurse is 10 feet away from the client, she can clearly hear the music from the radio headset. When the nurse calls the adolescent's name, she does not respond.

c. Mrs. James complains to the nurse about the tasteless hospital food. It has been noted in the medical record that the 80-year-old Mrs. James has very poor oral hygiene habits.

d. Mr. Gray has had to remain in bed for 3 days because of flulike symptoms. He cannot even get out of bed to go to the bathroom. Nursing interventions thus far have been limited to changing his position to prevent pressure sores. He is complaining of numbness in his extremities.

5. Clinical situation: nursing process for the client with sensory impairment

Mrs. Everett is an active 65-year-old woman who enters the hospital for eye surgery. The physician has indicated that Mrs. Everett will have bilateral eye patches for the first 24 hours after surgery and a left eye patch throughout her hospital stay.

a. What nursing interventions related to Mrs. Everett's sensory function would be appropriate during the preoperative period?

b. Develop a postoperative nursing care plan for Mrs. Everett that focuses on her sensory needs.

ADDITIONAL READINGS

Blanco KM: The aphasic patient, *J Neurosurg Nurs* 14:34, 1982.

Defines and classifies neurological communication disorders. Presents detailed comparison of expressive and receptive aphasia. Provides general nursing management and communication methods appropriate for aphasic clients.

Downs FS: Bedrest and sensory disturbances, *Am J Nurs* 74:435, 1974.

Describes a study in which healthy young adults experienced moderate social isolation for limited periods. Discusses distortions in sensory processes experienced. Makes recommendations to reduce sensory distortion associated with bedrest.

Kopac CA: Sensory loss in the aged: the role of the nurse and the family, *Nurs Clin North Am* 18:373, 1983.

Describes the effect of the hospital on clients who enter with a sensory loss. Identifies common problems of vision, hearing, touch, taste, and smell found in the older adult. Presents areas for assessment and specific interventions for sensory deficits. Identifies support of sensory function as an area for active family participation. Describes ways that family members can provide meaningful stimuli for sensory-impaired older persons. Can be applied to other clients with sensory loss.

Primental PA: Alterations in communication, *Nurs Clin North Am* 21(2):321, 1986.

Describes the neurophysiological effects of stroke on communication. Provides guidelines for the assessment and care of clients with aphasia, dysarthria, and right-sided hemisphere syndromes.

Rubin M: How bedrest changes perception, *Am J Nurs* 88:55, 1988.

Describes alterations in sensory stimuli associated with bed rest. Discusses perceptual changes that may occur in clients on bed rest and offers suggestions for approaches to minimize alterations in perception.

Walsh C: Common sense nursing care for the patient with poor vision, *RN* 49(10):24, 1986.

Provides practical guidelines for maintaining the safety and comfort of clients with visual impairment.

Chapter 46
Substance Abuse

PREREQUISITE READING
Chapter 46, pp. 1572 to 1597

OBJECTIVES
Mastery of content in this chapter will enable the student to:
- Define selected terms associated with substance abuse and chemical dependency.
- Discuss the general health risks related to the abuse of any substance.
- Compare and contrast physiological and psychological dependence.
- List nine major groups of drugs and substances and their signs and symptoms of intoxication.
- Describe several psychosocial causative variables in substance abuse.
- Describe the disease of chemical dependency and its progression.
- Discuss signs and symptoms of chemical dependency and physical, psychological, and social outcomes to the disease.
- Describe the typical course of substance abuse.
- State at least three special groups particularly at risk for substance abuse.
- Describe special assessment approaches for clients with substance abuse problems.
- List examples of nursing diagnoses related to substance abuse.
- List and discuss seven general types of interventions appropriate for substance abusers.
- Describe major characteristics of the evaluation process for nursing care of substance abusers.

REVIEW OF KEY CONCEPTS
1. Define substance.
2. Current research supports the hereditary nature of chemical dependency. (True or false?)
3. Differentiate among the meaning of the following: drug use, drug misuse, and drug abuse.
4. A condition in which an individual experiences withdrawal syndrome when a substance is abruptly stopped is:
   a. psychological dependence.
   b. physiological dependence.
   c. drug misuse.
   d. drug abuse.
5. An emotional reliance on a drug is _____ .
6. Define FAS.
7. Which statement concerning substance abuse is accurate?
   a. The majority of substance abusers come from lower socioeconomic levels.
   b. Knowledge of the dangers of abuse will prevent addiction.
   c. Continued abuse may be avoided through use of willpower.
   d. Once addicted to a substance, an individual will be addicted to that substance for life.
8. Match the pattern of alcohol and drug use with the description.

Pattern
a. Recreational use _____
b. Circumstantial use _____
c. Intensified use _____
d. Compulsive use _____

Description
1. Use of high doses of drugs or alcohol to the exclusion of other meaningful life activities
2. Use of drugs or alcohol inspired by the intent to obtain a specific effect within the context of a certain situation
3. Use of drugs or alcohol in social settings for the purpose of experiencing effects of the substance
4. Use of alcohol or drugs daily in small to moderate amounts; motivated by desire for relief from a problem or desire to improve or maintain a level of performance
9. Over-the-counter analgesics such as aspirin and acetaminophen may be abused. (True or false?)
10. All of the following statements regarding alcohol withdrawal are true except:
    a. signs and symptoms may occur within 6 to 12 hours after drinking has ceased.

b. respiratory depression and hypotension are common during withdrawal.
c. seizures and hallucinations may occur during withdrawal.
d. delirium tremens (DTs) may occur during the second to fourth day after drinking has stopped.

11. Describe the psychological effect produced by each of the substances listed.

Substance	Psychological Effect
Alcohol	
Sedatives-hypnotics	
Benzodiazepines (tranquilizers)	
CNS sympathomimetics	
Hallucinogens	
Marijuana	
Inhalants	

12. List two motivations that may explain why a person first misuses a substance.

a.

b.

13. List and briefly describe four major theories of substance abuse.

a.

b.

c.

d.

14. Define addiction.

15. The primary defense mechanism used by chemical dependents is:
a. suppression.
b. projection.
c. denial.
d. rationalization.

16. Children who grow up in homes with an alcoholic parent often:
a. are at high risk for abuse.
b. blame themselves for their parent's emotional neglect.
c. are at greater risk of becoming substance abusers.
d. all of the above.

17. Alcohol consumption by pregnant women may have adverse effects on the fetus even when the mother is not an alcoholic. (True or false?)

18. Briefly describe the nursing focus for each level of chemical dependency care listed.
a. Primary prevention
b. Secondary care
c. Tertiary care

19. List four goals of care appropriate for clients with chemical dependency.

a.

b.

c.

d.

20. Identify the three major goals of chemical dependence treatment based on the principles of Alcoholics Anonymous (AA).

a.

b.

c.

21. Removal of mood-altering chemicals from the chemically dependent person's body is _____ .

22. Rapid removal of mood-altering chemicals from a chemically dependent person's body may cause:
a. seizures.
b. DTs.
c. death.
d. all of the above.

23. Mr. Jones is an alcoholic. The most appropriate self-help group to assist his wife would be:
a. Alateen.
b. Al-Anon.
c. Alcoholics Anonymous.

24. List seven general interventions the nurse may use in assisting chemically dependent clients during their treatment program.

a.

b.

c.

d.

e.

f.

g.

25. Mr. North, a heroin addict who has undergone extensive rehabilitation therapy, is being discharged from the care unit. What are four forms of ongoing support that may be provided by the nurse?

a.

b.

c.

d.

26. The most appropriate goal of care for any individual with a chemical dependence would be to maintain long-term abstinence. (True or false?)

CRITICAL THINKING AND EXPERIENTIAL EXERCISES

1. Primary prevention of drug abuse
a. Select a specific developmental age group.
b. Identify conditions and situations predisposing persons in the developmental level to drug abuse.
c. Identify the types of substances most commonly abused by this population.

d. Identify community resources supporting substance abuse prevention in the selected population.

e. Formulate a developmentally appropriate teaching plan for the identified population. Share this teaching plan with your instructor. If possible, arrange to present this information to the target audience or your clinical group.

2. Clinical situation: substance abuse in special groups

One evening you are one of two registered nurses (RNs) working on a busy clinical unit. While you are taking your dinner break, one of your clients requests diazepam (Valium) for anxiety. Ms. Samuels, RN, reports that she administered the diazepam, but you assess that the client still is very anxious. You observe that Ms. Samuels appears slightly euphoric and that her speech is slurred.

a. What action should you take in relation to your client's anxiety?

b. What action should you take in relation to Ms. Samuels' behavior?

3. Clinical situation: nursing process for clients with chemical dependence

Mr. West is admitted to the hospital for evaluation and treatment of duodenal ulcers. The physician indicates that the ulcers are related to long-term alcohol abuse.

During assessment, Mr. West's wife tells the nurse that Mr. West has been fired from his job as a sales representative because of poor attendance, appearance, and belligerence with clients. She reports that lately Mr. West has not been eating and that most of the grocery money for family food purchases has been spent on whiskey and beer. Mr. West reports difficulty sleeping but denies more than occasional social drinking.

a. What interviewing techniques would be appropriate to use in obtaining accurate information from Mr. West? (If possible, role play this interview with another student, incorporating the interviewing techniques appropriate for the chemically dependent client.)

b. Describe at least four behaviors expected with alcohol abuse.

c. Describe at least four clinical manifestations that would be expected if Mr. West were to experience withdrawal syndrome.

d. Based on the information presented in the clinical situation and your understanding of chemical dependence, formulate nursing diagnoses appropriate for Mr. West.

e. Formulate at least three goals for Mr. West's care related to his chemical dependence.

f. For each area of nursing intervention, describe actions appropriate for Mr. West's care.

(1) Acute care period

(2) Verbal abuse to the hospital staff

(3) Family support

(4) Teaching and counseling

(5) Involvement in community programs (client and family)

ADDITIONAL READINGS

Adams F: Drug dependency in hospital patients, *Am J Nurs* 88:4767, 1988.

Describes approaches to the care of the chemically dependent client from initial interview through hospital discharge. Emphasizes the importance of health care team members' ongoing interaction and consistency in care. Includes a chart summarizing controlled substances, actions, medicinal use (if any), common effects, and withdrawal characteristics.

House MA: Cardiovascular effects of cocaine, *J Cardiovasc Nurs* 6(2):1, 1992.

Reviews the chemical action and metabolism of cocaine. Includes a detailed presentation of clinical manifestations of drug use and its clinical complications. Presents treatment protocols focusing on symptom management.

Hughes T: Models and perspectives of addiction: implication for treatment, *Nurs Clin North Am* 24(1):1, 1989.

Provides an overview of popular theories regarding chemical addictions and discusses implications for care derived from these theories.

Lawrence F et al: Admitting the intoxicated patient, *Am J Nurs* 84:617, 1984.

Describes the complex problems associated with the care of the intoxicated client. Explores characteristic behaviors and makes recommendations for effective strategies in working with intoxicated clients. Although the focus is on admission, strategies can be applied to any health care setting in which the nurse encounters intoxicated clients.

Powell A, Minick M: Alcohol withdrawal syndrome, *Am J Nurs* 88:312, 1988.

Overviews the pathophysiological basis of alcohol withdrawal syndrome. Describes the characteristic symptoms and common medical treatment. Discusses nursing interventions to promote client safety during withdrawal.

Throwe AN: Families and alcohol, *Crit Care Q* 8(4):79, 1986.

Explores the effect of alcoholism on the entire family. Discusses family responses often encountered by the nurse in the acute care setting and offers approaches for assisting them.

Tweed SH: Identifying the alcoholic client, *Nurs Clin North Am* 24(1):13, 1989.

Emphasizes the importance of assessment in all client care settings to identify alcoholism. Includes physiological, psychological, and behavioral manifestations.

Zahourek R: Identification of the alcoholic in the acute care setting, *Crit Care Q* 8(4):1, 1986.

Defines and describes the extent of alcoholism in the acute care population. Describes characteristic signs of chemical dependence and additional subtle signs of alcoholism. Details assessment strategies and selected tools and explores the psychodynamics of alcoholism. Includes interventions appropriate to the acute care setting.

Zerwekh J, Michaels B: Co-dependency: assessment and recovery, *Nurs Clin North Am* 24(1):109, 1989.

Presents the concept of co-dependency and its characteristic manifestations. Presents interventions in dealing with co-dependency.

Chapter 47
Surgical Client

PREREQUISITE READING
Chapter 47, pp. 1600 to 1651

OBJECTIVES
Mastery of content in this chapter will enable the student to:
- Define selected terms associated with care of the surgical client.
- Explain the concept of perioperative nursing care.
- Differentiate among classifications of surgery.
- List factors to include in the preoperative assessment of the surgical client.
- Describe how to correctly witness a client's informed consent for surgery.
- Demonstrate postoperative exercises: diaphragmatic breathing, coughing, turning, and leg exercises.
- Design a preoperative teaching program.
- Prepare a client on the morning of a scheduled surgery.
- Compare and contrast the actions and side effects of general, regional, and local anesthesia.
- Explain the nurse's role in the operating room.
- Describe the nurse's role in phase I and II recovery.
- Identify factors to include in the postoperative assessment of a client in recovery.
- Describe the rationale for nursing interventions designed to prevent postoperative complications.
- Explain the difference and similarities in caring for outpatient versus inpatient surgical clients.

REVIEW OF KEY CONCEPTS
1. Define perioperative nursing.
2. List the three major classifications for all surgical procedures.

   a.

   b.

   c.
3. Match the following surgical procedure classifications with the most accurate description.

Description
a. Extensive reconstruction or alteration in body parts _____
b. Minimal alteration in body parts, often to correct deformities _____
c. Surgery performed on the basis of the client's choice _____
d. Surgery necessary for client health but not an emergency _____
e. Surgery that must be done immediately to save a life or preserve a body part _____
f. Surgical exploration to confirm a diagnosis _____
g. Excision or removal of a diseased body part _____
h. Relief or reduction of the intensity of disease symptoms but procedure that will not produce a cure _____
i. Restoration of the function or appearance of tissues _____
j. Replacement of malfunctioning organs or structures _____
k. Restoration of function lost or reduced because of congenital anomalies _____

Classification
1. Palliative
2. Ablative
3. Emergency
4. Minor
5. Urgent
6. Major
7. Reconstructive
8. Constructive
9. Elective
10. Transplant
11. Diagnostic

4. Describe four nursing responsibilities during the preoperative phase.

   a.

   b.

   c.

   d.

5. Describe how each condition increases the risk associated with surgery.
   a. Bleeding disorders
   b. Diabetes mellitus
   c. Heart disease
   d. Respiratory infections
   e. Liver disease
   f. Fever
   g. Chronic respiratory disease
   h. Immunological disorders
6. Prescription drugs taken before surgery are automatically continued after surgery. (True or false?)
7. Explain why a client who smokes is at greater risk for pulmonary complications after surgery.
8. The client who habitually uses alcohol requires lower doses of postoperative analgesics to avoid excess CNS depression. (True or false?)
9. Which preoperative assessment parameter would be particularly important for clients anticipating spinal anesthesia?
   a. Level of hydration
   b. Self-concept
   c. Smoking habits
   d. Motor function
10. List and briefly describe three conditions that increase surgical risk.

    a.

    b.

    c.
11. A risk factor that can directly interfere with postoperative wound healing is:
    a. the use of preoperative antibiotics.
    b. smoking.
    c. low serum potassium levels.
    d. poor nutrient intake.
12. In an older client, surgery poses a risk because:
    a. there is a stiffening of the rib cage and reduced range of diaphragmatic movement.
    b. blood flow to the liver is reduced, increasing bleeding tendencies.
    c. the client has increased sensitivity to painful stimuli.
    d. the basal metabolic rate is increased.
13. Which preoperative diagnostic study would provide the most useful information about the risk of postoperative bleeding?
    a. Serum electrolyte analysis
    b. Complete blood count (CBC)
    c. Prothrombin time (PT) and partial thromboplastin time (PTT)
    d. Electrocardiogram (ECG)
14. Which preoperative diagnostic test would be most important for a client at risk for losing a large amount of blood during surgery.
    a. Type and cross match tests
    b. Sputum tests for culture and sensitivity

    c. Serum creatinine analysis
    d. Serum sodium analysis
15. List six goals appropriate for the care of the preoperative client.

    a.

    b.

    c.

    d.

    e.

    f.
16. The primary responsiblity for informing the client about the surgical procedure rests with the nurse. (True or false?)
17. A client's signature on a consent form means that:
    a. the client understands the procedure that will be performed.
    b. the physician is not liable for errors made during the procedure.
    c. the client has been informed about the procedure.
    d. the client has read the information on the consent form.
18. Which of the following clients would be able to give consent?
    a. A 24-year-old who is illiterate
    b. A 24-year-old who has just received a sedative
    c. A 78-year-old who has a nursing diagnosis of confusion
    d. A 16-year-old who lives at home with the parents
19. Describe the four ways in which structured preoperative teaching may influence a client's postoperative recovery.

    a.

    b.

    c.

    d.
20. The best time to initiate preoperative teaching is:
    a. the night before surgery.
    b. the day of surgery.
    c. a few days before surgery.
    d. after the preoperative orders are written.
21. Describe six of the criteria developed by the Association of Operating Room Nurses (AORN) that may be used in determining the client's understanding of the surgical procedure.

    a.

    b.

    c.

    d.

    e.

    f.

22. State the basic rationale that supports the performance of each of the following postoperative exercises:
    a. Turning
    b. Coughing
    c. Deep breathing
    d. Leg exercises
23. Briefly discuss the purpose of each of the following orders.
    a. NPO after midnight
    b. Shower with antimicrobial soap the evening before surgery
    c. Soapsuds enema the evening before surgery
    d. Dalmane, 15 mg PO, at bedtime (night before surgery)
24. Shaving the surgical site before surgery decreases the risk of postoperative infection. (True or false?)
25. An effective way to reduce postoperative wound infection is to keep the client's preoperative hospital stay short. (True or false?)
26. Why does the nurse complete a preoperative checklist?
27. List the 11 responsibilities of a nurse caring for a client the morning of surgery.

    a.

    b.

    c.

    d.

    e.

    f.

    g.

    h.

    i.

    j.

    k.
28. Match the purpose of nasogastric (NG) intubation with the correct description.

Description

    a. Removal of secretions and substances, relief of

        distention _____
    b. Instillation of liquid nutrients when the client is

        unable to swallow _____
    c. Internal application of pressure to prevent internal

        hemorrhage _____
    d. Irrigation of the stomach for active bleeding, poisoning, or gastric dilation _____

Purpose

    1. Lavage
    2. Decompression
    3. Gavage
    4. Compression
29. The NG tube of choice for gastric decompression is the:
    a. Miller-Abbott.
    b. Levin.
    c. Dobhoff.
    d. Salem sump.
30. The NG tube of choice for gavage is the:
    a. Dobhoff.
    b. Miller-Abbott.
    c. Salem sump.
    d. Sengstaken-Blakemore.
31. List nine pieces of equipment that should be present in the postoperative bedside unit.

    a.

    b.

    c.

    d.

    e.

    f.

    g.

    h.

    i.
32. During which stage of anesthesia does the surgeon perform the operation?
    a. Stage 1
    b. Stage 2
    c. Stage 3
    d. Stage 4
33. Epidural anesthesia is an example of which type of anesthesia?
    a. Local
    b. Regional
    c. General
    d. Nerve block
34. Which method of anesthesia is most commonly used for minor procedures in an ambulatory surgical setting?
    a. General
    b. Spinal
    c. Caudal
    d. Local
35. The circulating nurse in the operating room performs all of the following except:
    a. disposing of soiled equipment.
    b. keeping an accurate instrument count.
    c. helping reposition a client.
    d. handling the surgeon's surgical instruments.
36. Who is responsible for informing the family about complications arising from the surgical procedure?
    a. Primary nurse
    b. Recovery room nurse
    c. Anesthesiologist
    d. Surgeon

37. List six areas of assessment to determine the respiratory status of a postoperative client.

a.

b.

c.

d.

e.

f.

38. List three major causes of airway obstruction in the postoperative client.

a.

b.

c.

39. The preferred position for recovery of the postoperative client is:
   a. supine with head turned to the side
   b. side-lying with neck flexed forward
   c. side-lying with face down and neck extended.
   d. semi-Fowler's with neck extended.

40. Before removing an artificial airway in the recovering postoperative client, the back of the airway should be suctioned. (True or false?)

41. How soon in the recovery period should the client begin coughing and deep-breathing exercises?
   a. When responsive
   b. When fully awake
   c. When vital signs are stable
   d. When preparing to leave the recovery room

42. List four areas for assessment to determine a postoperative client's circulatory status.

a.

b.

c.

d.

43. In the table, describe the characteristic findings associated with postoperative hemorrhage.

Area of Assessment	Characteristic Finding
Blood pressure	
Heart rate	
Respiratory rate	
Pulse volume	
Skin	
Client behavior	

44. Which of the following could be signs of hemorrhage?
   a. Increased bloody drainage from an incisional drain
   b. Incisional dressings saturated with blood
   c. Swollen, tight incisional site
   d. All of the above

45. Signs of internal hemorrhage include:
   a. swelling of affected body part with elevation in blood pressure and pulse rate.
   b. swelling of body part with fall in blood pressure and elevation in pulse rate.
   c. presence of bloody drainage from wound with fall in blood pressure and pulse rate.
   d. fall in blood pressure, elevation in pulse, and appearance of bloody drainage on dressing.

46. Postoperative shivering is always a sign of hypothermia. (True or false?)

47. When assessing the client's level of consciousness on arrival in the recovery room, the nurse should first:
   a. apply a painful stimulus.
   b. touch or gently move a body part.
   c. call the client by name in a moderate tone.
   d. call the client by name in a loud tone.

48. What action would be appropriate if the client requires painful stimuli for arousal in the recovery room?
   a. Take no action for this expected response
   b. Notify the anesthesiologist
   c. Attempt to stimulate the gag reflex
   d. Increase the intensity of the pain stimulus

49. How would the amount of drainage from a surgical wound be estimated?

50. After anesthesia, return of voluntary control over urinary function may require up to 8 hours. (True or false?)

51. What is the minimum expected urine output in a catheterized post-operative client weighing 154 pounds?

52. Nausea in the Phase I postoperative client may be minimized by all of the following except:
   a. avoiding sudden movements.
   b. irrigating NG tube (if present).
   c. offering sips of water.
   d. preventing NG tube kinking (if present).

53. Mucus suctioned from airways should be included in the client's output measurements. (True or false?)

54. Pain can be perceived before the recovering client is fully conscious. (True or false?)

55. The preferred route for analgesic administration in the immediate postoperative period is:
   a. oral.
   b. subcutaneous.
   c. intramuscular.
   d. intravenous.

56. During which phase of postoperative care should the nurse initiate client teaching?
   a. Phase I
   b. Phase II

57. Describe five pieces of information that must be presented to postoperative ambulatory surgical clients before discharge.

a.

b.

c.

d.

e.

58. List nine criteria for evaluating recovery room discharge readiness.

a.

b.

c.

d.

e.

f.

g.

h.

i.

59. What task must the division nurse perform before the recovery room nurse leaves the client in the room?

60. A nurse may modify the frequency of ordered postoperative vital signs if the client appears normal during the initial assessment. (True or false?)

61. List four goals appropriate for the postoperative client.

a.

b.

c.

d.

62. The respiratory complication in which alveoli collapse and mucous secretions are retained is:
a. pneumonia.
b. pulmonary embolism.
c. atelectasis.
d. hypoxia.

63. Identify three nursing interventions for each of the following areas of need in the postoperative client.

Area of Need	Nursing Interventions
Maintaining respiratory function	
Preventing circulatory stasis	
Promoting normal bowel elimination	
Promoting adequate nutrition	
Promoting normal urinary elimination	

64. Wound dehiscence is characterized by:
a. an invasion of wound tissue by pathogenic microorganisms.
b. separation of wound edges at the suture line.

c. protrusion of internal organs and tissue through the incision.
d. inflammation, purulent exudate, and fever.

65. A postoperative client complaining of sudden chest pain with dyspnea, cyanosis, tachycardia, and hypotension is mostly likely experiencing:
a. pneumonia.
b. hypovolemic shock.
c. pulmonary embolism.
d. wound infection.

66. A clean surgical wound usually regains strength against normal stress within:
a. 24 to 48 hours.
b. 3 to 6 days.
c. 15 to 20 days.
d. 4 to 6 weeks.

67. Describe five measures to maintain a client's self-concept during the postoperative period.

a.

b.

c.

d.

e.

CRITICAL THINKING AND EXPERIENTIAL EXERCISES

1. Preoperative assessment
   a. Complete a preoperative assessment of an assigned client using a standardized or modified preoperative assessment tool.
   b. Based on the data elicited, formulate a list of nursing needs related to preoperative, intraoperative, and postoperative care.
   c. Identify the need for additional resources or referrals to assist the client during the perioperative period. With the assistance of your instructor or a co-assigned staff nurse, initiate the needed referrals.
   d. Formulate a preoperative teaching plan for the client, individualized to the client's unique characteristics or requirements.
   e. Before initiating your preoperative teaching plan, validate your interventions with a staff nurse or your instructor.

2. Preoperative diagnostic screening
   Complete the table describing common diagnostic tests for a preoperative client.

Diagnositc Test	Normal Values	Significance to the preoperative client
Urinalysis		
CBC		
Chemistry profile		
Chest x-ray film		
ECG		

3. Preoperative teaching

  a. If possible, arrange for an observational experience that encompasses the three phases of perioperative care. As you observe, attempt to identify all of the sensory experiences that the client would be exposed to in the course of a surgical experience (sight, sound, smell, touch, and taste).

  b. Outline a preoperative teaching plan for a client that addresses:

    (1) routine preoperative preparation.

    (2) perioperative sensory experiences.

    (3) prevention of postoperative complications.

    (4) return to normal or optimal physical functioning.

  c. Present the preoperative teaching plan to a peer for critique and feedback.

  d. Elicit instructor evaluation of your teaching plan before using it in an actual client-care situation.

  e. Implement the teaching plan and request client feedback before surgery and during the postoperative period.

  f. Care for the client during the postoperative period to evaluate the effectiveness of your teaching and its effect on the postoperative course.

4. Intraoperative anesthesia

  Complete the table.

	General Anesthesia	Regional Anesthesia
Vital sign changes		
Level of consciousness		
Nature of surgical procedure		
Postoperative nursing assessment		

5. Clinical situation: surgical risks

For each client situation, identify the risk factors for surgical complications and describe the physiological basis of the identified risk. Discuss nursing actions to minimize the risks identified. Describe conditions that assist in recovery.

  a. Mrs. Burns is a 36-year-old woman who previously had surgery for a benign tumor of the uterus. She is scheduled to have surgery for cancer of the colon after receiving a course of radiation treatments. Mrs. Burns smokes a pack of cigarettes daily and drinks only an occasional glass of wine when dining out.

  b. Mrs. Rush, a 78-year-old woman with a history of degenerative joint disease, is admitted for a total knee replacement. Although she experiences pain in more than one joint, she takes indomethacin (Indocin) and aspirin only for her knee pain. She is allergic to penicillin and shellfish. She is able to describe the procedure for replacing her knee joint and hopes that she will be able to walk again without pain. Mrs. Rush is 63 inches tall and weighs 150 pounds. Her family reports that she has at least two bourbon and soda drinks every evening before dinner and has a nightcap at bedtime.

  c. Mr. Gregory is a 50-year-old man who has been hospitalized for 7 days after an automobile accident. During this time, he has lost 15 pounds. He is receiving antibiotics for an infection from an abcess that developed in a wound suffered during the accident. Mr. Gregory is receiving intravenous fluids and has a Foley catheter in place. The surgeon is planning additional exploratory surgery to determine whether Mr. Gregroy has further internal injuries. Mr. Gregory has a history of hypertension and has been receiving hydrodiuril (Esidrex) and methyldopa (Aldomet) regularly for the past 3 years.

6. Clinical situation: perioperative client care

Mrs. Wilson, 43 years old, is scheduled for a cholecystectomy tomorrow. She is approximately 50 pounds overweight and smokes a pack of cigarettes every day. She has two children, 13 and 8 years. Her husband is supportive and will be present on the day of surgery.

  a. What special considerations will be involved in conducting Mrs. Wilson's preoperative teaching?

  b. Why will it be important for Mrs. Wilson to be able to cough frequently?

  c. List at least five topics the nurse should discuss with Mrs. Wilson's family in preparing them for her surgery.

  d. What steps should be taken with Mrs. Wilson on the morning of surgery in relation to:

    (1) her partial plate (partial dentures)?

    (2) her wedding ring?

    (3) her religious medal?

    (4) her shoulder-length hair?

    (5) her nail polish?

    (6) her complaints of thirst?

  e. Complete the following table, which outlines common postoperative complications and the related nursing care for Mrs. Wilson.

Complications	Preventive intervention	Rationale
Thrombophlebitis		
Nausea/vomiting		
Atelectasis		
Urinary retention		
Wound infection		

  f. Mrs. Wilson is experiencing acute incisional pain after surgery. Her incision line extends from the upper right abdominal quadrant and is approximately 12 cm (5 inches) long. Her dressing is intact, but she states that it feels as if it is pulling on the incision. A drainage tube containing bile secretions extends from the wound site to a drainage bag. Describe at least four specific interventions for promoting Mrs. Wilson's comfort.

g. Mrs. Wilson has just examined her incision for the first time and expresses concern about "how ugly it looks, especially with that nasty green drainage." Develop one goal, two outcome criteria, and four interventions to address Mrs. Wilson's alteration in self-concept.

SKILL AND TECHNIQUE ACTIVITIES

1. NG intubation and irrigation
   a. Review your institution's procedure for NG intubation and irrigation.
   b. In the nursing laboratory or in the clinical unit, examine the various NG tubes and related equipment used in your institution.
   c. Formulate a list of all the equipment needed to insert an NG tube. Locate this equipment on your clinical unit.
   d. In the nursing laboratory, using a demonstration mannequin or simulation model, practice inserting, irrigating and changing the tape on an NG tube while another student observes and critiques your performance.
   e. Elicit an instructor's evaluation of your technique for NG intubation and maintenance.

2. Preoperative client preparation
   a. Review your institution's policies regarding client preparation for surgery.
   b. Review policies regarding nurses' and student nurses' responsibilities in obtaining or witnessing informed consent.
   c. Obtain a preoperative checklist and review the tasks that must be performed to complete it correctly.
   d. Observe, assist, or provide care to a client before surgery. Identify care unique to the preoperative client. Compare the care provided to that described in your text. Share your perceptions with your instructor.

3. Perioperative experience
   a. If possible, schedule an observational experience involving preoperative, intraoperative, and postoperative (recovery room) client care.
   b. Identify the nursing roles unique to each of these settings.
   c. Identify specific sensory stimuli that the client encounters in each phase of the perioperative experience.
   d. If possible, schedule an observational experience in an ambulatory surgical care area. Compare the role of the nurse and the client experiences to those observed in an inpatient setting.

4. Postoperative exercises
   a. In the nursing laboratory, practice teaching and

performing the major postoperative exercises with a partner. Be sure to include methods of turning, coughing, deep breathing, and performing leg exercises.
   b. In the client care setting, with an instructor's supervision, provide preoperative teaching to a client that focuses on these postoperative exercises. Obtain feedback though demonstration and document the client's response to the teaching session.

ADDITIONAL READINGS
Other resources describing perioperative client care in relation to pain control, mobility, and wound healing can be found in Chapters 37, 43, and 48.

Blackwood S: Back to basics: the preop exam, *Am J Nurs* 86:39, 1986.
   Describes essential elements of the preoperative nursing assessment. Presents information in table form, summarizing areas to examine, examination techniques, and normal and abnormal findings.

Lepczyk M et al: Timing of preoperative patient teaching, *J Adv Nurs* 15:300, 1990.
   Describes a study revealing little difference in knowledge and anxiety levels related to the time of preoperative teaching. Provides direction for additional readings.

Lindeman C, VanAernman B: Nursing intervention with the presurgical patient: effects of structured and unstructured preoperative teaching, *Nurs Res* 20:319, 1971.
   A classic article, cited frequently in works related to patient teaching. Explores the influence of preoperative teaching on variables in the client's postoperative course.

McConnell, EA: *Clinical considerations in perioperative nursing: preventive aspects of care*, Philadelphia, 1987, Lippincott.
   Overviews the perioperative experience for nurses caring for surgical clients. Describes client needs from physical and emotional perspectives. Identifies nursing interventions specific to each phase of the perioperative experience directed toward prevention of complications and promotion of optimal recovery. Very useful for individuals unfamiliar with the perioperative experience.

McHigh NG et al: Preparatory information: what helps and why, *Am J Nurs* 82:780, 1982.
   Discusses client education before diagnostic or therapeutic procedures. Describes studies in which sensory information was found to be the most critical in preparing clients. Provides several guidelines to follow when giving clients preparatory information or initiating preoperative teaching.

Meeker MH, Rothrock JC: *Alexander's care of the patient in surgery*, ed 8, St Louis, 1991, Mosby–Year Book.
   Comprehensively addresses care of the client through all phases of the operative experience. An excellent reference frequently cited in nursing literature.

Wells N: The effect of relaxation on postoperative muscle tension and pain, *Nurs Res* 31:236, 1982.
   Presents a study revealing a reduction in pain distress for postoperative clients using relaxation techniques. Reinforces the importance of preoperative instruction about relaxation techniques to promote postoperative comfort.

Chapter 48
Clients with Wounds

PREREQUISITE READING

Chapter 48, pp. 1652 to 1696

OBJECTIVES

Mastery of content in this chapter will enable the student to:

- Define selected terms associated with wounds and wound care.
- Discuss normal stages of wound healing by primary intention.
- Describe complications of wound healing and their usual time of occurrence.
- Explain the factors that impair or promote wound healing.
- Describe differences in assessing a wound in a stable versus emergency setting.
- Conduct an assessment of a closed and open wound.
- Identify nursing diagnoses related to clients with wounds.
- Discuss principles of first aid in wound care.
- Explain nursing care implications in the use of dressings.
- Apply sterile dry or wet-to-dry dressings.
- Discuss the purpose of bandages and binders.
- Describe the effects of heat and cold on wound healing.
- Apply warm and cold applications safely to an injured body part.

REVIEW OF KEY CONCEPTS

1. Match the classification of wound type with the most accurate description.

Description

- a. Wound involving a break in the skin or mucous membranes _____
- b. Wound involving no break in skin integrity _____
- c. Wound resulting from therapy _____
- d. Wound occurring unexpectedly _____
- e. Superficial wound involving scraping by friction _____
- f. Wound involving a break in the epidermal, dermal, and deeper tissue layers _____
- g. Penetrating wound from the entry and exit of a foreign object through an internal organ _____
- h. Wound containing no pathogens _____
- i. Wound made under aseptic conditions but involving entrance into organs normally harboring microorganisms _____
- j. Closed wound caused by a blow to the body (a bruise) _____
- k. Bacterial organisms present in a wound site (greater than 10^5 organisms per gram of tissue) _____
- l. Wound containing microorganisms _____
- m. Tearing of tissues with irregular edges _____
- n. Wound condition in which the presence of microorganisms is likely _____
- o. Wound involving only the epidermal layer of skin _____

Type

1. Clean-contaminated
2. Unintentional
3. Open
4. Perforating
5. Infected
6. Closed
7. Laceration
8. Contusion
9. Intentional
10. Clean
11. Colonized
12. Contaminated
13. Superficial
14. Abrasion
15. Penetrating

2. A surgical wound such as an appendectomy incision is mostly likely to heal by:
   a. primary intention.
   b. secondary intention.
3. Which type of wound is most likely to heal by secondary intention?
   a. A cholecystectomy incision
   b. A laceration on a finger from a knife cut
   c. A scalp laceration that requires suturing
   d. A deep burn on a hand
4. List in sequence and briefly describe the four stages of healing by primary intention.

   a.

   b.

   c.

   d.
5. The cells responsible for cleaning a wound and preparing it for tissue repair are:
   a. neutrophils.
   b. macrophages.
   c. platelets.
   d. epithelial cells.
6. List at least four components necessary for fibroblast collagen synthesis.

   a.

   b.

   c.

   d.
7. When healing occurs by secondary intention:
   a. inflammation is more acute.
   b. tissue defects are filled with granulation tissue rather than collagen.
   c. collagen is an essential component in the process of wound contraction.
   d. connective tissue scarring is minimized.
8. A localized collection of blood under tissues is a _____ .
9. According to the Centers for Disease Control, what is the most important finding that indicates an infected wound?
   a. Purulent material draining from a wound
   b. A positive wound culture
10. Typically, a surgical wound infection develops around:
    a. the seventh postoperative day.
    b. the fourth or fifth postoperative day.
    c. the second or third postoperative day.
    d. within 24 to 48 hours.
11. Describe four signs and symptoms of wound infection.

    a.

    b.

    c.

    d.
12. Mr. Swan, an obese client, had abdominal surgery 2 days ago. After a severe bout of coughing, he calls for the nurse, stating that he feels "as though something has come loose under my dressing." The nurse observes Mr. Swan's wound; the sutures are intact, but there is an increase in serosanguineous drainage. What complication of wound healing could Mr. Swan be experiencing?
    a. Infection
    b. Dehiscence
    c. Evisceration
    d. Fistula
13. What action should the nurse take when a client's wound eviscerates?
14. An abnormal passage between two organs or between an organ the outside of the body is a _____ .
15. Which form of chronic fluid drainage would place the client at highest risk for skin breakdown?
    a. Urine
    b. Stool
    c. Pancreatic drainage
    d. Bile drainage
16. Define third-intention wound healing.
17. List the five nutrients needed for wound healing and describe their contribution to the healing process.

    a.

    b.

    c.

    d.

    e.
18. Describe how each factor impairs wound healing.
    a. Age
    b. Malnutrition
    c. Obesity
    d. Impaired oxygenation
    e. Smoking
    f. Steroids
    g. Antibiotics
    h. Chemotherapeutic drugs
    i. Diabetes
    j. Radiation
    k. Wound stress
19. List six areas for assessment of a wound in a stable setting (for example, after surgery or treatment).

    a.

    b.

    c.

    d.

e.

f.

20. Which wound description would most likely indicate a complication?
  a. Inflammation along the outer edges of the wound on the second postoperative day
  b. Bluish discoloration of tissue around the incision site
  c. Yellowish brown discoloration of the skin around the incision site
  d. Redness and swelling around wound edges on the seventh postoperative day

21. Fill in the correct term describing the characteristic type of wound drainage.
  a. Thick and yellow, green, or brown

  _____

  b. Clear, watery, and straw colored

  _____

  c. Pale, pink tinged, and watery

  _____

  d. Fresh bleeding _____

22. Before collecting a wound culture, the nurse first cleans the wound to remove skin flora. (True or false?)

23. Compare the techniques used to obtain an aerobic and anaerobic wound culture.

24. List six goals appropriate for the client with a wound.

  a.

  b.

  c.

  d.

  e.

  f.

25. List, in order of priority, the four first aid interventions for clients with a traumatic wound.

  a.

  b.

  c.

  d.

26. Application of pressure to an injury site in which the potential for blood loss is high fulfills which objective of wound care?
  a. Promotion of hemostasis
  b. Promotion of wound healing
  c. Prevention of infection
  d. Prevention of further trauma

27. Which wound type should be allowed to bleed to remove contaminants?
  a. Abrasion
  b. Laceration

  c. Contusion
  d. Puncture

28. Match the topical cleansing agent with the characteristics described.

Agent

  a. Povidone-iodine solutions (Iodophor) _____
  b. Dakin's solution _____
  c. Acetic acid solution _____
  d. Hydrogen peroxide _____
  e. Saline _____

Characteristic

  1. Effective against gram positive and gram-negative organisms; does not impact tissue healing
  2. Contains sodium hypochlorite and boric acid; must be diluted to avoid skin irritation
  3. Primarily used as debriding agent; no antimicrobial action; destroys granulation tissue
  4. Bactericidal; will not harm fibroblasts; antiseptic effect inactivated in presence of exudative wounds
  5. Maintains moist surface needed to promote development and migration of epithelial tissue

29. List six purposes of dressings.

  a.

  b.

  c.

  d.

  e.

  f.

30. List and briefly describe the purpose of each of the three layers of a surgical dressing.

  a.

  b.

  c.

31. When changing a dressing that adheres to a wound surface healing by primary intention, the nurse should:
  a. irrigate the dressing with warm tap water.
  b. gently pull off the dressing.
  c. moisten the dressing with sterile normal saline.
  d. leave the contact dressing in place and reinforce outer layers.

32. Which dressing type is most appropriate for wounds requiring debridement?
  a. Self-adhesive transparent film (second skin)
  b. Nonadherent gauze (Telfa)
  c. Hydrogel
  d. Wet-to-dry

33. What is the meaning of the the order, "reinforce dressing prn"?
34. List the four guidelines for the dressing-change procedure recommended by the CDC.

    a.

    b.

    c.

    d.

35. List four nursing actions appropriate in preparing a client for a dressing change.

    a.

    b.

    c.

    d.

36. To safely remove tape securing dressings, the nurse does all of the following except:
    a. gently pull the outer end parallel with the skin.
    b. pulls the tape in the direction of hair growth.
    c. apples light traction to the skin toward the wound.
    d. pulls the tape gently toward the wound.

37. The most effective antiseptic solutions for skin cleansing are:
    a. tincture of chlorhexidine (Hibiclens) and iodophors (Betadine).
    b. 70% alcohol and Betadine.
    c. chlorhexidine and peroxide.
    d. peroxide and 70% alcohol.

38. The nurse uses all of the following principles when cleansing a draining wound except:
    a. cleaning in the direction from the least contaminated area to the most contaminated.
    b. using gentle friction when applying antiseptics to the skin.
    c. irrigating from the least contaminated area to the most contaminated area.
    d. cleaning from a drain site toward the incision area.

39. List the three purposes of wound irrigation.

    a.

    b.

    c.

40. Irrigation of an open wound requires sterile technique. (True or false?)
41. Correct technique for wound irrigation includes:
    a. occluding the wound opening with the syringe.
    b. irrigating with the syringe tip in the actual drainage site.
    c. flushing the outer edges and contaminated areas first.
    d. using slow, continuous pressure to flush the wound.

42. Disposable gloves should be used to remove soiled dressings. (True or false?)

43. Threads or wires used to sew body tissues together are _____ .
44. Describe a drainage evacuator.
45. Soft, waferlike, plastic materials applied to the skin with adhesive to prevent drainage from interfering with wound healing are _____ .
46. List five purposes for the use of a binder or bandage.

    a.

    b.

    c.

    d.

    e.

47. Describe four nursing responsibilities that must be performed before applying a bandage or binder.

    a.

    b.

    c.

    d.

48. The nurse should have a physician's order before loosening or removing a bandage applied by a physician. (True or false?)
49. Using Montgomery ties to secure a dressing is advantageous because:
    a. pressure on the incision is reduced.
    b. skin irritation from frequent dressing changes is reduced.
    c. infection to the incision is reduced.
    d. drainage from the wound is reduced.

50. Identify whether heat (H) or cold (C) applications produce the physiological response described.

    a. Vasodilation _____

    b. Local anesthesia _____

    c. Reduced muscle tension _____

    d. Reduced cellular metabolism _____

    e. Increased capillary permeability _____

    f. Increased blood viscosity _____

51. List five conditions that increase the risk of injury from heat or cold applications.

    a.

    b.

    c.

    d.

    e.

52. List six factors that influence the body's response to heat and cold therapies.

    a.

    b.

c.

d.

e

f.

53. Describe the four areas to assess before applying heat or cold therapies.

a.

b.

c.

d.

54. Complete the safety chart describing "do's and don'ts" for application of heat or cold therapy.

Do's	Don'ts
a.	a.
b.	b.
c.	c.

55. Application of heat or cold requires a physician's order. (True or false?)

56. Moist heat:
   a. has less risk of burn to skin than dry heat.
   b. does not cause skin maceration.
   c. penetrates deeply into tissue layers.
   d. retains temperature longer.

57. Fill in the appropriate term for the heat or cold application described.
   a. Piece of gauze dressing moistened with a cool, prescribed solution _____
   b. Immersion of a body part in a warmed solution _____
   c. Immersion of the peritoneal area in warm fluid in a special tub, chair, or basin

      _____
   d. Exposure of superficial layers of the skin to a 40- to 74-watt light bulb _____

58. Identify the appropriate temperature for each of the following:
   a. Cold compresses or soaks
   b. Hot, moist compresses
   c. Warm soaks
   d. Aquathermic pads

59. A client has an inflamed area on the right forearm from an infiltrated intravenous line. The client states that there is considerable discomfort. The nurse should obtain an order for:
   a. warm, moist compresses.
   b. an Ace bandage.
   c. a Telfa dressing.
   d. ice compresses.

60. When wrapping an extremity, apply a bandage first at the proximal end and progress distally. (True or false?)

CRITICAL THINKING AND EXPERIENTIAL EXERCISES

1. Factors influencing wound healing
   a. Conduct a comprehensive assessment of an assigned client.
   b. Based on the data obtained, identify factors that would facilitate or inhibit wound healing in this client.
   c. For factors known to inhibit wound healing, identify nursing actions that could alleviate or minimize the client's risk.

2. Wound assessment
   a. With the assistance of a designated staff nurse or your instructor and the permission of clients, observe surgical or traumatic wounds of clients in the clinical setting.
   b. Formulate your own description of the wound using the following criteria.
      (1) Wound classification: status of skin integrity, cause, severity, cleanliness, and other descriptive qualities
      (2) Stable wound assessment: appearance, characteristic drainage, presence of drains, wound closure, pain, and cultures
      (3) Nature of healing (primary or secondary intention)
   c. Submit your description to your instructor for critique.

3. Clinical situation: wound care in the emergency setting

   You are on a camping trip with a group of friends. The group leader falls and sustains an 8-cm laceration on the right forearm on a jagged rock. The group leader is right handed. You are about a 2-hour hike away from the campground and a 4-hour drive from any health care facility.
   a. Describe each assessment area that you should evaluate related to the group leader's injury.
   b. Discuss the emergency care you would provide for the laceration. Include actions for each of the following areas:
      (1) Hemostasis
      (2) Cleansing
      (3) Protection

4. Clinical situation: application of heat and cold

   Ms. Claire is a 43-year-old teacher with a deep vein thrombosis in her left leg. The physician's orders include strict bed rest, leg elevation at all times, and aquathermic pad prn.
   a. What therapeutic benefits will an aquathermic pad have on Ms. Claire's condition?
   b. What factors would you assess before instituting the use of an aquathermic pad?
   c. What information will you present to Ms. Claire concerning:
      (1) the purpose of the treatment?
      (2) the symptoms she may experience with temperature exposure?
      (3) the precautions to take to prevent injury?

d. Which form of heat (moist or dry) would be preferable for Ms. Claire? Why?

e. What aquathermic pad termperature setting would be safe for Ms. Claire?

f. What schedule would you design for application and removal of the pad to optimize client comfort and therapeutic effect?

5. Clinical situation: nursing process for a client requiring wound care

Mrs. Tucker, a 48-year-old nurse, has been hospitalized for the past 3 weeks. Initially she was admitted for a cholecystectomy, but she developed several complications in the postoperative period.

At this time, she is being treated for multiple abscesses under her incision. She has severe skin breakdown around the incision line and drain sites. Her dressing must be changed every 3 to 4 hours because there is a large amount of purulent drainage.

Every time a nurse changes her dressing, Mrs. Tucker turns her face away and states that she "can't look at that ugly mess." Mrs. Tucker's appetite is steadily decreasing. She has asked her husband to not bring the children to visit.

a. Formulate a list of nursing diagnoses for Mrs. Tucker. Place them in order of priority.

b. Select the three priority diagnoses, and formulate a goal for each.

c. For each goal, identify at least one outcome criterion that will measure goal achievement.

d. For each goal, describe two nursing interventions and their rationale.

SKILL AND TECHNIQUE ACTIVITIES

1. Wound management

a. Review your institution's policies regarding wound care and dressing changes.

b. In the nursing laboratory or on the assigned clinical area, examine supplies and equipment used for wound management.

c. On the assigned clinical area, visit clients with traumatic or surgical wounds and observe the care that they receive. Compare the techniques for wound care and dressing changes used by the staff with those described in your text. If you note modifications in technique, attempt to determine the rationale or these changes. Discuss your analysis with your instructor.

2. Dressing changes

a. In the nursing laboratory, practice each of the following dressing techniques using a demonstration mannequin or simulation model while a peer observes and and critiques your performance.

(1) Removing a soiled dressing

(2) Cleansing a surgical wound with a drain in place

(3) Applying a dry, sterile dressing

(4) Applying a wet-to-dry dressing

(5) Irrigating a wound

b. Elicit an instructor's evaluation of your technique.

3. Special dressing applications

a. In the nursing laboratory, practice application of each of the following binders on a demonstration mannequin while a peer observes and critiques your performance.

(1) Abdominal binder

(2) T binder (single or double)

(3) Breast binder

b. In the nursing laboratory, practice application of each of the following on a partner:

(1) Arm sling (personally or commercially made)

(2) Elastic bandage (arm, leg, and head) to practice the various circling techniques described in your text.

4. Application of heat and cold

a. Review your institution's policies regarding application of heat and cold.

b. In the nursing laboratory or on the clinical unit, examine supplies and equipment used for heat or cold applications.

c. In the nursing laboratory, with an instructor's supervision, practice application of the following thermal treatments with a partner. Be sure to assess and initiate the actions with regard to client safety and therapeutic effect.

(1) Cold compress

(2) Heat lamp

(3) Warm soak

(4) Aquathermic pad

d. In the nursing laboratory or on the clinical unit, gather and set up the equipment needed to provide a sitz bath for a client.

ADDITIONAL READINGS

Other resources addressing related topics of aseptic technique, nutritional support, and surgical trauma are found in Chapters 18, 35, and 47.

Cooper D: Optimizing wound healing: a practice within nursing's domain, *Nurs Clin North Am* 25(1):165, 1990.

Emphasizes the importance of nurses understanding the healing process to provide informed, holistic care. Details the stages of the healing process and factors affecting healing. Briefly describes the ineffectiveness of current treatment modalities.

Cuzzell J: Artful solutions to chronic problems, *Am J Nurs* 85:163, 1985.

Identifies appropriate goals for chronic wound management. Describes selected wound-care techniques appropriate for specific types of wounds and the rationale for their use. Analyzes the pros and cons of the various wound care techniques described.

Garvin G: Wound healing in pediatrics, *Nurs Clin North Am* 25(1):181, 1990.

Comprehensive presentation of the physiological and psychological differences in the pediatric client and the influence of these on the healing process. Describes specific macronutrients and micronutrients necessary for wound healing in pediatric clients.

Hotter AN: Wound healing and immunocompromise, *Nurs Clin North Am* 25(1):193, 1990.

Describes basic concepts of immunity related to stages of wound healing. Explores common problems influencing resistance to infection and wound healing. Presents nursing interventions to promote wound healing.

Jones PL, Millman A: Wound healing and the aged patient, *Nurs Clin North Am,* 25(1):263, 1990.

Presents physiological changes accompanying the aging process. Explores physical and emotional care to optimize wound healing in this high-risk population.

Young M: Malnutrition and wound healing, *Heart Lung* 17(1):60, 1988.

Discusses stages of wound healing and nutritional requirements necessary for normal healing. Overviews causes and physiological effect of malnutrition. Includes assessment criteria for identifying the client at high risk. Discusses nutritional support for the postoperative client.

Answers to Review of Key Concepts

NB: number in parentheses refers to page on which concept is presented

CHAPTER 1

1. According to ICN: profession that assists an individual to perform activities contributing to health, recovery, or peaceful death (4). According to ANA: profession concerned with diagnosis and treatment of human responses to actual and potential health problems (15). According to CNA: profession concerned with promotion, maintenance, and restoration of health; prevention of illness; alleviation of suffering; and ensurance of a peaceful death when life can no longer be sustained (15).
2. False (4)
3. True (4)
4. d (4,5)
5. a. 4 (6)
   b. 6 (6)
   c. 1 (7)
   d. 2 (6)
   e. 3 (6)
   f. 5 (6)
6. Goldmark report (7)
7. Lysaught report (7)
8. Any seven (8):
   a. Guide research to establish empirical knowledge base for nursing.
   b. Identify area to be studied.
   c. Identify research techniques and tools that will be used to validate nursing interventions.
   d. Identify nature of contribution that research will make to advancement of knowledge.
   e. Formulate legislation governing nursing practice, research, and education.
   f. Formulate regulations interpreting nurse practice acts so that nurses and others better understand laws.
   g. Develop curriculum plans for nursing education.
   h. Establish criteria for measuring quality of nursing care, education, and research
   i. Prepare job descriptions used by employers of nurses.
   j. Guide development of nursing care delivery systems.
   k. Provide knowledge to improve nursing administration, practice, education, and research.
   l. Provide systematic structure and rationale for nursing activities.
   m. Identify domain and goals of nursing.
9. a. 5 (12)
   b. 7 (12)
   c. 6 (12)
   d. 3 (12)
   e. 4 (13)
   f. 8 (11)
   g. 2 (13)
   h. 1 (13)
   i. 10 (13)
   j. 9 (8)
10. Refer to table below (16):
11. True (16)
12. To prepare nurse clinicians capable of improving nursing care through advancement of nursing theory and sciences (16)
13. Any three (17):
    a. To improve and maintain nursing practice
    b. To promote and exercise leadership in effecting change in health care delivery systems
    c. To fulfill professional learning needs

	Length of Program	Educational Institution	Degree Granted	Program Focus
Associate degree program	2 years	College, junior college	AD	Theoretical and practical course related to nursing practice
Diploma program*	2-3 years	Hospital based	Diploma	Same as AD
Baccalaureate program	4 years	College, university	BSN, BScN, BS, BN	Same as AD but with courses in the social sciences, basic sciences, and humanities to support nursing theory

*In Canada the diploma programs are offered in community colleges or hospitals and are 2- or 3-year programs comparable to associate degree programs in the United States.

d. To help nurses become specialized in a particular area of practice

e. To teach nurses new skills and techniques

14. True (17)

15. Instruction or training provided by a health care agency or institution within the institution, designed to increase knowledge, skills, and competencies of nurses and other personnel (17)

16. Clinical ladder (18)

17. a. Establish standards of practice to serve as guidelines for providing care and criteria for evaluating care (18).

b. Regulate licensure and define scope of nursing practice (20).

c. Establish institutional/agency policies and procedures for nursing practice (21).

18. True (21)

19. Any three (21):

a. New disease entities

b. New forms of supportive therapy

c. Opportunistic infections associated with acquired immunodeficiency syndrome (AIDS)

d. Increased critical care technology

e. Increased frequency of organ transplantation

20. (22):

a. Increased number of older adults

b. Increased number of clients with chronic illnesses

c. Increased number of clients with functional impairments

21. Any four (22):

a. Health promotion

b. Health maintenance

c. Health education

d. Health management

e. Coordination and continuity of care in the community

22. a. Function with high level of independence; provide a variety of health-related services within a designated community (22)

b. Provide health education, care for clients with nonemergency illnesses, and make referrals for more specialized health care (22)

c. Develops programs to increase worker health and safety; treats nonemergency acute illness; provides first aid; in emergencies, provides immediate care and arranges hospital transport; and makes referrals to health resources (22)

d. Provide home-based nursing care, with particular attention to teaching the client and family to perform nursing activities.

23. a. Care giver (23)

b. Teacher (24)

c. Manager (23)

d. Comforter (23)

e. Rehabilitator (23)

f. Protector (24)

g. Decision maker (23)

24. Communicator (24)

25. a. 3 (24)

b. 7 (24)

c. 4 (24)

d. 2 (25)

e. 5 (25)

f. 1 (25)

g. 6 (25)

26. a. Physician (MD [doctor of medicine] or DO [doctor of osteopathy]) (25)

b. Physician assistant (26)

c. Physical therapist (26)

d. Occupational therapist (26)

e. Respiratory therapist (26)

f. Pharmacist (26)

g. Social worker (26)

h. Spiritual advisor (26)

27. a. A profession requires an extended education of its members and a basic liberal foundation; nursing requires that its members possess an appropriate education incorporating current scientific and technological advances (27).

b. A profession has a theoretical body of knowledge leading to defined skills, abilities, and norms; several theoretical models of nursing serve as frameworks for nursing curricula and clinical practice (27).

c. A profession provides a specific service; nursing is a vital component of the current health care delivery system (27).

d. Members of a profession have autonomy in decision making and practice; nurses are taking on independent practice roles in various settings and regulate accountability through nursing audits and standards of practice (27).

e. The profession as a whole has a code of ethics for practice; nursing has a code of ethics that defines the principles by which nurses function (28).

28. a. American Nurses Association: to improve standards of health and availability of health care, to foster high standards for nursing, and to promote the professional development and general and economic welfare of nurses (28)

b. Canadian Nurses Association: to improve standards of health and availability of health care, to foster high standards for nursing, and to promote the professional development and general and economic welfare of nurses (28)

c. National League for Nursing: to improve nursing education, nursing service, and health care delivery in the United States (28)

d. ICN: to promote national associations of nurses, improve standards of nursing practice, seek a higher status for nurses, and provide an international power base for nurses (28)

e. National Student Nurses Association: to consider issues of importance to nursing students and often cooperate in activities and programs with the professional organizations (United States) (28)

f. Canadian Student Nurses Association: to consider issues of importance to nursing students and often cooperate in activities and programs with the professional organizations (Canada) (28)

29. Any four (28-29):
   a. Technological advances
   b. Demographic changes
   c. Consumer movement
   d. Health promotion
   e. Women's movement
   f. Human rights movement

30. Any three (30):
   a. Learn about social needs.
   b. Become activists in influencing policies to meet social needs.
   c. Contribute time and money to nursing, professional organizations, and political candidates.
   d. Become active in development of health care policies and practices.

31. A document supporting creation of a health care system ensuring access, quality, and services at an affordable cost. The plan focuses on primary health care services and the promotion, restoration, and maintenance of health (31)

CHAPTER 2

1. A dynamic state in which the individual adapts to changes in internal and external environments to maintain a state of well-being in all dimensions (39)
2. A person's ideas, convictions, and attitudes about health and illness (39)
3. Any three (39):
   a. Immunizations
   b. Adequate sleep patterns
   c. Adequate exercise
   d. Adequate nutrition
4. Any three (39):
   a. Smoking
   b. Drug abuse or alcohol abuse
   c. Poor diet
   d. Refusal to take prescribed medications
5. a. 2 (39)
   b. 4 (44)
   c. 5 (41)
   d. 3 (41)
   e. 1 (42)
   f. 6 (40)
6. d (41)
7. c (45, 46)
8. Health promotion activities (47)
9. Illness prevention activities (47)
10. d (47)
11. False (48)
12. Any seven (48):
   a. Smoking
   b. Nutrition
   c. Alcohol use
   d. Habituating drug use
   e. Driving

f. Exercise
g. Sexuality and contraceptive or barrier use
h. Family relationships
i. Risk factor modification
j. Coping and adaptation

13. a. 2 (50)
   b. 3 (50)
   c. 1 (49)
   d. 2 (50)
   e. 1 (49)
14. b (50)
15. Any two for each category (51):
   a. Genetic and physiological factors: pregnancy, obesity, and family history of diabetes mellitus, cancer, coronary disease, renal disease
   b. Age: Advancing age increasing risk of cardiovascular disease, cancer, birth defects, and complications of pregnancy; advancing age accentuating other risk factors already present
   c. Environment: prolonged exposure to chemicals or toxic wastes; air, water, or noise pollution; living in high crime areas; poor living conditions and overcrowding; and family conflicts and problems
   d. Lifestyle: negative health practices such as overeating or poor nutrition, insufficient rest and sleep, poor personal hygiene, smoking, alcohol or drug abuse, and involvement in dangerous activities (for example, skydiving); overexposure to the sun; and severe or prolonged emotional stress
16. False (53)
17. A state of diminished or impaired physical, emotional, intellectual, social, developmental, or spiritual functioning when compared with the person's previous experience (53)
18. b (53)
19. True (53)
20. False (53, 54)
21. Any five (55):
   a. Visibility of and familiarity with symptoms
   b. Person's perception of symptoms as serious (estimate of present and future risks)
   c. Person's information, knowledge, and cultural assumptions and understanding related to perceived symptoms
   d. Extent to which symptoms disrupt family, work, and social activities
   e. Frequency of appearance of symptoms and their persistence
   f. Extent to which others exposed to the person tolerate the symptoms
   g. Extent to which basic needs are denied due to illness
   h. Extent to which meeting other needs competes with illness responses
   i. Extent to which the person gives other interpretations to the symptoms
   j. Availability and physical proximity of treatment

resources; psychological and monetary costs of taking action (such as costs related to time and effort, stigma, social distance, and feelings of humiliation)

22. **a.** Stage 1: Symptom experience—person becomes aware something is wrong and acknowledges the presence of a health problem (55).
   b. Stage 2: Assumption of the sick role—person seeks confirmation of illness from family and social group and permission to be excused from normal duties and role expectations (56).
   c. Stage 3: Medical care contact—person becomes the client, seeking expert validation and treatment of illness (56).
   d. Stage 4: Dependent client role—client depends on health professionals for relief of symptoms and accepts care, sympathy, and protection from life's stresses and demands (56).
   e. Stage 5: Recovery and rehabilitation—client relinquishes sick role and resumes an optimal level of functioning or (with chronic illness) makes necessary adjustment to prolonged reduction in level of health and functioning (57).

23. False (57)
24. c (57, 58)
25. Body image (58)
26. Self-concept (59)
27. All four (58, 59):
   a. Type of change
   b. Adaptive capacity of client and family
   c. Rate at which the change takes place
   d. Supportive services available to client and family

CHAPTER 3

1. d (66)
2. Medicare (66)
3. Medicaid (66)
4. True (67)
5. a (67)
6. c (67)
7. Both responses (67)
   a. Escalating health care costs
   b. Availability of quality health care services
8. d (67, 68)
9. a (67, 68)
10. b (68)
11. Restoration of a client to normal or near-normal function after a physical or mental illness, injury, or chemical addiction (69)
12. a (69)
13. **a.** 2 (69, 70)
   b. 6 (72)
   c. 5 (73)
   d. 7 (73)
   e. 4 (70)
   f. 3 (74)
   g. 1 (74)
14. **a.** Extended care facility offering apartments or condominiums for relatively independent clients

in a partially protective setting; provides food service, laundry, social activities, transportation, emergency medical care, and nursing care; bridges gap between independent living and nursing home placement (71)
   b. Provides care and supervision, during the day, to specific client populations such as older clients or clients with emotional illnesses (72)
   c. Provides emergency psychiatric care and counseling to clients experiencing extreme stress or conflict, often involving suicide attempts or drug or alcohol abuse (73)
   d. Also referred to as a skilled care facility. Offers skilled care from a licensed nursing staff; services are usually covered by third-party payers (71)
   e. Often referred to as nursing home care. Provides 24-hour intermediate and custodial care to clients with chronic or debilitating illnesses (71)

15. a (75)
16. All five (75-77):
   a. Society and the consumer movement
   b. New knowledge and technology
   c. Legal and ethical issues
   d. Economics
   e. Politics
17. All three (77):
   a. Increased poverty, resulting in less preventive care: leads to more premature and low-birth-weight infants and increased infant morbidity and mortality
   b. Rapid increase in number of clients with AIDS and AIDS-related illnesses: results in much higher costs for care, which must be absorbed through public or private insurance
   c. Modern technology: results in better treatment for victims of accident and disease, increasing survival and life expectancy and creating greater cost to public and private sectors
18. False (77)
19. Informed consent (77)
20. **a.** 4 (79)
   b. 1 (79)
   c. 3 (80)
   d. 2 (80)
   e. 5 (80)
21. Any four:
   a. Cost control—Health care costs continue to rise as reimbursement for services declines; agencies are challenged to reduce costs without sacrificing quality care (83).
   b. Specialization—Advanced knowledge and technology have increased specialization in specific health care areas. Although specialization provides sophisticated care, care is often fragmented because no one provides care for the family or the person as a whole unit (83).
   c. Older adult population—Chronic illness most often affects older adults; as people live longer,

the number of clients with chronic disease increases and the quality vs. quantity of life issue becomes more prevalent (84).
d. Access—Although the United States spends a considerable percentage of the Gross National Product (GNP) on health care, a significant portion of the population has limited access to health care providers (84).
e. Quality—As public awareness about health care improves and statistics about health care system performance become available, facilities need to demonstrate positive client outcomes to maintain accreditation and government funding (84).

22. Any four:
a. Managed care and case management: allows one care giver to coordinate care from admission through discharge, facilitating multidisciplinary planning and enhancing the quality of services delivered (84-85)
b. National health care plan: provides all Americans with health insurance, financing health and illness care (87)
c. Nursing services: Nurses can provide services at a more reasonable, cost-effective, and qualitative level than other providers. Nursing, which focuses on preventive and primary care, can reduce costs associated with illness.
d. Gerontological care: Rapidly growing population of older adults requires specialized knowledge in maintaining health and optimal function. Gerontological nurses can provide primary care to this population and coordinate services to optimize care of the chronically ill or disabled older adult (88)
e. Quality improvement: provides a coordinated way to improve continually health care practices and services to guarantee favorable outcomes for clients (89)

CHAPTER 4

1. Interaction occurring when each person attempts to understand the other's point of view from each person's own cultural frame of reference (96)

2. Areas of commonalities (96)
3. a (97)
4. True (97)
5. Melting pot theory proposes that people of varied ethnic background are acculturated into the dominant culture while heritage consistency theory examines acculturation on a continuum of traditional and dominant cultures (97).
6. True (97)
7. Culture (98)
8. Ethnicity (98)
9. Religion (98)
10. Refer to table below:
11. All six:
a. Environmental control—ability of members to plan activities controlling nature or the environment (100)
b. Biological variation—unique physical and genetic traits (100)
c. Social organization—family units and group with which clients and family identify (100)
d. Communication—language differences, verbal and nonverbal behaviors and silence (100-102)
e. Space—personal space (behaviors and attitudes about space around self) and territoriality (attitude about an area claimed and response to encroachment by others) (103)
f. Time orientation—cultural tendency related to valuing time commitments (focusing on present or the immediate or long-range future) (103)
12. All four (103):
a. Intimate zone—extends up to 1½ feet; allows adults the most body contacts for perception of breath and odor, not acceptable in public places; visual distortions are also present (103).
b. Personal distance—extends from 1½ feet to 4 feet; extension of self (like having a "bubble" of space surrounding the body). At this distance, the voice can be moderate, body odors may not be apparent, and visual distortions may disappear.
c. Social distance—extends from 4 to 12 feet. The distance reserved for impersonal business trans-

Heritage Consistent	Heritage Inconsistent
a. Childhood development in country of origin or U.S. neighborhood of like ethnic group	Childhood development not in country of origin or like ethnic group
b. Frequent visits to country of origin or the "old (ethnic) neighborhood"	No visits to country of origin or "old neighborhood"
c. Family home in ethnic community	Family not in ethnic community
d. Individual raised in extended family setting	Individual not raised in extended family setting
e. Name not Americanized	Name Americanized
f. Educated in nonpublic school with religious or ethnic philosophy	Educated in public schools
g. Knowledgeable of ethnic culture and language	Not knowledgeable of ethnic culture or language
h. Participates in traditional religious or cultural activities	Does not participate in these activities
i. Incorporates elements of historical beliefs and practices into present philosophy	Does not incorporate these beliefs and practices into present philosophy

actions. Perceptual information is much less detailed.

d. Public distance—extends 12 feet or more; individuals interact impersonally; Communicators' voices must be projected, and subtle facial expressions may be lost.

13. The cause of illness within a belief system influenced by cultural, ethnic, or religious background (104)
14. a (100)
15. Folk medicine (104)
16. Traditional healers are aware of cultural and personal needs of the client and are able to understand the client in the context of personal problems in today's world (105).
a. Traditional healers maintain informal, friendly, affective relationship with entire family; physicians deal primarily with the client.
b. Traditional healers come to the house at any time; physicians usually see clients in an office or clinic. Traditional healers use a consultative approach during the diagnostic process by interacting with the head of the house and other family members, building rapport and expectation of cure.
c. Physicians deal primarily with the ill person, often dealing only with the person's illness and sometimes creating fear through an authoritarian manner.
d. Traditional healers are generally less expensive than physicians.
e. Traditional healers have rapport with the symbolic, spiritual, creative, or holy force; physicians are primarily secular, paying little attention to the religious beliefs of a client or the meanings that illness holds.
f. Traditional healers understand the lifestyle of the client, often speaking the same language and living in the same neighborhood or in similar socioeconomic condition; this may or may not be true of physicians.
17. False (106)
18. a. 3 (109)
b. 5 (111)
c. 2 (106)
d. 1 (108)
e. 4 (107, 108)
f. 5 (110)
g. 1 (109)
h. 3 (110)
i. 4 (107)
j. 2 (106)
19. b (111)
20. True (114)

CHAPTER 5

1. True (122)
2. Act included Patient Self Determination Act (effective December 1991). Requires clients to receive information about their rights to formulate advance directives such as living wills (124)

3. All four (124, 127):
a. Client and family understand diagnosis, level of function, discharge medications, and medical follow-up
b. Specialized training or instruction provided to the client and family for care after discharge
c. Community support systems coordinated
d. Relocation of client and coordination of support systems or transfer to another health care facility
4. Any six (124):
a. Lack of knowledge of treatment plan
b. Newly diagnosed chronic disease
c. Major surgery
d. Radical surgery
e. Prolonged recuperation from major surgery or illness
f. Social isolation
g. Emotional or mental instability
h. Complex home care regimen
i. Lack of financial resources
j. Lack of available or appropriate referral sources
k. Terminal illness
5. d (124)
6. False (127)
7. Client choosing to leave hospital against medical advice usually at risk for complications associated with premature discharge. Requires health professional to present all risks and inform client of possible outcomes. Requires completion of form with client signature releasing physician and hospital from legal liability (129)
8. The provision of medically related professional and paraprofessional services and equipment to clients and families in their homes (129)
9. To promote client and family independence through teaching of self-care (129)
10. a. Home health agencies—provide skilled, intermittent professional and home health aide services, which allows clients to live independently, usually with the help of family members; reimbursement is through government, private insurance, and private payers (132).
b. Private duty agencies provide professional and paraprofessional home health care services on a more continuous basis than is provided by home health care agencies; reimbursement is provided primarily by private insurance and private payers (132).
c. Durable medical equipment companies provide medical equipment and supplies; reimbursement is through government and private insurance, with stringent guidelines for determining amount of reimbursement (132).
11. Any four (132, 133):
a. Decreased hospital funding caused by changing government health care payment systems
b. Higher acuity level of clients at hospital discharge
c. Increased number of older and chronically ill clients
d. Advances in home health care technology

e. Breakdown of the extended family
f. More households requiring more than one source of income (fewer family members at home to care for older and disabled family members)
12. True (134)
13. All three (134):
    a. Insurance coverage
    b. Health care needs
    c. Family and home situation
14. Any five (135):
    a. Physical assessment and history of body systems with emphasis on present illness
    b. Psychosocial assessment
    c. Family dynamics
    d. Community resources
    e. Environmental factors
    f. Functional limitations
    g. Client and family knowledge and attitudes toward illness and health behaviors and the impact on lifestyle
15. False (135)
16. True (136)
17. c (137)
18. b (137-138)
19. Any three (139):
    a. Emphasis on preventive care and personal responsibility for health
    b. Managed health care systems and government pressure to meet needs of poor and catastrophically ill clients
    c. Growth of hospital-based agencies
    d. Expansion of computerization and high technology in home health care industry

CHAPTER 6

1. One of the following:
   a. A method for organizing and delivering care (146)
   b. A systematic method for assessing health status, diagnosing health care needs, formulating a plan of care, initiating the plan, and evaluating the effectiveness of the plan (147).
2. (146):
   a. Assessment
   b. Nursing diagnosis
   c. Planning
   d. Implementation
   e. Evaluation
3. (146):
   a. Planning
   b. Assessment
   c. Evaluation
   d. Implementation
   e. Nursing diagnosis
4. Observations or measurements made by the data collector, based on an accepted standard (150)
5. Clients' perceptions about their health problems (150)

6. d (150)
7. Any five (151):
   a. Client
   b. Family member or significant others
   c. Health team members
   d. Health/medical records
   e. Other records
   f. Pertinent nursing and medical literature
8. a (151)
9. All four (151, 154):
   a. Interview
   b. Nursing history
   c. Physical examination
   d. Results of laboratory and diagnostic tests
10. a (153)
11. a (153)
12. b (153)
13. a. Orientation phase—to familiarize the client, the nurse reviews the purposes for the interview, the type of questions that will be asked, the client's role in the interview, and the amount of time it will take; part of the orientation phase also involves spending a few minutes getting acquainted with the client (153).
    b. Working phase—the nurse asks specific questions to formulate a data base from which the nursing care plan will be developed; this involves use of interviewing techniques and communication strategies (154).
    c. Termination phase—the nurse provides direct clues that the interview will be ending and provides specific information about when there will be additional contact; it is important to ensure that the termination phase is positive and reflects concern for the client (154).
14. (154):
    a. 4
    b. 6
    c. 1
    d. 9
    e. 8
    f. 3
    g. 10
    h. 5
    i. 7
    j. 2
15. All four: To identify (155):
    a. Patterns of health and illness
    b. Presence of risk factors for physical and behavioral health problems
    c. Any deviations from normal
    d. Available resources for adaptation
16. False (156)
17. All of the following (157):
    a. Nature of the onset (sudden versus gradual)
    b. Duration (always present or intermittent and time seconds, minutes, or hours)
    c. Location of the pain

d. Intensity of the pain

e. Quality of the pain

f. Actions that precipitate the pain

g. Actions that make the pain worse

h. Actions that relieve the pain

18. Determines client's expectation of outcomes (cured, pain-free, or independent in self-care). Helps establish goals of care and expectations of self and the health care team. Gives information about the client's perceptions about illness or lifestyle changes (157)

19. The specific reactions that occurred (signs and symptoms) and the treatment (if any) that was given for the reaction (157)

20. Lifestyle patterns or habits may place the client at risk for a variety of diseases (157).

21. When possible, these aspects of the client's lifestyle may be incorporated into the nursing care plan (the nurse may also identify areas for education concerning positive health habits) (157).

22. b (158)

23. To verify information obtained during interview and collect further data, which are compared with the standards to determine whether the findings are normal or abnormal (158).

24. a. Auscultation (162)

b. Palpation (158)

c. Inspection (158)

d. Percussion (162)

25. Any two (162):

a. Verify alterations identified in the nursing health history and physical examination.

b. Provide baseline information about the client's response to illness and treatment.

c. Evaluate positive or negative outcomes of nursing or medical care.

d. Identify actual or potential health care problems not identified by the client or examiner.

26. Data validation (162)

27. Data clustering (163)

28. All three (162-163):

a. Consulting another source

b. Physical examination

c. Results of laboratory and diagnostic tests

29. True (163)

CHAPTER 7

1. A statement of the client's actual or potential response to a health problem that the nurse is licensed and competent to treat (172)

2. Part 1: the diagnostic statement; the client's actual or potential health problem or need that can be affected by nursing interventions (173)
Part 2: the etiology or cause: the reason for the client's health problem (represented by the phrase "related to") (173)

3. The etiology (represented by the phrase "related to") (173)

4. Refer to table (174):

	Medical diagnosis	Nursing diagnosis
Nature of diagnosis	Identification of disease condition	Statement of potential or actual health problem the nurse is licensed and competent to treat
Goal	Identify and design treatment plan for curing disease	Identify actual and potential client response
Objective	Prescribe treatment	Develop plan of care to enable client and family to adapt to changes resulting from health problems

5. (174):

a. Analysis and interpretation of data

b. Identification of general health care problems

c. Formulation of nursing diagnoses

6. The clinical criteria resulting from data clustering that supports the presence of the nursing diagnosis (174)

7. False (174)

8. False (177)

9. Any three (180-181):

a. Facilitates communication among nurses about client's level of wellness and discharge plan

b. Serves as a focus for quality assurance and peer review

c. Eliminates potential problems in giving care

d. Maintains a focus on meeting the client's health care goals

e. Helps to ensure high-quality care for clients and families

f. Promotes continuity of care

g. Promotes organizational skills used in charting

10. Any two (181):

a. Verbose and may contain jargon

b. Potential for incorrectly "labeling" a client

c. Confusion about the language of the diagnostic label

d. Not well understood by other health care professionals

e. Limited by the present taxonomy of nursing diagnoses

11. c (176-178)

12. d (176-178)

13. a (178-179)

14. b (178-179)

CHAPTER 8

1. (188):

a. Setting priorities

b. Determining goals

   c. Projecting outcomes

   d. Formulating the nursing care plan

2. (188, 189):

   a. 2

   b. 1

   c. 2

   d. 3

   e. 1

   f. 1

3. Specific statements of client behaviors or responses that the nurse anticipates from nursing care (189)

4. Both responses (189):

   a. Provides direction for individualized nursing intervention

   b. Provides way to determine effectiveness of interventions

5. c (189)

6. d (189)

7. Short-term goals are achieved in a short period (usually less than one week) and direct the immediate care plan. Long-term goals are achieved in the future (often address problem resolution after discharge) and tend to focus on prevention, rehabilitation, and health education (189).

8. Desired measurable behavior changes in the client in response to nursing care (189; other acceptable definitions: 189-190)

9. Any three (190, 191):

   a. Provide direction for nursing activities

   b. Provide observable client behaviors and measurable outcomes for each goal

   c. Provide a projected time for goal attainment

   d. Provide an opportunity to state any additional resources required

   e. Serve as criteria to evaluate effectiveness of nursing activities

10. All seven (191-192):

   a. Client centered: reflect expected client behaviors and responses to nursing care

   b. Singular factors: each addresses only one behavioral response

   c. Observable factors: desired outcome must be observable through interview or physical assessment

   d. Measurable factors: standard against which to measure client response; allows more objective quantification of client response

   e. Time limited: describes when expected response should occur

   f. Mutual factors: client and nurse agree on direction and time limits of care

   g. Realistic factors: allows short, realistic outcomes to provide a sense of accomplishment for client and nurse

11. b (189)

12. d (190)

13. c (190)

14. c (192)

15. d (193)

16. a (193)

17. False (193)

18. All three (194):

   a. Deliberation: review of client needs, priorities, and previous experiences for possible interventions

   b. Research: review of standardized care plans, texts, and nursing and related literature for problems and usual nursing actions

   c. Collaboration: interaction of nurse with client and other appropriate persons to individualize interventions

19. Any four (194):

   a. Document the client's health care needs

   b. Coordinate nursing care

   c. Promote continuity of care

   d. Provide outcome criteria for evaluation of nursing care

   e. Provide a means for communication with other nurses and health care professionals

20. a. Unique institutional format for writing and recording a nursing care plan; often involves the Kardex system (195).

   b. Forms created for a specific clinical area in which care is provided for a particular type of client; requires the nurse to individualize standardized form to the specific client; helps to conserve nursing time (195).

   c. An elaborate, detailed plan intended to teach care planning; includes scientific rationale for nursing actions (198).

21. b (198)

22. All four (199):

   a. What is the intervention?

   b. When should each intervention be implemented?

   c. How should the intervention be performed?

   d. Who should be involved in each aspect of the intervention?

23. c (199)

24. Both responses (200):

   a. When the nurse has identified a problem that cannot be solved using personal knowledge, skills, and resources

   b. When the exact problem in a nursing situation remains unclear

25. All six (200, 201):

   a. Identifying the general problem area

   b. Identifying the appropriate professional for consultation

   c. Providing the consultant with pertinent information and resources about the problem area

   d. Avoiding consultant bias by eliminating the nurse's subjective and emotional conclusions about the client and the problem

   e. Remaining available to discuss the consultant's findings and recommendations

   f. Incorporating the consultant's recommendations into the nursing care plan

CHAPTER 9

1. True (206)
2. Standing orders (206)
3. Protocol (206)
4. False (206)
5. (207):
   a. Identify all possible nursing actions.
   b. List all possible consequences associated with each nursing action.
   c. Determine the probability that the consequences will occur.
   d. Make a judgment based on the value of that consequence to the client.
6. a. Reassessing the client: a partial assessment focusing on a specific dimension (physical, psychological, spiritual, social, or cultural) or body system, with the purpose of gathering new data that can affect implementation or outcome of care (207-208).
   b. Reviewing and modifying the existing care plan: the client's status may change, requiring changes in the plan to provide appropriate nursing care (208).
   c. Identifying areas of assistance: to implement the care plan, the nurse may require certain types of assistance (additional personnel, additional knowledge, or additional nursing skills) (209).
   d. Implementing nursing interventions: activities requiring cognitive, interpersonal, and psychomotor skills directed toward achievement of the client-centered goals (210).
   e. Communicating nursing interventions: verbal interaction and written documentation concerning the need for nursing care (assessment data), the care plan, and the client's response to care (211).
7. All three responses (209,210):
   a. Additional personnel
   b. Additional knowledge
   c. Additional nursing skills
8. Any five:
   a. Assisting with activities of daily living (ADL): helping the client or performing for the client activities usually performed in the course of a normal day such as eating, dressing, bathing, oral hygiene, and grooming.
   b. Counseling: assisting the client in using problem-solving process to recognize and manage stress and other "normal" adjustment difficulties or enhance interpersonal relationships (211, 212).
   c. Teaching: presenting principles, procedures, and techniques of health care to the client and family, or providing information about the health status of the client and family (212).
   d. Giving care to achieve therapeutic goals: initiating interventions to compensate for adverse reactions, using precautionary and preventive measures in providing care, applying correct techniques in administering care and preparing the client for special procedures, and initiating life-saving measures in emergency situations (212-213).
   e. Giving care to facilitate client attainment of health goals: providing an environment conducive to attainment of health care goals, adjusting care in accordance with the client's needs, stimulating and motivating the client to achieve self-care and independence, and encouraging the client to accept care or adhere to the treatment regimen (214).
   f. Supervising and evaluating the work of other staff members: delegating appropriate nursing interventions to other health care team members; requires the nurse to ensure that the assigned team member is capable of performing and completing the task according to the standard of care (215).
9. True (215)

CHAPTER 10

1. The nurse's measurement of client response to nursing actions and the client's progress toward goal achievement (220)
2. True (220)
3. b (220)
4. (220)
   a. Examine goal statement to identify the exact desired client behavior or response.
   b. Assess client for that behavior or response.
   c. Compare the established outcome criteria with the behavior or response.
   d. Judge the degree of agreement between outcome criteria and the behavior or response.
5. b (221)
6. Expected outcomes are statements of the progressive, step-by-step responses or behaviors that the client needs to accomplish to remove or modify the etiology of the nursing diagnosis. The goal of care is a summary statement of behavior or response that indicates resolution of a nursing diagnosis or maintenance of a health state (222, 223).
7. a (223)
8. A planned systematic process for monitoring and evaluating the quality and appropriateness of client care and for resolving identified problems (226)
9. d (226,227)
10. a. 5 (228)
    b. 7 (228)
    c. 1 (227)
    d. 10 (229)
    e. 2 (228)
    f. 8 (229)
    g. 4 (228)
    h. 9 (229)
    i. 3 (228)
    j. 6 (228)

CHAPTER 11

1. (236):
   a. 2
   b. 5

  c. 3
  d. 4
  e. 1
2. All five (237):
  a. The investigation is planned and conducted in a systematic and orderly fashion.
  b. External factors not under direct investigation, which may influence the relationship among phenomena, are controlled.
  c. Empirical data are gathered directly or indirectly through human senses.
  d. The goal is to understand phenomena so that knowledge may be applied generally, not just to isolated cases or circumstances.
  e. Investigations are conducted to test or develop theories and thereby advance knowledge.
3. Systematic, controlled, empirical, and critical investigation of natural phenomena guided by theory and hypotheses about the presumed relationship among the phenomena (Kerlinger, 1986, cited 237)
4. Develops knowledge about health and health promotion throughout the life span, care of persons with health problems and disabilities, and nursing action to enhance the ability of individuals to respond effectively to actual or potential health problems (ANA Commission on Nursing Research, 1981, cited 237)
5. d (237)
6. (238):
  a. 4
  b. 7
  c. 2
  d. 6
  e. 5
  f. 1
  g. 3
7. a (238)
8. Quantitative research is concerned with information as statistics and with interpretation of statistical data. Qualitative research invites discovery of important characteristics and the way they might be related (239).
9. (239):
  a. 4
  b. 3
  c. 5
  d. 2
  e. 1
10. b (240)
11. Any five (240):
  a. Promote health, well-being, and ability for self-care among all health care consumers.
  b. Minimize and prevent behaviorally and environmentally induced health problems.
  c. Minimize the negative effects of new health technologies.
  d. Ensure that the care needs of particularly vulnerable groups are met effectively and acceptably.
  e. Classify nursing practice phenomena.

  f. Ensure that principles of ethics guide nursing research.
  g. Develop instruments to measure nursing outcomes.
  h. Develop integrative methods for the holistic study of people.
  i. Design and evaluate alternative models for delivering health care and administering health care systems.
  j. Evaluate the effectiveness of alternative approaches to nursing education.
  k. Identify and analyze historical and contemporary factors influencing nursing's professional involvement in national health policy development.
12. b (241)
13. True (242)
14. d (241)
15. c (243)
16. b (243)
17. d (243)
18. a (244)
19. c (245)
20. Any three (245):
  a. It should reflect something that could be improved in clinical practice.
  b. It should be a problem that occurs frequently in a particular client group.
  c. It should be able to be consistently and accurately measured.
  d. It should have the potential to change how nursing care is delivered.
  e. It may describe client phenomena (responses).
  f. It may assist in devising measurement tools for research (246).
21. All four (250):
  a. How much substantiating evidence is provided by other scientific studies that have yielded similar results?
  b. Were the subjects and environment in the study similar to those in which the nurse practices?
  c. What is the theoretical basis for present nursing care and its present effectiveness in solving clinical nursing problems?
  d. How feasible is it to apply the findings in the nurse's clinical setting based on ethical and legal limitations, institutional policy, changes in nursing services that might be required, and potential costs (personnel, time, money, and equipment)?
22. Half of what a nurse learns today may be out of date within 5 years. To remain current in nursing, it is important to develop skills to read and understand nursing research studies and to continue life-long learning (251).

CHAPTER 12

1. Personal belief about the worth of a given idea or behavior upon which a person acts; a standard that influences behavior (258)

2. Feelings about a person, object, or idea (258)
3. True (258)
4. b (258, 259)
5. All five (260):
   a. Modeling: individual learns to behave by observing action of others
   b. Moralizing: individual holds to a rigid standard of right and wrong prescribed by others
   c. Laissez-faire: individual acquires values informally through unrestricted behavior
   d. Responsible choice: individual is allowed choices in value selection in an environment that promotes freedom but that has specific restrictions
   e. Reward and punishment: individual is offered rewards for valued behavior and punishment for noncompliance with valued behavior
6. Responsible choice (260)
7. a (260)
8. c (261)
9. True (261)
10. All four (262):
    a. Caring must be viewed as an ultimate or overriding value to guide one's actions.
    b. Caring must be considered a universal value and, therefore, must be applied to all persons in similar circumstances.
    c. Caring must be considered prescriptive, in that certain behaviors (for example, empathy, support, compassion, and protection) are preferred.
    d. Caring must regard the needs of the people; it must consider the human flourishing of others and not just one's own welfare.
11. All seven (263):
    a. Altruism: concern for the welfare of other people
    b. Equality: having the same rights, privileges, or status
    c. Esthetics: qualities of objects, events, and persons that provide satisfaction
    d. Freedom: capacity to exercise choice
    e. Human dignity: inherent worth and uniqueness of an individual
    f. Justice: upholding moral and legal principles
    g. Truth: faithfulness to fact or reality
12. Values clarification (264)
13. (264):
    a. Choosing one's beliefs and behaviors
    b. Prizing one's beliefs and behaviors
    c. Acting on one's beliefs and behaviors
14. False (256)
15. Any one (265-266):
    a. Completing unfinished sentences—individual completes sentences that address certain values; through sentence completion, the individual explores attitudes, beliefs, interests, and goals that are indicators of values; completed sentences can be shared to enhance communication and affirm values.

b. Rank ordering—individual selects priorities among values listed; priority assignment assists in identification and affirmation of values held.
c. Health values scale: individual places 10 values in order of importance; the placement of health in the rank order assists in determining the client's value of health; when the nurse is aware of the value that the client places on health, a more effective client teaching plan may be developed.
16. Any three (267):
    a. Brief
    b. Selective
    c. Nonjudgmental
    d. Thought provoking
    e. Spontaneous
17. b (267-268)

CHAPTER 13

1. Study of principles or standards governing appropriate professional conduct (274)
2. One of the following (274):
   a. A situation in which there is a conflict in values and the person is unsure what constitutes proper conduct
   b. A situation in which a choice must be made between equally undesirable or unsatisfactory alternatives
3. d (274, 275)
4. c (275)
5. a. Self-determination (275, 278)
   b. Doing good (275, 280)
   c. Avoiding harm (275, 280)
   d. Treating people fairly (275, 280)
   e. Truth telling (275, 281)
   f. Keeping promises (275, 281)
   g. Respecting privileged information (275, 281)
6. Responsibility refers to the appropriate performance of duties associated with the nurse's particular role. Accountability means being answerable for one's actions. The nurse is accountable to self, client, profession, employer, and society (277).
7. c (278)
8. A law requiring that all persons receiving Medicare and Medicaid be given written information about their rights under state law to make decisions about medical care, including the right to accept or refuse medical or surgical treatment.
   Information, such as the right to formulate advanced directives (a living will) or to appoint someone to speak for the patient through durable power of attorney, must be provided at admission. This information must be documented and reviewed periodically (279).
9. d (280)
10. (282-283):
    a. Identify the important factors—list everyone involved in the decision-making process.

b. Presume good will—everyone involved is concerned with providing comfort and care.

c. Gather relevant and factual information—include preferences of the client, family systems, social considerations, daily life, planned medical intervention, community surroundings, care givers' input, and the "ideal picture" perceived in solving the dilemma.

d. State values (principles)—related to beneficence, nonmaleficence, and fidelity.

e. Rank values identified.

f. Take action based on the ranking.

11. a (283, 284)

CHAPTER 14

1. All three (292):
   a. Nurse practice acts
   b. Professional organizations
   c. Institutional policies
2. False (292)
3. True (293)
4. c (293)
5. (293):
   a. 3
   b. 4
   c. 1
   d. 2 (293)
6. Tort (293)
7. Carelessness or failure through action or inaction to meet appropriate nursing care standards, resulting in client injury (294)
8. (294):
   a. Nurse owed a duty to the client.
   b. Nurse did not perform the duty.
   c. Client was injured.
   d. Client's injury was a result of the nurse's failure to perform the duty.
9. Follow standards of care, give competent health care, develop empathetic rapport with clients, complete objective documentation, keep current with practice, and know and follow institutional policies and procedures (294).
10. False (294)
11. d (294)
12. b (294)
13. a (295)
14. b (294)
15. All four (296):
   a. Person giving consent must be mentally and physically competent and legally an adult.
   b. Person must give consent voluntarily.
   c. Person giving consent must thoroughly understand the procedures, risks, benefits, and alternatives.
   d. Person giving consent must have an opportunity to have all questions answered satisfactorily.
16. d (296)
17. False (296)
18. c (296)

19. Absence of brain function (297)
20. True (297)
21. True (298)
22. c (299)
23. To document the situation that was not consistent with good care and could actually or potentially cause injury; also used for institutional quality assurance and risk management (299)
24. To encourage health care professionals to assist in emergency situation by limiting liability and offering legal immunity, provided reasonable care was given (300)
25. True (300)
26. a (301)

CHAPTER 15

1. The complex, multifaceted, dynamic series of events that involves transmission of information or feelings between two or more people through the use of verbal and nonverbal behaviors (310)
2. (310):
   a. Intrapersonal: communication within the individual (self-talk).
   b. Interpersonal: communication between two people or a small group.
   c. Public: communication with large groups of people.
3. d (310)
4. **a.** Receiver (312)
   b. Feedback (312)
   c. Message (311)
   d. Channels (312)
   e. Sender (311)
   f. Referent (311)
5. b (312)
6. **a.** 4 (312)
   b. 2 (313)
   c. 1 (312)
   d. 3 (313)
7. Both verbal and nonverbal communication involve transmission of a message. Verbal communication uses spoken or written words. Nonverbal communication occurs through actions, without use of words (312, 314).
8. b (314)
9. b (313, 314)
10. Any five:
   a. Metacommunication (314)
   b. Personal appearance (314)
   c. Intonation (315)
   d. Facial expression (315)
   e. Posture and gait (316)
   f. Gesture (316)
   g. Touch (316)
11. Any five:
   a. Development—relates to neurological ability and intellectual development (312)
   b. Perceptions—individual's personal view of events (317)

c. Values—standards that influence behavior (317)
d. Emotions—subjective feelings about events (317)
e. Sociocultural background—cultural origin (318)
f. Gender—varied communication styles between men and women (318)
g. Knowledge: ability to understand words used (318)
h. Roles and relationships—societal expectation of behavior in specific situations (319)
i. Environment—setting in which communication occurs (319)
j. Space and territoriality—distances maintained by individuals during interaction (319)

12. False (310)
13. True (319)
14. d (319)
15. (319):
   a. Intimate distance: 18 inches or less
   b. Personal distance: 18 inches to 4 feet
   c. Social distance: 4 to 12 feet
16. a (319)
17. False (320)
18. Any four (320):
   a. Face the client while he or she is speaking.
   b. Maintain natural eye contact to show willingness to listen.
   c. Assume an attentive posture (avoid crossing legs and arms).
   d. Avoid distracting body movements.
   e. Nod in acknowledgment when client talks about an important point or looks for feedback.
   f. Lean toward the speaker to communicate involvement.
19. Any two:
   a. Listen without interrupting (320)
   b. Provide verbal feedback that demonstrates understanding (320)
   c. Be sure nonverbal cues match verbal communication (321)
   d. Avoid arguing, expressing doubts, or attempting to change the client's mind (321)
20. False (320)
21. b (321)
22. a. 4 (322)
   b. 1 (321)
   c. 3 (322)
   d. 2 (322)
23. Any four:
   a. Giving an opinion—takes decision making away from client, inhibits spontaneity and problem solving, creates doubt (323).
   b. Offering false reassurance—discourages open communication (324).
   c. Being defensive—suggests that the client has no right to an opinion, erodes client trust (324).
   d. Showing approval or disapproval—praise implies that the behavior is the only acceptable one; disapproval implies that the client must meet the

nurse's expectations, possibly making the client feel rejected (325).
   e. Stereotyping—inhibits uniqueness and oversimplifies the situation (325).
   f. Asking why—may be interpreted as an accusation, causes resentment, insecurity, and mistrust (325).
   g. Changing the subject inappropriately—displays rudeness and lack of empathy (325).
24. a (324)
25. Any four (324):
   a. There is hope
   b. The nurse is listening
   c. Care is available
   d. Certain undesirable changes can be expected
   e. The client will be treated like a persons
   f. The client's problem is understood
26. Relationship focusing on client needs and promoting a psychological climate to facilitate positive change and growth in the client (326)
27. All five:
   a. Trust—feeling that other individuals will be able and willing to assist (326).
   b. Empathy—ability to understand and accept another person and accurately perceive that person's feelings (326).
   c. Caring—having a positive regard for another person (327).
   d. Autonomy—ability to be self-directed (327).
   e. Mutuality—ability to share with another person (327).
28. Empathy is a fair, sensitive, and objective look at another person's experiences. Sympathy is subjective; it involves thinking or feeling as another person does. Empathy is therapeutic; sympathy is not (326).
29. a. 1 (328)
   b. 3 (330)
   c. 2 (329)
   d. 2 (329)
   e. 4 (332)
   f. 3 (330)
   g. 2 (329)
30. b (332)
31. Any two:
   a. Confrontation—nurse makes client aware of inconsistencies in behavior or thought (331).
   b. Immediacy—nurse focuses interaction on present situation, drawing attention to client's behavior or statements (331).
   c. Self-disclosure—nurse reveals personal experiences, thoughts, ideas, values, or feelings in the context of the relationship (331).
32. d (329)
33. b (328)
34. False (332)
35. d (334)
36. Any five (337):
   a. Pad and felt-tipped pen or magic slate

b. Communication board with words, letters, or pictures
c. Call bells or alarms
d. Sign language
e. Use of eye blinks or movements of fingers for simple responses
f. Flash cards with common words or phrases the client may use

37. Any three (337):
a. Regulating room temperature to a comfortable level
b. Eliminating or reducing loud noises in the room
c. Making the client comfortable
d. Asking other staff or family (if appropriate) not to enter the room during the interaction
e. Reducing bright or glaring light

38. d (338, 339)

39. Any three (339):
a. Be sure hearing aid is clean and inserted properly and has a functioning battery.
b. Adjust volume of hearing aid to a comfortable level.
c. Speak slowly and articulate clearly.
d. Stand in front of the client to provide opportunity for lip reading.
e. Talk toward the client's best ear.
f. Reduce background noise.

40. c (339)

41. False (339, 340)

CHAPTER 16

1. All three:
a. Maintaining health and illness prevention (348)
b. Restoring health (350)
c. Coping with impaired function (351)

2. An interactive process consisting of a deliberate set of actions that helps individuals gain knowledge or perform new skills (351)

3. Acquisition of knowledge or skills through reinforcement, practice, and experience (351)

4. True (348)

5. (352):
a. 2
b. 6
c. 3
d. 1
e. 7
f. 5
g. 8
h. 4

6. False (353)

7. a. Affective (354)
b. Psychomotor (354)
c. Cognitive (353)

8. All three:
a. Motivation to learn—the individual is willing to take action to become involved in learning (355)
b. Ability to learn—the individual has the physical, developmental, and cognitive capabilities necessary for learning to take place (358)

c. Learning environment—conditions supporting learning and interpersonal communication exist in the learning setting (358)

9. c (355, 356)

10. b (355)

11. Client fulfills the prescribed course of therapy (356).

12. All four (356):
a. Person believes there is a susceptibility to the disease in question
b. Person believes there would be serious effects on life or lifestyle
c. Person believes that actions can be taken to reduce the chance of contracting the disease or lessen its severity
d. Person believes that the threat of taking these actions is not as great as the threat of the disease

13. d (356, 357)

14. a (356, 357)

15. All three (358):
a. Developmental level
b. Age group
c. Physical ability

16. b (358)

17. b (358)

18. Any five (358-360):
a. Number of persons
b. Need for privacy
c. Lighting
d. Temperature
e. Noise
f. Ventilation
g. Furniture
h. Room size

19. a. 3
b. 1
c. 4
d. 2
e. 5 (361, 362)

20. All five:
a. Learning needs (361)
b. Motivation to learn (361)
c. Ability to learn (362)
d. Teaching environment (362)
e. Resources for learning (362)

21. d (364)

22. All three (366):
a. Behavior—learner's ability to do something after the learning experience (involves an action verb)
b. Content to be learned—what is to be learned
c. Conditions and timing—situation under which the learned behavior will occur or when the behavior will be achieved

23. c (366)

24. b (366)

25. To promote continuity of the teaching plan, particularly when several nurses are involved or several teaching sessions are needed (368)

26. Teaching approach involves the nurse's task and relationship behaviors with the client. Teaching methodology refers to the techniques used to convey information (370).

27. Any seven (366-370):
    a. Know the client's learning needs.
    b. Select a time that coincides with the client's readiness and ability to learn.
    c. Know the client's ability to comprehend.
    d. Select a teaching method that fits the learning domain for the client's learning needs.
    e. Select and establish priorities for content.
    f. Actively involve the client and family in the teaching plan.
    g. Be aware of personal teaching abilities.
    h. Use appropriate teaching aids and resources.
    i. Control the environment so that it is conducive to learning.
    j. Use repetition and reinforcement appropriately.
    k. Give the client feedback.

28. b (372)
29. a (372)
30. At least six (375):
    a. Use slow pace of presentation.
    b. Give small amounts of information.
    c. Repeat information frequently.
    d. Reinforce oral teaching with audiovisual material, written exercises, and practice.
    e. Use analogies and examples.
    f. Reduce interruptions.
    g. Allow time for learners to express themselves.
    h. Establish reachable short-term goals.
    i. Apply teaching to present situation.
    j. Base new information on what the client already knows.

31. c (375)
32. d (366-370)
33. b (367)
34. All three (377):
    a. Specific content (what was taught)
    b. Evaluation of learning (behaviors demonstrated by the client indicating that learning has occurred)
    c. Method of teaching (how teaching was implemented)

CHAPTER 17

1. Leadership is the ability to influence other people toward accomplishment of a goal; management is the direction, coordination, and supervision of a group's activities (384).
2. a. 3 (384)
   b. 6 (385)
   c. 2 (385)
   d. 1 (385)
   e. 4 (385, 386)
   f. 5 (386)
3. (388):
   a. Leader provides specific instructions and supervises task accomplishment.
   b. Leader directs and closely supervises task ac-

complishment; leader also explains decisions, seeks suggestions, and supports progress.
   c. Leader facilitates and supports the efforts of subordinates toward task accomplishment.
   d. Leader gives the responsibility for decision making and problem solving to subordinates.
4. c (387)
5. d (388)
6. b (387)
7. a (387)
8. (389):
   a. Unfreezing—disturbing the equilibrium, creating awareness of needed change.
   b. Change—selecting and implementing alternatives, creating a change in behavior.
   c. Refreezing—integration of changes into the system, making them the usual procedure or method of operation (389).
9. d (389, 390)
10. All four categories, two behaviors for each category (390):
    a. Skills of personal behavior
       (1) Sensitive to feelings of the group
       (2) Identifies self with the needs of the group
       (3) Listens attentively
       (4) Does not ridicule or criticize another person's suggestions
       (5) Helps other people feel important and needed
       (6) Does not argue
    b. Skills of communication
       (1) Makes sure everyone understands what is needed and why it is needed
       (2) Establishes positive communication with the group as a routine part of the job
       (3) Recognizes that everyone's contributions are important
    c. Skills of organization
       (1) Develops long- and short-range objectives
       (2) Breaks big problems into small ones
       (3) Shares responsibilities and opportunities
       (4) Plans, acts, follows up, and evaluates
       (5) Attentive to details
    d. Skills of self-examination
       (1) Aware of personal motivation
       (2) Aware of group members' level of hostility so that appropriate measures to counteract it can be taken
       (3) Makes group members aware of their attitudes and values.

CHAPTER 18

1. Invasion of the body by pathogens or microorganisms capable of producing disease (398)
2. (398):
   a. Infectious agent or pathogen
   b. Reservoir or source for pathogen growth
   c. Portal of exit from reservoir
   d. Mode of transmission or vehicle
   e. Portal of entry to the host
   f. Susceptible host

3. **a.** 4 (398)
   b. 5 (399)
   c. 6 (400)
   d. 2 (398)
   e. 7 (400)
   f. 1 (398)
   g. 3 (402)
4. True (401)
5. (401):
   a. Contact—direct physical transfer, indirect contact with contaminated inanimate object, and droplet (coming in contact, within 3 feet, through sneezing or coughing).
   b. Air—droplet nuclei or residue of evaporated droplets suspended in air or dust.
   c. Vehicle—contaminated items such as liquids and food.
   d. Vectors—insects and animals.
6. d
7. (402):
   a. 3
   b. 1
   c. 4
   d. 2
8. **a.** Normal flora (403)
   b. Body system's unique defenses (403)
   c. Inflammation (403)
   d. Immune response (405)
9. b (403)
10. Refer to Table 18-3, p. 404.
11. Body's cellular response to injury or infection; a protective vascular reaction delivering fluid, blood products, and nutrients to interstitial tissues in an area of injury. Process neutralizes and eliminates pathogens or necrotic tissues and establishes a means of repairing body cells and tissues (403).
12. True (403)
13. (403, 404):
   a. Redness
   b. Localized warmth (heat)
   c. Swelling (edema)
   d. Pain or tenderness
   e. Loss of function
14. **a.** Vascular and cellular responses: dilation of arterioles increasing local circulation; white blood cells (WBCs) arrive at the site (403).
   b. Formation of inflammatory exudate: accumulation of fluid and dead tissue cells and WBCs (404).
   c. Tissue repair: defensive, reconstructive, and maturative stages (405).
15. (403):
   a. Fever
   b. Leukocytosis
   c. Malaise
   d. Anorexia
   e. Nausea
   f. Vomiting

   g. Lymph node enlargement
16. **a.** 3 (405)
   b. 4 (405)
   c. 2 (406)
   d. 5 (406)
   e. 1 (405)
   f. 7 (406)
   g. 6 (406)
17. (405, 406):
   a. 2
   b. 4
   c. 1
   d. 3
   e. 5
18. c (406)
19. **a.** Nosocomial
   b. Iatrogenic
   c. Exogenous
   d. Endogenous
20. Any three (407):
   a. Number of health care employees having direct contact with the client
   b. Number of invasive procedures
   c. Type of invasive procedures
   d. Medications
   e. Treatments
   f. Length of stay
21. a (408)
22. **a.** Age (408)
   b. Nutritional status (409)
   c. Stress (409)
   d. Heredity (410)
   e. Disease process (410)
   f. Medical therapies (410)
23. b (408)
24. b (409)
25. **a.** 3 (407)
   b. 7 (407)
   c. 5 (407)
   d. 2 (407)
   e. 1 (407)
   f. 6 (415)
   g. 8 (400)
   h. 4 (400)
26. Hand washing (417)
27. Any six (417):
   a. Before contact with client who is susceptible to infection
   b. After caring for infected client
   c. After touching organic material
   d. Before performing invasive procedure
   e. Before and after handling dressing or touching open wound
   f. After handling contaminated equipment
   g. Between contact with different clients in high-risk units
28. (413-422):
   a. 6

b. 5
c. 2
d. 4
e. 1
f. 3
g. 2
h. 3
i. 4

29. Any three (412):
   a. Preventing exposure to infectious organisms
   b. Controlling or reducing the extent of infection
   c. Understanding infection-control self-care practices
   d. Maintaining resistance to infection

30. Both responses (413):
   a. Preventing the onset and spread of infection
   b. Promoting measures for the treatment of infection

31. All four (414):
   a. Protective apparel—mask, eyewear, and water-proof gloves
   b. Stiff brush
   c. Detergent or soap
   d. Running water (cool to rinse, warm to wash)

32. c (418)

33. c (421)

34. (421):
   a. Body substance isolation—system using generic infection precautions for all clients; emphasizes potential infectiousness of all moist body substances.
   b. Specific guidelines—disease-specific practices followed for each disease; less costly and time consuming because certain diseases require only minimal protection; category-specific practices based on methods of organism transmission

35. (424, 425):
   a. Prevents transmission of highly contagious or virulent infections spread by air and contact
   b. Prevents transmission of highly contagious infections spread by close or direct contact (that do not warrant strict precautions)
   c. Prevents transmission of infectious diseases over short distances via air droplets
   d. Prevents infections transmitted by direct or indirect contact with feces
   e. Special category for clients with pulmonary tuberculosis who have positive results on sputum or chest x-ray films indicating active disease
   f. Prevent infections transmitted by direct or indirect contact with purulent material or drainage from an infected body site
   g. Prevent infections transmitted by direct or indirect contact with infected blood or body fluids
   h. Protects an uninfected client with lowered immunity and resistance from acquiring infectious organisms

36. (424, 425):

Type of Isolation	Room	Gown	Gloves	Mask
Strict	X	X	X	X
Contact	X	X	X	X
Respiratory	X			X
Enteric precautions	If poor hygiene	X	X	
Tuberculosis isolation	X			X
Drainage and secretion precautions		X	X	
Universal blood and body fluid precautions	If poor hygiene	X	X	If droplet splattering likely
Care of the severely compromised client	X	X	X	X

37. False (422)

38. **a.** Universal precautions (424, 425):
   (1) Universal precautions apply to blood and other body fluids containing visible blood.
   (2) Gloves should be worn for touching blood and body fluids suspected of containing blood, nonintact skin, and mucous membranes of all clients.
   (3) Gloves should be worn for handling items or surfaces soiled with blood or body fluids and for performing venipuncture and other vascular access procedures.
   (4) Gloves should be changed after contact with each client.
   (5) Masks and protective eyewear or face shields should be worn during procedures that are likely to generate droplets of blood or other body fluids containing blood to prevent exposure of mucous membranes of the mouth, nose, and eyes.
   (6) Gowns should be worn during procedures that are likely to generate splashes of blood or other body fluids containing blood.
   (7) Hands and other skin surfaces should be washed immediately and thoroughly if contaminated with blood or other body fluids.
   (8) To prevent needlestick injuries, needles should not be recapped, or purposely bent, broken, or removed from disposable syringes; used needles should be placed in puncture-resistant containers near the work area.

(9) To reduce the need for mouth-to-mouth resuscitation, mouthpieces, resuscitator bags, or other ventilation devices should be used.

(10) Health care workers who have exudative lesions should refrain from all direct client care and from handling care equipment.

(11) Universal precautions do not apply to feces, saliva, nasal secretions, sputum, sweat, tears, urine, or vomitus unless it is visibly contaminated with blood.

b. Body substance isolation (422):

(1) Clean, disposable gloves should be worn before contact with mucous membranes, nonintact skin, or moist body substances.

(2) Gloves should change between clients and between activities with the same clients when gloves become excessively soiled.

(3) Hands should be washed for at least 10 seconds when the hands are soiled, before each new client contact, and after gloves are removed.

(4) Additional barriers such as gowns or plastic aprons, masks, goggles or glasses, hair covers, and shoe covers should be used as needed to keep moist body substances off clothing, skin, and mucous membranes of wearer.

(5) All sharp instruments and needles should be discarded uncapped in a rigid, puncture-proof container at the point of use, such as a client room or treatment area.

(6) Laboratory specimens from all clients should be handled as if they are infectious.

(7) Handling and reprocessing practices should be uniform for all articles and equipment used on all clients.

(8) Soiled linen should be bagged securely before transport.

(9) Private rooms should be used for clients with communicable diseases transmitted via the air or clients who soil their environment uncontrollably with body substances, and a large, red sign reading "Stop" should be placed at the door of the client's room. For certain diseases, people entering the client's room should wear masks. Roommates who are immune to the client's disease or who are infected with the same disease may share rooms (based on institutional policy).

39. All four (423):

a. Hands should be washed thoroughly before entering and leaving the room of a client who is isolated.

b. Contaminated supplies and equipment should be disposed of in a manner that prevents the spread of microorganisms to other people.

c. Knowledge of the disease process and the means of infection transmission should be applied when using protective barriers.

d. Measures should be implemented to protect other people who might be exposed to the client in locations outside of the isolated room.

40. Both responses (423):

a. Family education about the client's condition, need for isolation, and method of performing needed precautions

b. Provision of meaningful stimuli

41. a (423)
42. d (426)
43. True (430)
44. a (426)
45. b (426)
46. True (431)
47. (429):

a. 2
b. 4
c. 1
d. 5
e. 3

48. Any five (433):

a. Provide staff education for infection control.
b. Review infection-control policies and procedures.
c. Recommend appropriate isolation procedures.
d. Screen client records for community-acquired infections.
e. Consult with employee health departments about recommendations to prevent spread of infection among personnel.
f. Gather statistics about epidemiology of nosocomial infections.
g. Notify public health department of incidences of communicable diseases.
h. Confer with all hospital departments to investigate unusual events or clusters of infection.
i. Educate clients and families.
j. Identify infection-control problems with equipment.
k. Check microorganism sensitivity to antibiotics and confer with medical staff about resistance.

49. False (435)
50. All three (435):

a. Avoid sudden movements of body parts covered by sterile drapes.
b. Refrain from touching sterile supplies, drapes, or the nurse's gloves and gown.
c. Avoid coughing, sneezing, or talking over a sterile area.

51. (435-437):

a. C
b. S

c. C
d. C
e. S
f. C
52. d (435)
53. (441-443):
   a. 2
   b. 4
   c. 1
   d. 3
54. c (436)
55. (441-442):
   a. Remove all jewelry.
   b. Keep nails short and clean; do not wear nail polish.
   c. Wash from fingertips to 2 inches above elbow.
   d. Wash for at least 5 minutes (based on institutional policy).
   e. Use brush, orange stick or nail file, antiseptic solution, and sterile towel.
   f. Hold fingers and hands up and elbows down.
   g. Dry from fingers to elbows, using a rotating motion.
56. False (437)
57. True (437)
58. False (438, 439)
59. b (438, 440)
60. b (438)
61. (439):
   a. Grasp the corner of the drape with the dominant hand, touching only the 1-inch margin at the corner.
   b. Lift the drape straight up with one hand and allow it to gently unfold (do not shake or allow the drape to touch the uniform).
   c. With the nondominant hand, grasp the adjacent corner of the drape and hold it straight.
   d. Approach the area to be draped, being careful not to touch any contaminated surfaces with the drape.
   e. First position the bottom half of the drape over the area.
   f. Position the top half of the drape last to avoid reaching over the sterile area.
   g. Grasp the 1-inch border around the drape edge to position as needed.
62. True (434)
63. (434):
   a. Client susceptibility to infection
   b. Chain of infection, with emphasis on the means of organism transmission
   c. Basic handwashing techniques
   d. Hygienic practices to minimize organism growth and spread
   e. Preventive health care (diet, immunizations, exercise, and rest)
   f. Proper methods for handling and storing food
   g. Family members at risk for acquiring infection

CHAPTER 19

1. Any five (457):
   a. On admission to the health care facility
   b. On routine schedule according to physician's order or hospital policy
   c. Before and after surgical procedures
   d. Before and after invasive diagnostic procedures
   e. Before and after administration of certain medications affecting cardiovascular, respiratory, or temperature control functions
   f. With changes in the client's general physical condition
   g. Before and after nursing interventions influencing vital signs
   h. When client reports nonspecific symptoms of physical distress
2. True (457)
3. Hypothalamus (458)
4. d (458)
5. a. Metabolism (459)
   b. Muscle activity (459)
   c. Thyroid hormone (459)
   d. Sympathetic stimulation (vasoconstriction, shivering, and piloerection) (459)
6. (460):
   a. 2
   b. 1
   c. 4
   d. 3
7. (461):
   a. Infants: thermoregulatory mechanisms not fully developed, temperature influenced greatly by environment.
   b. Older adults: thermoregulatory mechanisms deteriorating, vasomotor control unstable, subcutaneous tissue reduced, sweat gland activity reduced, metabolism reduced; may also lack physical ability to take action to control environmental temperature exposure.
   c. Clients with decreased level of consciousness or impaired thought processes: illness or injury that may alter awareness of the environment or ability to think rationally, potentially inhibiting the individual's ability to control environmental temperature exposures.
8. d (462)
9. Body temperature above 38° C (100.4° F) measured rectally under resting conditions. (Although this definition is commonly accepted, determination of fever must be considered in light of the client's actual hypothalamic set point.)
10. a (462, 464)
11. False (464)
12. Febrile seizures (or dehydration) (464)
13. At least five (465):
   a. Measure vital signs when fever is suspected and on an ongoing basis as ordered (for example,

every 2 to 4 hours) until body temperature returns to normal.
b. Inspect and palpate skin and check turgor.
c. Ask how the client feels.
d. Note the presence of vomiting or diarrhea.
e. Observe the client for behavioral changes.
f. Monitor test results for electrolyte levels.
g. Inspect the oral mucosa for dryness and lesions.
h. Monitor intake and output.
14. Prevent the hypothalamus from synthesizing prostaglandin E, which is responsible for elevating the hypothalamic set point (467).
15. d (466)
16. Any three (467):
  a. Attaining a sense of comfort and rest
  b. Returning to normal body temperature
  c. Maintaining adequate nutrition
  d. Maintaining fluid and electrolyte balance
17. c (467, 468)
18. d (469)
19. (*T*, tympanic not available in all settings) (469):
  a. A
  b. R, A, T
  c. R, A, T
  d. A, T
  e. O, T
20. True (472, 473)
21. See the table below (469-476):
22. (471):
  a. $(100.4 - 32) \times 5/9 = $ degrees C
     $68.4 - 32 = $ degrees C
     $38 = $ degrees C
     ANSWER $ = 38°$ C
  b. $(38.3 \times 9/5) + 32 = $ degrees F
     $68.94 + 32 = $ degrees F
     $100.94 = $ degrees F
     ANSWER $ = 102°$ F

  c. $(98.0 - 32) \times 5/9 = $ degrees C
     $66 \times 5/9 = $ degrees C
     $36.66 = $ degrees C
     ANSWER $ = 36.6°$ C
  d. $(39.4 \times 9/5) + 32 = $ degrees F
     $70.92 + 32 = $ degrees F
     $102.9 = $ degrees F
     ANSWER $ = 103°$ F
23. d (477)
24. **a.** Pulse $= 72$
  b. Cardiac output $= 5760$ ml
  c. Yes
25. c (477)
26. Any three (477):
  a. Impaired peripheral blood flow
  b. Abnormal or inaccessible radial pulse
  c. Infant or child
  d. Medications affecting heart rate
  e. Irregular heart rhythm
27. d (477)
28. All four (482-484):
  a. Pulse rate*
  b. Rhythm*
  c. Strength
  d. Elasticity
  e. Equality
29. d (483)
30. (483):
  a. 4
  b. 6 (483)
  c. 2 (483)
  d. 5 (483)
  e. 1 (478)
  f. 7 (482)
  g. 8 (482)
  h. 3 (482)

Site	Type of Glass Thermometer	Time Left in Place	Client's Position	Special Precautions
Oral	Slim tipped or stubby; may have blue tip	2 min (or based on agency policy)	Comfortable; mouth accessible	Not used for clients who are unable to hold thermometer in mouth or might bite thermometer; infants; small children; confused or unconscious clients; clients who have oral surgery, had face or mouth trauma, oral pain; mouth breathers; clients with history of convulsions; clients experiencing shaking chills
Rectal	Stubby or pear tip	2 min (or by agency policy)	Sims	Not used for clients after rectal surgery, clients with rectal disorders, clients who cannot be positioned for proper placement, or newborns. Expose only anal area; lubricate thermometer; never force thermometer; insert in direction of umbilicus 1.2 cm (½ inch) in infants, 3.5 cm (1½ inches) in adults; and hold in place
Axillary	Stubby or slim tip	5-10 min	Lying supine; sitting	Expose shoulder and arm, with arm placed across client's chest. Hold thermometer in position.

31. (479-481):

Site	Equipment Needed	Length of Time	Indications	Special Techniques or Precautions
Radial	Pen, vital sign graphic, wristwatch with second hand or digital display	Regular: 15 sec Irregular: 1 min	Usual nonemergency pulse site	Arm relaxed with wrist extended
Apical	All of the above, plus stethoscope and alcohol wipes	Regular: 30 sec Irregular: 1 min	See answer 26.	Expose left side of chest, locate PMI, warm diaphragm in hand
Apical-radial	All of the above	1 min	Irregular pulse	Simultaneous assessment of apical and radial pulses by two nurses using the same time for measurement and the same watch

32. (484):
  a. 3
  b. 5
  c. 2
  d. 6
  e. 4
  f. 1
33. b (484)
34. (484):
  a. Decreased oxygen levels.
  b. Chronic lung conditions characterized by elevation of carbon dioxide levels in the arterial blood, causing loss of carbon dioxide as the normal stimulus for ventilation.
35. (485):
  a. Client splints or inhibits chest wall expansion breaths are shallow.
  b. Less oxygen is carried in the blood; client breathes faster to increase delivery of available oxygen.
  c. Collapse of lung reduces chest wall movement on involved side and causes asymmetrical chest wall movement.
  d. Chest appears barrel shaped; client actively uses neck and chest wall muscles to forcibly exhale.
36. (485):
  a. Rate
  b. Depth
  c. Rhythm
37. d (487)
38. **a.** Dyspnea (488, 489)
  b. Respiratory stridor (489)
  c. Tachypnea (488, 489)
  d. Apnea (487, 488)
  e. Orthopnea (488)
39. **a.** Hyperventilation (or Kussmaul) (488)
  b. Normal (487, 488)
  c. Cheyne-Stokes (488)

40. (487):
  a. 30 to 35 breaths/min
  b. 20 to 25 breaths/min
  c. 12 to 20 breaths/min
41. (489):
  a. Skin color
  b. Level of consciousness
  c. Difficulty breathing/ease of breathing
  d. Sounds of breathing
42. (489):
  a. The force exerted by the blood against a vessel wall.
  b. The maximal pressure exerted against the arterial walls, which occurs as the left ventricle pumps blood into the aorta.
  c. The minimal pressure exerted against the arterial walls at all times, which occurs as the ventricles relax.
43. **a.** 59
  b. 116
  c. 57
44. (489-491):
  a. ↓
  b. ↓
  c. ↑
  d. ↑
  e. ↑
  f. ↑
  g. ↓
  h. ↑
  i. ↑
45. When an average of two or more diastolic readings on at least two subsequent visits is 90 mm Hg or higher or when the average of multiple systolic blood pressures on two or more subsequent visits is consistently higher than 140 mm Hg (491)
46. a (497)
47. b (492, 499)

48. (497, 498):
  a. 156/88
  b. No, the systolic pressure is higher than normal.
49. (494-497):
  a. 2
  b. 6
  c. 1
  d. 4
  e. 8
  f. 5
  g. 3
  h. 7
50. c (498, 499)
51. Temporary disappearance of sound between first and second Korotkoff sound, may be seen in client with hypertension (498)
52. (498):
  a. Palpation
  b. Doppler
53. True (499)

CHAPTER 20

1. (508):
  a. Gather baseline data about the client's health.
  b. Supplement, confirm, or refute data obtained in the nursing history.
  c. Confirm and identify nursing diagnoses.
  d. Make clinical judgments about a client's changing health status and management.
  e. Evaluate the physiological outcomes of care.
2. False (508)
3. Any four: Have good lighting. Position and expose body parts so all surfaces can be viewed. Inspect each area for size, shape, color, symmetry, position, and abnormalities. Compare each area inspected with the same area on the opposite side of the body. Use additional light (Penlight or flashlight) to inspect body cavities (510).
4. c (510)
5. (510)
  a. Dorsum of hand and fingers;
  b. Pads of fingertips;
  c. Palm of hand;
  d. Fingertips (grasping body part)
6. The sensing hand is relaxed and placed lightly over the client's skin. The active hand applies pressure to the sensing hand. The lower hand does not exert pressure directly and is able to retain the sensitivity needed to detect organ characteristics (510).
7. Location, size, and density of underlying structures (511)
8. c (512)
9. (512):
  a. 4
  b. 1
  c. 3
  d. 2
10. b (513)
11. True (514)

12. Any three (514):
  a. Privacy
  b. Adequate lighting
  c. Soundproof, which eliminates sources of extraneous noise
  d. Steps to prevent interruptions
  e. Warmth
  f. Necessary equipment
13. d (517)
14. (516, 517):
  a. 1, 3, 5
  b. 1
  c. 5
  d. 2, 4
  e. 2, 4
15. b (517)
16. One per age group:
  a. Infants and younger children: Gather all or part of the information from parent or guardian. Offer parents support during the examination; do not pass judgment. Call children by first name; address parent beginning with "Mr.," "Mrs.," or "Ms." (517).
  b. Older children: Interview older child; observe parent-child interaction. Allow older child to provide information about health and current symptoms (518).
  c. Adolescents: Treat as adults and individuals. Assure of right to confidentiality. Confirm history with parents. Speak alone with adolescent (518).
  d. Older adults: Do not stereotype. Recognize effect of aging on sensory or physical status and modify sessions as indicated. Allow additional time or plan additional sessions (518).
17. (519, 520):
  a. General appearance and behavior
  b. Vital signs
  c. Height and weight
18. Any eight (519):
  a. Gender and race
  b. Signs of distress
  c. Body type
  d. Posture
  e. Bait
  f. Body movements
  g. Age
  h. Hygiene and grooming
  i. Dress (reflecting culture, lifestyle, socioeconomic level, and personal preferences)
  j. Body odor
  k. Affect and mood
  l. Speech
  m. Client abuse or neglect
19. d (520)
20. (520):
  a. Weigh at same time
  b. Weigh on same scale
  c. Weigh in same or equivalent clothes

21. Position supine on firm surface with legs extended straight and soles of the feet supported upright. Measure with a tape measure from the soles of the feet to the vertex of the head (521).
22. See the table below (521-523):
23. Hyperpigmentation (521)
24. a (524)
25. Turgor is a measure of the skin's elasticity assessed by grasping and then releasing a fold of the client's skin. Normally, the skin snaps back immediately to its original (resting) position (524).
26. Petechiae (525)
27. Any six: Color, location, size, type, grouping, distribution, mobility, contour, consistency (525)
28. (526):
    a. Ulcer
    b. Atrophy
    c. Macule
    d. Pustule
    e. Vesicle
    f. Wheal
    g. Papule
    h. Nodule
29. (525):
    a. The nurse applies firm pressure over the edematous area with the thumb for 5 seconds.
    b. The client has edema that, when pressure has been applied to the area, pits to a depth of 2 cm.
30. Any two (523):
    a. Wear wide-brimmed hats and long sleeves to avoid over-exposure to the sun.
    b. Use sunscreens (with a sun protection factor of 15 or greater) before going into the sun and after swimming or perspiring.
    c. Avoid tanning under direct sun (from 11 AM to 3 PM).
    d. Do not use indoor sunlamps or tanning pills; do not patronize tanning parlors.
31. Endocrine disorder (526)
32. b (527)
33. Baldness or hair loss (527)
34. True (527)
35. d (529)
36. Acromegaly (530)
37. a. Visual acuity (530)
    b. Extraocular movements (532)
    c. Visual fields (532)
    d. Pupil reflex (534)
38. (531):
    a. 6
    b. 3
    c. 1
    d. 5
    e. 4
    f. 2
39. Ask the client to read printed material under adequate lighting (530).
40. Without correction (glasses or contact lenses), the client standing 20 feet away can read a line that a person with normal vision can read at 60 feet (532).
41. d (531)
42. a. Nystagmus (532)
    b. Exophthalmos (532)
    c. Ptosis (533)
    d. Conjunctivitis (534)
    e. Arcus senilis (534)
    f. Red reflex (536)
    g. Photophobia (531)
43. Pupils equal, round, and reactive to light and accommodation (535)
44. False (534)
45. Any three (536):
    a. Clear
    b. Yellow optic nerve disc
    c. Red-pink retina (European Americans)
    d. Darkened retina (African Americans)
    e. Light-red artery and dark-red veins
    f. A3:2 vein-artery ratio in size; avascular macula
46. d (536)
47. Any three (538):
    a. Hypoxia at birth
    b. Meningitis

Skin Color	Mechanisms	Causes	Assessment Sites
Cyanosis	Increased deoxygenated hemoglobin, associated with hypoxia	Heart or lung disease, cold environment	Nail beds, lips, mouth, skin (severe cases)
Pallor	Reduced amount of oxyhemoglobin	Anemia	Face, conjunctivae, nail beds, skin
	Reduced visibility of oxyhemoglobin from decreased blood flow	Shock	
	Congenital or autoimmune condition causing lack of pigmentation	Vitiligo	
Jaundice	Increased deposit of bilirubin in tissues	Liver disease, destruction of red blood cells	Sclera, mucous membranes, skin
Erythema	Increased visibility of oxyhemoglobin caused by dilation or increased blood flow	Fever, direct blushing, alcohol intake	Face, areas of trauma

Assessment Finding	Assessment Skill Used	Explanation or Possible Cause
Bulging	Inspection of ribs and intercostal spaces on expiration	Client using great effort to breathe
Reduced tactile fremitus	Palpation of chest wall	Mucous secretions, lung lesions, or collapsed lung tissue blocking vibrations
Reduced excursion	Palpation of lower rib cage: hands parallel with thumbs 5 cm (2 in) apart, pressing toward spine	Client not breathing deeply because of disease state or changes associated with aging
Resonance over posterior aspect of thorax	Percussion	Normal finding
Retraction	Inspection of ribs and intercostal spaces on inspiration	Client using great effort to breathe
Anteroposterior diameter 1:1	Inspection of chest contour	Aging, chronic lung disease; normal finding in infants

c. Birth weight less than 1500 g
d. Family history of hearing loss
e. Congenital anomalies of skull or face
f. Intrauterine viral infection
g. Exposure to high noise levels

48. (537):
  a. 4
  b. 2
  c. 1
  d. 5
  e. 3
49. False (537)
50. c (538, 539)
51. (538):
  a. Pull auricle back and down; insert speculum into ear canal slightly down and forward.
  b. Pull auricle gently up, back, and slightly out; insert speculum into ear canal slightly down and forward.
52. a. Conduction hearing loss—interruption of sound waves traveling from the outer ear to the cochlea of the inner ear (539).
  b. Sensorineural hearing loss—failure of the inner ear, auditory nerve, or hearing center of the brain to transmit or interpret sound waves (540).

  c. Mixed hearing loss—combination of conduction and sensorineural loss (540).
53. True (540)
54. Bone conduction can be heard after air conduction sound becomes inaudible—a sign of conduction deafness (540).
55. False (541)
56. a. Light pink, moist, and smooth (545).
  b. Medium red or pink, moist, slightly rough on top surface, smooth along lateral margins, midline with protrusion, undersurface highly vascular (544).
  c. Smooth, white, shiny (544).
  d. Pink, moist, and smooth (in African Americans patchy pigmentation) (544).
57. (544):
  a. Sore that bleeds easily and does not heal
  b. Lump or thickening
  c. Persistent red or white patch (leukoplakia) on the mucosa, especially under the tongue
58. d (547)
59. a (548)
60. See the table above (549-557):
61. c (554)
62. See the table below (555):

Sound	Site of Auscultation	Cause	Character
Pleural friction rub	Anterior lateral lung field (client upright)	Inflamed pleura	Grating quality heard on inspiration; does not clear with cough
Rhonchi	Primarily over trachea and bronchi; if loud, over most lung fields	Fluid or mucus in larger airways	Low pitched, continuous, musical; loudest on expiration; may clear with cough
Wheezes	Over all lung fields	Severely narrowed bronchus	High pitched, continuous, musical; heard on inspiration or expiration; do not clear with cough
Crackles	Most common in dependent lobes, right and left bases	Sudden reinflation of groups of alveoli	Fine, short, interrupted crackling; during inspiration, expiration, or both; vary in pitch; may or may not clear with cough

63. a. Point of maximal impulse, the point at which the apex of the heart actually touches the anterior chest wall (557).
  b. Third or fourth intercostal space, just to the left of the midclavicular line (557).
  c. Fourth to fifth intercostal space, midclavicular line (557, 558).
  d. (559, 560):
   (1) Locate the angle of Louis between the sternal body and the manubrium; this is the second intercostal space. Count down to the fifth intercostal space on the left (by locating each intercostal space with the fingers), and locate the point lateral to this space in the midclavicular line.
   (2) Gently place the palm of the hand (or fingertips) over the left part of the chest in the area of the fifth intercostal space and midclavicular line and attempt to feel the apical impulse against the chest wall.
   (3) When it is difficult to locate the PMI with the client in a supine position, assisting the client to the left side-lying position will move the heart closer to the chest wall.

64. a. *A*, Aortic area: S_2 louder than S_1
  b. *P*, Pulmonic area: S_2 louder than S_1
  c. *T*, Tricuspid area: S_1 louder than S_2
  d. *M*, Mitral area (apex): S_1 louder than S_2, S_3 and S_4 (if present) audible

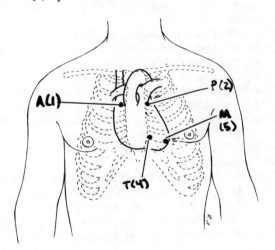

65. a (560, 561)
66. (561):
  a. Timing (place in the cardiac cycle)
  b. Location (place best heard)
  c. Radiation
  d. Intensity (loudness)
  e. Pitch
  f. Quality (561)
67. Thrill (562)
68. Bruit (564)
69. (563):
  a. Examine one artery at a time; if both arteries are occluded during palpation, client could lose con-

sciousness because of inadequate circulation to the brain.
  b. Do not vigorously palpate or massage artery; carotid sinus in upper third of the neck may be stimulated and cause a reflex drop in heart rate and blood pressure.
70. False (564)
71. False (564)
72. c (566)
73. (569):
  a. A
  b. V
  c. A
  d. V
  e. V
  f. A
74. (570):
  a. Inspection: Calf appears red and swollen.
  b. Palpation: Calf muscle is tender and firm. Homan's sign (pain in calf with forceful dorsiflexion of the foot) is positive.
75. True (570)
76. b (574, 575)
77. (573-576):
  a. N
  b. A
  c. N
  d. A
  e. A
  f. N
78. Any five (576):
  a. Location
  b. Size in centimeters
  c. Shape
  d. Consistency
  e. Tenderness
  f. Mobility
  g. Discreteness (detectable boundaries of the mass)
79.

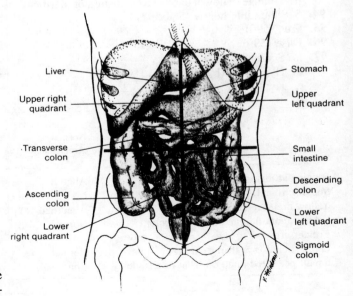

80. Costovertebral angle (581)
81. Any four (577, 579):
   a. Encourage client to empty bladder.
   b. Keep room warm.
   c. Keep client's upper chest and legs draped.
   d. Encourage client to remain supine with arms at side or folded across chest.
   e. Place small pillow under head or knees.
   f. Warm hands and stethoscope.
   g. Provide conversation to distract client.
   h. Work slowly and calmly.
   i. Ask client to report pain and point out tender areas.
82. d (579)
83. (579):
   a. 1
   b. 4
   c. 3
   d. 2
84. b (579, 580)
85. c (580)
86. Turn off the suction during auscultation (580).
87. 3 to 5 minutes (580)
88. Borborygmi (580)
89. c (581)
90. Guarding (581)
91. (582):
   a. Examiner presses hand slowly and deeply into tender area and releases quickly.
   b. Positive rebound tenderness test indicates inflammation of the abdominal cavity (peritonitis associated with any condition causing peritoneal injury or irritation such as appendicitis or pancreatitis).
92. Bladder distention (full bladder) (583)
93. Any three (591):
   a. Bleeding from rectum
   b. Black or tarry stools (melena)
   c. Rectal pain
   d. Change in bowel habits (constipation or diarrhea)
94. See the table below (584-592):
95. True (590)
96. False (590)
97. **a.** Scoliosis (593)
   b. Hypotonic (hypotonicity) (596)
   c. Kyphosis (593)

   d. Crepitus (595)
   e. Lordosis (593)
   f. Hypertonic (hypertonicity) (596)
98. b (595)
99. Any two maneuvers (596):
   a. Place hand firmly against client's upper jaw; ask client to turn head laterally against resistance (sternocleidomastoid).
   b. Place hand over midline of client's shoulder, exerting firm pressure; have client raise shoulders against resistance (trapezius).
   c. Pull down on forearm as client attempts to flex arm (biceps).
   d. As client flexes arm, apply pressure against the forearm; ask client to straighten arm (triceps).
   e. When client is sitting, apply downward pressure to the thigh; ask client to raise leg against resistance (quadriceps).
   f. Client sits, holding the shin of flexed leg; ask client to straighten the leg against resistance (gastrocnemius).
100. True (598)
101. Applying firm pressure with the thumb over the root of the fingernail (598)
102. c (599)
103. (599):
   a. 3
   b. 4
   c. 1
   d. 2
104. (600):
   a. IX, Glossopharyngeal
   b. XI, Spinal accessory
   c. V, Trigeminal
   d. II, Optic
   e. VII, Facial
   f. I, Olfactory
   g. X, Vagus
   h. III, Oculomotor
105. True (601)
106. Cerebellum (602)
107. **a.** Any maneuver: Client pats hand against thigh as rapidly as possible. Client alternately strikes thigh with the hand supinated and then pronated. Client touches each finger with the thumb of the same hand in rapid sequence. Client

Assessment Finding	Normal or Abnormal	Assessment Technique	Possible Cause (If Abnormal)
Bulging at inguinal ring	Abnormal	Inspection, palpation	Hernia
Smooth, round, firm prostate	Normal	Palpation	
Yellow drainage at cervical os	Abnormal	Inspection	Infection
Labia minora thin and darker in color than surrounding skin	Normal	Inspection	
Left testicle lower than right	Normal	Inspection, palpation	
Small, pea-sized lump on front of testicle	Abnormal	Palpation	Mass, possible testicular cancer

stands 2 feet away from nurse, alternately touching nurse's finger and client's nose. (602, 603)

    b. Any maneuver: Client performs Romberg test with feet together and eyes closed. Client closes eyes and stands on one foot and then the other. Client walks a straight line, placing heel of one foot directly in front of toes of the other foot. (603)

108. c (603)

109. b (605)

CHAPTER 21

1. (612):
    a. 4
    b. 1
    c. 2
    d. 3

2. d (612)

3. (613):
    a. Suspension
    b. Troche (lozenge)
    c. Capsule
    d. Ointment (salve)
    e. Syrup
    f. Enteric-coated tablet
    g. Lotion
    h. Tablet
    i. Paste
    j. Elixir
    k. Transdermal patch or disk

4. The nurse may be fined, imprisoned, and/or lose license (615).

5. The study of how drugs enter the body (absorption), reach their site of action (distribution), are metabolized, and exit the body (excretion) (616)

6. c (617)

7. a (617)

8. b (618)

9. d (618)

10. a (618)

11. Intended or predicted physiological response caused by a drug (618)

12. **a.** 5 (619)
    b. 4 (619)
    c. 2 (619)
    d. 3 (619)
    e. 1 (618)

13. The physiological action of two or more drugs given in combination is greater than the effects when given separately (619).

14. False (619)

15. The time it takes for the excretion process to lower the serum drug concentration by half (620)

16. (620)
    a. Plateau
    b. Peak
    c. Duration
    d. Onset

17. Any three (621, 622):
    a. Hormonal difference between men and women
    b. Age
    c. Nutritional status
    d. Disease states

18. True (622)

19. True (622)

20. c (622)

21. c (623)

22. d (623)

23. True (624)

24. Any two (623, 624):
    • Drug should not be chewed
    • Drug should not be swallowed
    • Drug should not be taken with liquids, and liquids should not be taken until the drug is completely dissolved
    • Sites should be alternated to avoid mucosal irritation

25. (625):
    a. Subcutaneous
    b. Intramuscular
    c. Intravenous
    d. Intradermal

26. Contamination of any of the materials or equipment may lead to infection (624).

27. (625):
    a. Meters (m or M)
    b. Grams (g or GM)
    c. Liter (l or L)

28. (625):
    a. Left
    b. Right

29. **a.** Deciliter = 0.1 l
    b. Milligram = 0.001 g
    c. Centimeter = 0.01 m
    d. Kiloliter = 1000 l

30. (625):
    a. Gram
    b. Ounce
    c. Fluid ounce
    d. Minim
    e. Dram

31. gr. iv (625)

32. (625):

Metric	Apothecary	Household
1 ml	15-16 minims	15 drops
15 ml	4 fluid drams	1 tablespoon
30 ml	1 fluid ounce	2 tablespoons
240 ml	8 fluid ounces	1 cup
480 ml	1 pint	1 pint (2 cups)
(approx. 0.5 l)		
960 ml	1 quart	1 quart
(approx. 1.0 l)		(2 pints, 4 cups)

33. (626):
    a. 5 grams of glucose dissolved in 100 milliliters of water

b. 1 milliliter of a liquid or 1 gram of a solid dissolved in 1000 milliliters of fluid

c. 250 milligrams in 1 milliliter of solution

34. (626):
   a. 0.1
   b. 2500
   c. 0.5
   d. 2
   e. ¼
   f. 2
   g. 10

35. (626): $\dfrac{\text{Dose ordered}}{\text{Dose on hand}} \times \text{Amount on hand}$

   $= \text{Amount to administer}$

36. (627): $\dfrac{\text{Surface area of child}}{1.7 \text{ M}^2} \times \text{Normal adult dose}$

   $= \text{Child's dose}$

37. a. One-half tablet

   $\left(\dfrac{0.125 \text{ mg}}{0.25 \text{ mg}} \times 1 \text{ tab} = 0.5 \text{ tab} \right)$

   b. TB syringe to ensure accuracy of the dose

38. a. 0.75 ml

   $\left(\text{gr. } \tfrac{1}{8} = 7.5 \text{ mg} \; \dfrac{7.5 \text{ mg}}{10 \text{ mg}} \times 1 \text{ ml} = 0.75 \text{ ml} \right)$

   b. TB syringe to ensure accuracy of the dose

39. a.
   $25 \text{ ml} \left(\dfrac{200 \text{ mg}}{400 \text{ mg}} \times 5 \text{ ml} = 2.5 \text{ ml} \right)$

   b. Draw up appropriate amount in a syringe to ensure accuracy of the dose.

40.
   $115 \text{ mg} \left(\dfrac{0.4 \text{ M}^2}{1.7 \text{ M}^2} \times 500 \text{ mg} = 115 \text{ mg} \right)$

   $\dfrac{0.4 \text{ M}^2}{1.7 \text{ M}^2} = 0.23$

41. (629):
   a. 4
   b. 3
   c. 1
   d. 2

42. a. Prescribes medications (628)
   b. Prepares, dispenses, and distributes prescribed medications (629)
   c. Determines whether the drug should be administered at a given time, assesses the client's ability to self-administer drugs, provides medications at the proper time, monitors the effects of prescribed medications, educates family and client about drug administration and monitoring (630)

43. c (630)

44. Any seven (631):
   a. Medical history: provides indications or contraindications for drug therapy
   b. History of allergies: potential allergic response to prescribed medications
   c. Purpose of drug order: determines whether a drug is needed or whether other interventions may be

as effective in creating the desired response

   d. Client's current condition: determines whether the drug should be given and how it should be administered
   e. Diet history: assists in planning dosage schedule more effectively
   f. Client's peceptual or coordination problems: determines whether self-administration is possible and provides clues that may be used in modifying approach to administering medications
   g. Client's knowledge and understanding of drug therapy: determines the willingness or ability to follow a drug regimen safely
   h. Client's attitude about the use of drugs: determines the level of client drug dependence
   i. Drug data: provides information needed by the nurse to safely administer medications
   Client's learning needs: determines client's need for instruction

45. True (633, 634)

46. Any five (635):
   a. Keep each drug in its original, labeled container.
   b. Be sure labels are legible.
   c. Discard any outdated medications.
   d. Always finish a prescribed drug unless otherwise instructed; never save a drug for future illnesses.
   e. Dispose of drugs in a sink or toilet (not the trash within reach or children).
   f. Do not give someone a drug prescribed for someone else.
   g. Refrigerate medications that require it.
   h. Read label carefully and follow all instructions.

47. b (635)

48. (637):
   a. Right drug
   b. Right dose
   c. Right client
   d. Right route
   e. Right time

49. (637):
   a. Before removing the container from the drawer or shelf
   b. As the amount of drug ordered is removed from the container
   c. Before returning the container to storage (with the unit dose system, the label is checked a third time with the medicine ticket or form even though there is no storage container)

50. d (637, 638)

51. (638):
   a. Check the medicine ticket or form against the client's identification bracelet.
   b. Ask the client to state name.

52. b (638)

53. a (640)

54. d (641)

55. (642-644):
   a. 6
   b. 4

c. 8
d. 1
e. 2
f. 5
g. 3
h. 7

56. False (643)
57. True (643)
58. (645):
   a. Bevel
   b. Shaft
   c. Hub
   d. Barrel
   e. Plunger
59. (646):
   a. Client size and weight
   b. Tissue to be injected
   c. Viscosity of fluid to be injected
60. d (646)
61. One milliliter of insulin solution contains 100 units of insulin (646).
62. (646):
   a. 2
   b. 4
   c. 3
   d. 1
63. Ampule (646)
64. Vial (650)
65. (652):
   a. Date solution was mixed
   b. Concentration of drug per milliliter
66. (650):
   a. Inject air into the vial.
   b. Between step 3 and 4.
67. (652):
   a. Vent vial A (being careful not to touch solution with the needle).
   b. Vent vial B and draw up the desired volume.
   c. Return to vial A and draw up the desired volume.
68. (652):
   a. Vent vial A (being careful not to touch solution with the needle).
   b. Vent vial B and draw up the desired volume.
   c. Apply new needle to the syringe.
   d. Draw up desired volume from vial A.
69. a (652)
70. c (652)
71. d (652, 653)
72. Any six (658):
   a. Use a sharp, beveled needle in the smallest suitable length and gauge.
   b. Position the client as comfortably as possible to reduce muscular tension.
   c. Select the proper injection site, using anatomical landmarks.
   d. Apply ice to the injection site to create local anesthesia before cleansing and needle insertion.
   e. Divert the client's attention from the injection through conversation.

   f. Insert the needls smoothly and quickly to minimize tissue pulling.
   g. Hold the syringe steady while the needle remains in tissues.
   h. Massage the injected area gently for several seconds unless contraindicated.
73. (649):

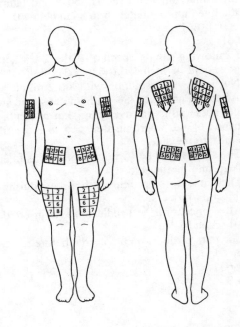

74. Abdomen (658)
75. b (658)
76. When using a 26 guage needle, if 5 cm (2 inches) of tissue can be grasped, the needle should be inserted at a 90 degree angle; if 2.5 cm (1 inch) of tissue can be grasped, the needle should be inserted at a 45 degree angle (659).
77. d (659)
78. (659):
   a. 3 ml
   b. Less than 2 ml
   c. No more than 1 ml
79. a (660-661)
80. c (661)
81. d (661)
82. a. Acromion process forms the base of a triangle in line with the midpoint of the lateral aspect of the upper arm. Injection site is in center of triangle (approximately 3 fingerbreadths below the acromion process) (662).
   b. Heel of hand is placed over the greater trochanter (right hand for left hip, left hand for right hip). Nurse points thumb toward client's groin and fingers toward the head, with the index finger over anterior superior iliac spine and middle finger along iliac crest toward the buttock. Injection site is in center of the V-shaped triangle formed by the fingers (660).

c. Handbreadth above the knee to handbreadth below the greater trochanter of the femur. Injection site is middle third of muscle, midline of top of the thigh to midline of the lateral aspect of the thigh (660).

d. Imaginary line is drawn between the posterior superior iliac spine and the greater trochanter of the femur. Injection site is above and lateral to the line (approximately 5 to 8 cm below the iliac crest) (661).

83. b (661)

84. The following points specific to the Z-track technique should be included (662, 663):

a. Nurse draws up solution with a 0.2 ml air lock.

b. After preparing the site with an antiseptic swab, the nurse pulls the overlying skin and subcutaneous tissues approximately 2.5 to 3.5 cm laterally to the side.

c. The skin is held taut while the needle is injected deep into the muscle.

d. The nurse does not release the tissue during the injection process.

e. After injection, the needle remains inserted for 10 seconds.

f. The nurse withdraws the needle before releasing the skin.

85. (654-657):

a. 6
b. 10
c. 3
d. 5
e. 1
f. 9
g. 2
h. 4
i. 8
j. 7

86. True (663)
87. b (664)
88. c (668)
89. b (668)
90. False (668)
91. Wear gloves (675).
92. False (678)
93. c (676)
94. a (678)
95. a (678)
96. b (680)
97. b (682)

CHAPTER 22

1. False (696)
2. Any order (698-700):
a. Factual
b. Accurate
c. Complete
d. Current
e. Organized
f. Confidential

3. Include first name, last name, and status (for example, Sally Blue, NS II) (698).
4. b (699)
5. 2205 (699)
6. c (700)
7. d (700)
8. a (700)
9. c (701, 702)
10. (702):
a. Background information
b. Assessment data
c. Nursing diagnoses
d. Teaching plan
e. Treatment
f. Family information
g. Discharge plan
h. Priority needs
11. (702):
a. Information communicated in a telephone report may not be permanently documented in written form.
b. Information should be repeated to the sender for verification.
12. c (703)
13. Any six (704):
a. Client information: name, age, primary physician, and medical diagnosis
b. Summary of medical progress up to time of transfer
c. Current health status (physical and psychological)
d. Current nursing diagnoses or problems and care plan
e. Critical assessments and interventions needed shortly after transfer
f. Special equipment needs
g. Questions
14. Any event that is not consistent with routine client care or routine activities on a health care unit (704)
15. False (704)
16. To identify and eliminate significant problems in nursing practice or delivery of health care (or, for institution use, to provide information for quality assurance and risk management) (704).
17. a. 4 (708)
b. 1 (706)
c. 5 (708)
d. 3 (709)
e. 6 (706)
f. 2 (706)
18. The federal government and private insurance carriers audit medical records to determine client and health care agency financial reimbursement for health care costs. Thorough documentation ensures that a maximal amount of money is recovered for the care delivered.
19. True (709)
20. False (709)
21. b (709)

22. a (711-713)

23. (713):
- **a.** Advantage: care giver can easily locate proper section for making charting entries.
- **b.** Disadvantage: Information is fragmented.

24. Any three (710):
- **a.** Emphasizes clients, their problems, an thier perceptions of their problems
- **b.** Requires continuous evaluation and revision of care plan
- **c.** Provides greater continuity of care
- **d.** Enhances effective communication among health care team members
- **e.** Increases efficiency in data gathering
- **f.** Provides easy-to-read information in chronological order
- **g.** Reinforces the use of the nursing process

25. (712):
- S: subjective data or information gathered from the client.
- O: objective data or information that may be observed or measured.
- A: assessment or conclusions drawn by the health care provider based on data obtained.
- P: plan of care, compared with plan in previous notes.

26. (713):
- P: problem or nursing diagnosis for the client.
- I: interventions or actions taken.
- E: evaluation of the outcomes of nursing interventions, and client's response to nursing therapies.

27. d (714)

28. a (715)

29. A documentation tool integrating standards of care from multiple disciplines (720).

30. b (721)

31. (720):
- **a.** Preprinted, established guidelines used to care for clients with similar health problems.
- **b.** Any three:
  - **(1)** Establishes sound standards of care for similar groups of clients
  - **(2)** Easily located in a client's record
  - **(3)** Educates nurses who become familiar with client care requirements
  - **(4)** Increases continuity of care
  - **(5)** Documentation less time consuming.
- **c.** Nurse must still individualize approaches to care and modify and update care plan on a routine basis.

CHAPTER 23

1. d (733)

2. **a.** 2 (733)
   b. 3 (733)
   c. 1 (733)

3. False (733)

4. c (734)

5. d (734)

6. False (735)

7. Any four (735):
- **a.** Communication among family members
- **b.** Goal setting
- **c.** Conflict resolution
- **d.** Nurturing
- **e.** Use of internal and external resources

8. (736):
- **a.** 4
- **b.** 6
- **c.** 5
- **d.** 1
- **e.** 3
- **f.** 2

9. True (737)

10. Any six (737):
- **a.** Relationships that foster problem solving and management of conflict
- **b.** Celebrations, or special events such as birthdays and religious holidays
- **c.** Communication, or ability to convey personal beliefs and emotions
- **d.** Good financial management
- **e.** Hardiness, or commitment to family and belief that members have control over their lives; health (physical and mental)
- **f.** Shared leisure activities
- **g.** Acceptance of each member's personality and behavior
- **h.** Social support network of relatives and friends
- **i.** Shared routines such as meals and chores
- **j.** Traditions that carry over from one generation to another

11. Nurses may approach the family as context or the family as client in providing effective nursing care. When the nurse views the family as context, the primary focus is on the health and development of an individual family member existing within the environment that is the family. When the nurse views the family as the client, care is directed toward each family member to achieve health and attain the developmental tasks of the family (738, 739).

12. b (738, 739)

13. False (739)

14. True (741, 742)

15. At least one for each area (743):
- **a.** **(1)** Observing family members performing care-centered activities
  - **(2)** Asking the client to identify ways to include family members in care.
- **b.** **(1)** Observing the manner in which the family adjusts to the hospitalized client's return home
  - **(2)** Asking the client to discuss ways to incorporate care measures within the family's lifestyle
  - **(3)** Observing family members' abilities to maintain current roles and relationships.
- **c.** **(1)** Observing family members regarding the nature and implications of the client's illness

   (2) Asking family members about the nature and implications of the client's illness.
  d. (1) Observing the client performing self-care activities at home
   (2) Observing the client discussing ways that care measures have been adapted to the home

CHAPTER 24

1. c (748)
2. True (748)
3. Maturation (749)
4. Development (749)
5. Growth (physical growth) (749)
6. All three (750):
   a. Individuals have adaptive potential for qualitative and quantitative changes by receiving stimuli from, and giving stimuli to, the environment.
   b. Individuals derive uniqueness from the interaction of heredity and environment.
   c. Primary goal of development is achievement of potential (self-realization or self-actualization).
7. All seven (750):
   a. Development is orderly and sequential.
   b. Development is directional and proceeds from cephalocaudal, proximodistal, and simple to complex.
   c. Development is complex yet predictable.
   d. Development is unique to individuals and their genetic potential.
   e. Development occurs through conflict and adaptation.
   f. Development involves challenges for individuals.
   g. Developmental tasks require practice and energy.
8. d (750)
9. False (750, 751)
10. (751):
    a. (1) Heredity*
       (2) Temperament*
    b. (1) Family*
       (2) Peer group*
       (3) Life experiences
       (4) Living environment
       (5) Health environment
11. a. 4 (753)
    b. 2 (752)
    c. 3 (753)
    d. 1 (752)
    e. 5 (754)
12. (755):
    a. Genetic factors
    b. Environmental factors
13. Any agent capable of producing adverse effects in the fetus including infection, drugs (including alcohol), and smoking (757).
14. The fetus is capable of life outside the uterus organ systems are complete and capable of functioning.

This usually occurs at the end of the second trimester (757).
15. Vernix caseosa (758)
16. Lanugo (758)
17. b (758)
18. a (758)
19. True (758)
20. (759):
    a. Patent airway
    b. Stabilization of body temperature
    c. Infection prevention
21. Ophthalmia conjunctivitis associated with gonorrhea and other bacterial infections (759)
22. c (759)
23. All five (759):
    a. Heart rate
    b. Respiratory effort
    c. Muscle tone
    d. Reflex irritability
    e. Color
24. c (759)
25. Parents and neonate are capable of exploring and responding to each other and desire to do so (759).
26. Parents and newborn elicit reciprocal and complementary behaviors (parental behaviors: attentiveness and physical contact; neonatal behavior: maintenance of contact with the parent) (760).
27. d (760-763)
28. b (764)
29. d (764)
30. c (765)
31. False (765)
32. Unsuccessful attempts at controlling the environment through independent actions (766)
33. d (766)
34. d (768, 769)
35. c (769)
36. True (769)
37. A return to earlier patterns of behavior, most often occurring in response to physical or emotional stress (770, 771)
38.

Play Pattern	Age Span	Characteristic Behaviors
Cooperative	Late preschool	Take turns, join efforts to produce desired outcomes (770)
Parallel	Toddler	Play next to not with another (767, 768)
Associative	Early preschool	Play with others in similar activity with no formal organization or distribution of responsibility, borrows and lends play materials (770)

39.

Stage	Age Span	Heart Rate	Respiratory Rate
Fetus	—	136-160	0
Neonate	0-1 months	120-140	30-50 (760)
Infant	1-12 months	80-130	30-35 (764)
Toddler	1-3 years	110	24-26 (766)
Preschooler	3-6 years	90	22-24 (768)

40. Any four (770):
  a. Developmental age
  b. Previous experiences with hospitalization
  c. Available support individuals
  d. Coping skills
  e. Seriousness of illness
41. Denver Developmental Screening Test (DDST) (771)
42. True (771)
43. Any four (774):
  a. Minimizing separation anxiety
  b. Establishing trust
  c. Reducing fear
  d. Minimizing physical discomfort
  e. Fostering normal growth and development
  f. Incorporating play and diversional activity into daily care
44. Any five (774):
  a. Parents should tell the child when they are leaving and when they will return in terms the child can comprehend. Then they should leave quickly.
  b. The primary nurse should be with the child when the parents leave to provide some support and distraction.
  c. The nurse should explain to the parents that protest is normal behavior and demonstrates strong relationship with the parents.
  d. Parents should leave some item that the child knows belongs to them because its presence will assure the child that they will return and provide comfort.
  e. A child should have favorite toys from home or familiar objects such as a "special blanket" that provides comfort.
  f. Parents should tape pictures of family members where the child can easily see them. Health care providers can discuss the photographs with the child.
  g. Telephone calls form family members provide a link between home and hospital.
  h. The child may be comforted by cassette recordings of family members reading stories, singing, or talking.
45. Any four (774, 775):
  a. Allow the child to observe friendly interaction between parents and the nurse before directly approaching the child.
  b. Approach the child at eye level.

  c. Communicate through a stuffed animal or doll before directly addressing the child.
  d. Allow the child to become accustomed to the nurse's presence through some type of play activity before touching the child.
  e. Avoid gestures such as broad smiles and extended eye contact.
  f. Speak in a clear manner that is unhurried and confident.
  g. Incorporate parents into initial assessment activities such as vital sign measurement.
46. (776):
  a. 3
  b. 4
  c. 1
  d. 2
47. Any four (776):
  a. Allow the child to sit up for assessments and procedures whenever possible.
  b. Demonstrate the exact steps of a procedure on a doll, another nurse, or parent before beginning the procedure on the child.
  c. Allow the child to see and handle equipment or use it on a doll.
  d. Describe sensations that the child will experience.
  e. Encourage parents' presence during procedures and treatments.
  f. Provide the child with the opportunity to "play through" experiences and release pent-up feelings of anger and frustration in an acceptable fashion.
  g. Allow the child to assist with the procedure.
  h. Plan with the child life worker for therapeutic play sessions.
48. Any five (776):
  a. Keep periods of restraint or immobility to a minimum.
  b. Comfort infants and toddlers by talking in a soft voice or singing and with physical contact such as holding and rocking, hugging, cuddling, and caressing.
  c. Provide young children with items that provide security and comfort.
  d. Reassure children that it is OK to cry, and emphasize the helpful things children do.
  e. Allow choices that are acceptable such as which finger to stick for a blood test.
  f. Encourage participation in a procedure that may result in discomfort.
  g. Provide incentives that encourage cooperation with uncomfortable nursing actions.
  h. Use a pain assessment tool that allows children to use colors to describe the degree of pain.
  i. Use a variety of techniques such as positioning, distraction, relaxation, and rhythmic breathing with imagery to alleviate pain.
  j. Provide adequate analgesic control of pain to pro-

vide comfort and promote cooperation with painful procedures.
49. Any four (777):
   a. Provide an environment of acceptance for re-
      gressive behavior.
   b. Provide favorite toys from home.
   c. Encourage participation in self-care activities.
   d. Provide intermittent auditory and visual stimu-
      lation.
   e. Provide opportunities for children to socially in-
      teract with other children.
   f. Provide toys and play equipment that promote
      development of fine and gross motor activities.
   g. Encourage development of new vocabulary by
      learning names for hospital items and personnel.
   h. Encourage participation in assessment and pro-
      cedures.
   i. Discuss the effects of hospitalization on growth
      and development with parents and explain how
      they can help children regain and attain optimal
      levels of growth and development.
50. Any six (777):
   a. Incorporate play into the daily activities of
      care.
   b. Provide opportunities for all children, especially
      those who are immobilized, to go to the play-
      room or engage in play with other children.
   c. Keep the playroom as a "safe" area by prohib-
      iting the administration of medications or per-
      formance of any procedures.
   d. Provide materials that encourage creativeness.
   e. Provide sense-pleasure play that allows infants
      and young children to enjoy sound, movement,
      smells, tastes, touch, and color through activities
      and objects.
   f. Promote motor development through skill play.
   g. Promote cognitive development through activi-
      ties such as reading, hiding and seeking of ob-
      jects, and counting games.
   h. Plan special activities for children whose activ-
      ities are limited by their health problems or med-
      ical regimen.
   i. When children are confined to their rooms, have
      parents select toys and games from the playroom
      to take to their child.
   j. Request visits by volunteers or the child life
      worker when children are confined.
   k. Prepare children for procedures through play
      with hospital equipment.
   l. Use children's cognitive levels as bases for
      choosing appropriate play activities for teaching
      purposes.
   m. Provide for judicious television watching.

CHAPTER 25

1. (785, 786):
   a. 2
   b. 2
   c. 1

   d. 2
   e. 1
   f. 2
   g. 1
   h. 1
2. c (784, 786)
3. (786):
   a. 70-90
   b. 19-21
   c. 110/70
4. b (789)
5. Provide nutritious snacks such as fruit, vegetables,
   and high-protein foods (789).
6. (790):
   a. 4
   b. 1
   c. 5
   d. 3
   e. 2
7. a (793)
8. d (793)
9. Adolescence (794)
10. Puberty (794)
11. Primary sex characteristics are the physical and hor-
    monal changes necessary for reproduction. Second-
    ary characteristics are the external changes differ-
    entiating males from females (794).
12. All four (794):
    a. Increased growth rate of skeleton, muscle, and
       viscera.
    b. Sex-specific changes such as changes in shoulder
       and hip width.
    c. Alteration in distribution of muscle and fat.
    d. Development of the reproductive system and sec-
       ondary sex characteristics.
13. True (795)
14. c (795)
15. True (796)
16. d (797)
17. True (797)
18. The time between achieving physical maturation and
    assumption of adult responsibilities; provides time
    for youth to try various roles before making a com-
    mitment (798)
19. a (798)
20. All six (798):
    a. Decreased school performance
    b. Withdrawal
    c. Loss of initiative
    d. Loneliness, sadness, and crying
    e. Appetite and sleep disturbances
    f. Verbalization of suicidal thoughts
21. Sexually transmitted diseases (798)
22. All five (799):
    a. Developmental level
    b. Response to care
    c. History of prior health care
    d. Medical history
    e. Available support persons

23. External support systems are significant others whom the child is able to use for support. Internal supports are those actions or behaviors that the child independently initiates to assist with coping (for example, reading, listening to music, and using relaxation techniques) (799).

CHAPTER 26

1. State in which individuals attain a balance of growth in physiological, psychosocial, and cognitive areas. Mature adults feel comfortable with themselves, look at work with a broad perspective, take on solvable problems, are open to suggestions, accept constructive criticism, learn from experience, acknowledge accomplishments and shortcomings, confront tasks openly; use decision-making techniques to solve problems, and are accountable and responsible for their actions (810).

2. All five (810):
   a. Early adult transition, age 18 to 20; person separates from family and desires independence.
   b. Entrance into the adult world, age 21 to 27; person tries out careers and lifestyles.
   c. Transition, age 28 to 32; person may modify life activities greatly.
   d. Settling down, age 33 to 39; person experiences greater stability.
   e. Pay-off years, age 45 to 65; person experiences maximal influence, self-direction, and self-appraisal.

3. True (810)
4. Issues of care and responsibility; relationships progress toward maturity of interdependence (810)
5. All five (810, 811):
   a. Achieve independence from parental controls.
   b. Begin development of strong friendships and intimate relationships outside the family.
   c. Establish a personal set of values.
   d. Develop a sense of personal identity.
   e. Prepare for life work and develop the capacity for intimacy.

6. a (811)
7. All seven (811):
   a. Achieving adult civic and social responsibility.
   b. Establishing and maintaining a standard of living.
   c. Helping teenage children become responsible and happy adults.
   d. Developing leisure activities.
   e. Relating to one's spouse as a person.
   f. Accepting and adjusting to the physiological changes of middle age.
   g. Adjusting to the needs of aging parents.

8. (813):
   a. Conception
   b. Pregnancy
   c. Birth
   d. Lactation

9. Any four (813):
   a. Make sure certain emotions are based on love rather than physical or sexual attraction.
   b. Explore motivation for wanting to marry.
   c. Develop clear communication.
   d. Understand that any annoying behavior patterns and habits are unlikely to change after marriage.
   e. Determine compatibility in important beliefs and values.

10. Any four (813):
    a. Establish an intimate relationship.
    b. Decide on and work toward mutual goals.
    c. Establish guidelines for power and decision-making issues.
    d. Set standards for interactions outside the family.
    e. Find companionship with other people for a social life.
    f. Choose morals, values, and ideologies acceptable to both partners.

11. Any six (814):
    a. A sense of meaning and direction in life.
    b. Successful negotiation through transitions.
    c. Absence of feelings of being cheated or disappointed by life.
    d. Attainment of several long-term goals.
    e. Satisfaction with personal growth and development.
    f. When married, feelings of mutual love for partner; when single, satisfaction with social interactions.
    g. Satisfaction with friendships.
    h. Generally cheerful attitude.
    i. No sensitivity to criticism.
    j. No unrealistic fears.

12. True (814)
13. b (814)
14. A man's, woman's, or couple's involuntary inability to conceive or the inability to conceive after a year or more of regular sexual intercourse (816)
15. True (816)
16. False (816)
17. (816-818):
    a. 3
    b. 1
    c. 2
    d. 2
    e. 1
    f. 1
18. A period of approximately 6 weeks after delivery during which the uterus returns to its approximate prepregnancy size (818)
19. b (818, 819)
20. c (819)
21. Disruption of the cycle of menstruation and ovulation, typically occurring between age 45 and 60 (819)
22. Decrease in the level of androgens occurring in men in their late 40s or early 50s, resulting in physiological changes in sexual response (820)

23. True (820)
24. Any four (822):
   a. Sex: female;
   b. Age: declines for women after their early 50s, increases for men after their late 50s
   c. Social isolation: absence of intimate, confiding relationships after a change in the nature of relationship with parents, children, or spouse
   d. Losses: parental deprivation or loss of a mother before age 14, other physical or emotional losses during midlife, and departure of the last child from home
   e. Family history: history of depression in the family of origin.
25. Any three (823):
   a. Improved knowledge about the effect of risk factors on a person's level of health.
   b. Improved health-promotion activities.
   c. Improved communication within family structures.
   d. Fewer reports of illnesses and inability to solve problems.
26. d (824)
27. (824):
   a. External: lack of facilities, materials, and social supports.
   b. Internal: lack of knowledge and motivation, insufficient skills to effect changes, undefined short- and long-range goals.

CHAPTER 27

1. Health specialty dealing with physiology and psychology of aging and with diagnosis and treatment of diseases affecting the aging adult (830)
2. The study of all aspects of the aging process and its consequences (830)
3. b (830, 831)
4. Discrimination against people because of their advancing age (831)
5. True (832)
6. (832-833):
   a. 2
   b. 5
   c. 1
   d. 6
   e. 4
   f. 3
7. Any five (833):
   a. Adjusting to decreasing health and physical strength
   b. Adjusting to retirement and reduced or fixed income
   c. Adjusting to the death of a spouse
   d. Accepting oneself as an aging person
   e. Maintaining satisfactory living arrangements
   f. Realigning relationships with adult children
   g. Finding meaning in life
8. (835):
   a. P
   b. E

   c. P
   d. E
   e. E
   f. E
   g. E
   h. P
   i. P
9. False (837)
10. True (837)
11. A syndrome involving progressive impairment of memory and other cognitive abilities, and personality change that may have a variety of causes (837).
12. Senile dementia of Alzheimer type (SDAT) (837)
13. Any three (837):
   a. Infection
   b. Drug reactions
   c. Metabolic disorders
   d. Depression
14. a (837)
15. False (837)
16. Any three (839):
   a. Attention difficulties
   b. Decreasing interest in life
   c. Indifference to ceremony and courtesy
   d. Forgetting nouns in speech
   e. Being vague, uncertain, and hesitant
17. c (839)
18. d (839)
19. True (840)
20. True (840)
21. Any four (840):
   a. Financial provisions for retirement income
   b. Available postretirement activities
   c. Living arrangements
   d. Role changes
   e. Health care needs
   f. Legal affairs
22. (841):
   a. Attitudinal: isolation occurring because society's bias against older adults prohibits social interaction with others.
   b. Presentational: isolation resulting from a person's unacceptable appearance or other factors involved in presenting oneself to others.
   c. Behavioral: isolation resulting from behaviors that are unacceptable to others.
   d. Geographical: isolation occurring because of distance from family, urban crime, and barriers within institutions.
23. False (843)
24. Any four (844):
   a. Activity level
   b. Financial status
   c. Accessibility of public transportation
   d. Community activities
   e. Environmental hazards
   f. Support systems
   g. Length of time arrangement will be appropriate
25. False (845)

26. (845):
  a. Cardiovascular disease
  b. Cancer
  c. Cerebrovascular disease
  d. Chronic obstructive pulmonary disease
27. Sundown syndrome (846)
28. b (846-847)
29. Have a physical examination including cardiac stress testing (847).
30. **a.** Therapeutic communication: effective communication establishing rapport and focusing on meeting the needs of the client (847).
  b. Touch: therapeutic tool that can provide stimulation, reduce anxiety, orient to reality, relieve physiological and emotional pain, and give comfort (847).
  c. Reality orientation: communication technique directed toward restoring reality, improving awareness, promoting socialization, elevating client's independent function, and minimizing confusion or disorientation and regression (847).
  d. Resocialization: identification and utilization of resources available to assist in expansion of the individual's social network (847-848).
31. b (848)
32. (848):
  a. Clarity
  b. Independence
  c. Reinforcement
  d. Realism
  e. Consistency
  f. Repetition
  g. Individualization
33. Any four (848):
  a. Select a small, quiet room that is well lit and has comfortable furniture.
  b. Keep meetings short enough (for example, 20 minutes) to promote learning without producing exhaustion.
  c. Choose participants who are able to participate.
  d. Consider sensory deficits when using audiovisual aids.
  e. Present one topic for discussion at each meeting.
  f. Make it clear that participation is voluntary.
34. (835):
  a. Home care
  b. Hospice
  c. Day care
  d. Respite care
  e. Long-term care

35. All three (851):
  a. Reflecting consideration of factors influencing normal aging
  b. Maintaining independence as much as possible
  c. Facilitating an optimal level of comfort and coping

CHAPTER 28

1. c (860)
2. **a.** Loss of external objects: loss of any possession that is worn out, misplaced, stolen, or ruined (860).
  b. Loss of a known environment: temporarily leaving a familiar setting or relocating permanently (861).
  c. Loss of significant others: loss of family, friends, acquaintances, or pets because of death, relocation, or job change (861).
  d. Loss of an aspect of self: loss of a body part or of physical or psychological function (861).
  e. Loss of life: fear of pain, dependence, and loss of control associated with the dying process; fear of death (861).
3. c (861)
4. (862):
  a. Accept reality of the loss.
  b. Accept grief as painful.
  c. Adjust to an environment that no longer includes the lost person, object, or aspect of self.
  d. Reinvest emotional energy into new relationships.
5. True (862)
6. See the table below (862-864):
7. False (864)
8. True (864)
9. (863-864):
  a. 2
  b. 5
  c. 4
  d. 1
  e. 3
10. True (864)
11. c (865)
12. (864-865):
  a. 6
  b. 4
  c. 7
  d. 2
  e. 1
  f. 3

Engle	Kübler-Ross	Martocchio
a. Shock and disbelief	**a.** Denial	**a.** Shock and disbelief
b. Developing awareness	**b.** Anger	**b.** Yearning and protest
c. Reorganization and restitution	**c.** Bargaining	**c.** Anguish, disorganization, and despair
	d. Depression	**d.** Identification in bereavement
	e. Acceptance	**e.** Reorganization and restitution

g. 8

h. 5

13. Any five (869):

 a. Need to be with the dying person

 b. Need to be helpful to the dying person

 c. Need for assurance of the spouse's comfort

 d. Need to be informed of the spouse's condition

 e. Need to be informed of the person's impending death

 f. Need to vent emotions

 g. Need for comfort and support of the family

 h. Need for acceptance, support, and comfort from health professionals

14. c (865)

15. All six (867-868):

 a. Affective: sensations and emotions that are part of hoping.

 b. Cognitive: processes of wishing, imagining, perceiving, thinking, learning, or judging in relation to hope.

 c. Behavioral: actions taken to achieve hope.

 d. Affiliative: involvement and relationships with others.

 e. Temporal: experience of time in relation to hoping.

 f. Contextual: perception of hope in relation to interpretation of life situations.

16. Any five (869):

 a. Low socioeconomic status

 b. Poor health

 c. Sudden death or short illness

 d. Perceived lack of available social support

 e. Lack of support from religious beliefs

 f. Lack of a supportive family or membership in a family that discourages grief expressions

 g. Strong tendency to cling to the person before death or preoccupation with the deceased person's image

 h. Strong reactions of distress, anger, and self-reproach

 i. History of psychiatric illness or suicidal intention

17. True (869)

18. Accomplishment of part of the grief work before the actual loss (869)

19. All four (872):

 a. Resolve grief.

 b. Accept the reality of the loss.

 c. Regain self-esteem.

 d. Renew normal activities or relationships.

20. All five (872):

 a. Gain and maintain comfort.

 b. Maintain independence.

 c. Maintain hope.

 d. Achieve spiritual comfort.

 e. Gain relief from loneliness or isolation.

21. All three (872):

 a. Control of pain

 b. Preservation of dignity and self-worth

 c. Love and affection

22. a (872-873)

23. One from each dimension (873): *Affective:* Convey empathetic understanding of client's worries, fears, and doubts; reduce the degree to which client becomes immobilized by concerns; build on client and family strengths of patience and courage. *Cognitive:* Clarify or modify hoping person's reality perceptions; offer information about the illnesses or treatment, correct misinformation, and share the experiences of other persons as a basis of comparison. *Behavioral:* Help client use personal and family resources in relation to hope; balance levels of independence, interdependence, and dependence when planning care; enhance client's self-esteem and capabilities; give praise and encouragement appropriately. *Affiliative:* Strengthen or foster relationships that provide hope.; help clients know that they are loved, cared for, and important to others. *Temporal:* Attend to client's experiences; use client's insights from past experiences and apply them to the present. *Contextual:* Provide the opportunity to communicate about life situations that influence hope; encourage discussion about desired goals, reminiscing, reviewing of values, and reflecting on the meaning of suffering, life, or death.

24. True (874)

25. Any four (877):

 a. Apply techniques of therapeutic communication.

 b. Express empathy.

 c. Pray with the client.

 d. Read inspirational literature.

 e. Play music.

26. Providing family-centered care to assist the terminally ill client in maintaining comfort and a satisfactory lifestyle through the phases of dying (878)

27. b (878)

28. (880):

 a. Algor mortis

 b. Livor mortis

 c. Rigor mortis

CHAPTER 29

1. Needs shared by all persons that are necessary for survival and health (890)

2. (890):

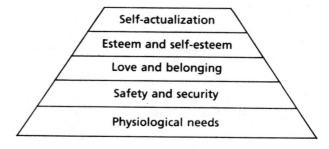

3. a (890)
4. (891):
  a. Oxygen*
  b. Fluid
  c. Nutrition
  d. Temperature
  e. Elimination
  f. Shelter
  g. Rest
  h. Sex
5. Any four (891):
  a. Very young (neonates and infants)
  b. Very old
  c. Poor
  d. Ill
  e. Handicapped
6. (892):
  a. Very old
  b. Very young
7. True (892)
8. False (895)
9. d (895)
10. True (896)
11. c (898)
12. Any six (899):
  a. Solves own problems
  b. Assists other persons in problem solving
  c. Accepts suggestions of others
  d. Possesses broad interests in work and social topics
  e. Possesses good communication skills as a listener and communicator
  f. Manages stress and assists other persons in managing stress
  g. Enjoys privacy
  h. Seeks new experiences and knowledge
  i. Is confident in abilities and decisions
  j. Anticipates problems and successes
  k. Likes self
13. True (900)
14. Any four (900-901):
  a. Life-threatening situations and unmet physiological needs
  b. Person's personality and mood
  c. Person's state of health
  d. Person's perception of need
  e. Person's family structure
  f. Interrelationship of needs
15. a. 1 (891)
  b. 2 (891-892)
  c. 13 (898-899)
  d. 8 (895)
  e. 9 (896)
  f. 7 (894-895)
  g. 3 (892-893)
  h. 6 (894)
  i. 12 (898)
  j. 5 (893-894)
  k. 10 (896-897)
  l. 11 (898)
  m. 4 (893)

CHAPTER 30

1. d (906)
2. a (907)
3. a. 3 (907)
  b. 2 (907)
  c. 4 (908)
  d. 1 (908)
4. b (907-908)
5. All four (908):
  a. Intensity of the stressor
  b. Scope of the stressor
  c. Duration of the stressor
  d. Number and nature of other stressors
6. All four (909):
  a. Good communication skills
  b. Mutual respect for all family members
  c. Adequate resources available for adaptation
  d. Previous experience with stressors
7. a. Physical-developmental dimension: physical body changes of LAS or GAS in response to internal or external environment; developmental task achievement (909).
  b. Emotional dimension: psychological coping mechanisms including task-oriented behaviors and ego-defense mechanisms (909).
  c. Intellectual dimension: gathering information, solving problems, and communicating with others (909).
  d. Social dimension: using individuals or organized groups to provide support, and using societal and community resources (909).
  e. Spiritual dimension: believing in a supreme being, unity with nature or positive sense of life's meaning and purpose (909).
8. Response of body tissue, organ, or part to the stress of trauma, illness, or other physiological change (910)
9. Defense response of the whole body to stress (911)
10. All four (910):
  a. Response is localized.
  b. Response is adaptive (meaning a stressor necessary to stimulate it).
  c. Response is short term.
  d. Response is restorative.
11. d (910)
12. All five (910):
  a. Localized pain
  b. Localized swelling
  c. Localized heat
  d. Localized redness,
  e. Changes in function
13. c (912)
14. (912):
  a. Alarm reaction: physiological changes that prepare a person to adapt to a stressor.
  b. Resistance stage: stabilization of the body to

allow the person to make an adaptive response.

   c. Exhaustion stage: energy insufficient for adaptation if the person is unable to alleviate the stress.

15. (912):
   a. 3
   b. 1
   c. 2
   d. 1
   e. 3
   f. 2
   g. 1
   h. 1

16. True (912)

17. Both responses (913):
   a. Task-oriented behaviors: use of direct problem-solving techniques.
   b. Ego-defense mechanisms: unconscious, indirect methods of coping with stress.

18. b (913)

19. All six (913):
   a. Compensation: making up for a deficiency in one aspect of self-image by strongly emphasizing a feature considered an asset.
   b. Conversion: unconsciously repressing an anxiety-producing emotional conflict and transforming it into nonorganic symptoms.
   c. Denial: avoiding emotional conflicts by refusing to consciously acknowledge anything that might cause intolerable emotional pain.
   d. Displacement: transferring emotions, ideas, or wishes from a stressful situation to a less anxiety-producing substitute.
   e. Identification: patterning behavior after that of another person and assuming that person's qualities, characteristics, and actions.
   f. Regression: coping with a stressor through actions and behaviors associated with an earlier developmental period.

20. Any eight (913):
   a. Elevated blood pressure
   b. Increased muscle tension in neck, shoulders, and back
   c. Elevated pulse and respiratory rate
   d. Sweaty palms
   e. Cold hands and feet
   f. Fatigue
   g. Slumped posture
   h. Tension headache
   i. Upset stomach
   j. Higher-pitched voice
   k. Nausea, vomiting, and diarrhea
   l. Change in appetite
   m. Change in weight
   n. Changes in urinary frequency
   o. Restlessness, difficulty falling asleep, or frequent awakening

   p. Dilated pupils
   q. Abnormal laboratory findings: elevated adrenocorticotropic hormones, cortisol, catecholamine levels and hyperglycemia

21. At least one behavior for each stage:
   a. Distrust, withdrawal, or limited interaction with other persons in later years.
   b. Excessive dependence on others.
   c. Passive, inactive behavior toward the environment.
   d. Inability and unwillingness to develop friendships.
   e. Rebelliousness, depression, and anxiety.
   f. Increased discord at home and work, extremes in social activities (excessive participation or withdrawal).
   g. Depression and anxiety.*
   h. Overdependence, strained family or social relationships.*

Refer to Answer 22 for additional responses. (914, 915)

22. Any 10 (915):
   a. Anxiety
   b. Depression
   c. Burnout
   d. Increased use of chemical substances
   e. Change in eating habits
   f. Change in sleep and activity patterns
   g. Mental exhaustion
   h. Feelings of inadequacy
   i. Loss of self-esteem
   j. Increased irritability
   k. Loss of motivation
   l. Emotional outbursts and crying
   m. Decreased productivity and quality of job performance
   n. Tendency to make mistakes and poor judgment
   o. Forgetfulness and blocking
   p. Diminished attention to detail
   q. Preoccupation—daydreaming or "spacing out"
   r. Inability to concentrate on tasks
   s. Increased absenteeism and illness
   t. Lethargy
   u. Loss of interest
   v. Increased tendency to have accidents

23. Any four (916):
   a. Decreased ability to learn
   b. Reduced role performance
   c. Impaired communication
   d. Inability to resolve conflict
   e. Decreased ability to solve problems
   f. Increased dependence on others

24. Any two (916):
   a. Anger with supreme being
   b. View of stressor as punishment
   c. Questions about meaning of life
   d. Spiritual depression

25. (917-921):

Reducing Stressful Situations	Decreasing Physiological Responses	Improving Responses to Stress
a. Habituation	**a.** Regular exercise	**a.** Support systems
b. Change avoidance	**b.** Humor	**b.** Crisis intervention
c. Time blocking	**c.** Nutrition and diet	**e.** Enhancing self-esteem
d. Time management	**d.** Rest	
e. Environmental modification	**e.** Relaxation techniques	

26. All three (920):
  a. Perceiving the stressful event realistically
  b. Having adequate support
  c. Using adequate coping mechanisms

CHAPTER 31

1. The person's subjective image of the self; the perception of physical, emotional, and social attributes or qualities (928)
2. Any five (928):
  a. Reactions of other persons to the infant's or child's body and behavior
  b. Ongoing perceptions of other peoples' reactions to self
  c. Experiences with self and other persons
  d. Personality structure
  e. Perceptions of physiological and sensory stimuli that affect self
  f. Prior and new experiences
  g. Present feelings about physical, emotional, and social self
  h. Expectations about self
3. The mental picture of one's body, including the external, internal, and postural image of the body (928)
4. False (928)
5. Either definition (929):
  a. The evaluation that individuals maintain about themselves and convey to other persons verbally or through behaviors.
  b. The acceptance of self because of basic worth, despite weaknesses, limitations, or deficiencies.
6. (929):
  a. Identity
  b. Body image
  c. Self-esteem
  d. Roles
7. c (929)
8. False (929)
9. A person's image of self as male or female and the meaning that this has for the person (929)
10. c (929, 930)
11. True (930)
12. Socialization (931)
13. (931):
  a. Reinforcement-extinction: behaviors that become common or avoided, depending on whether they are approved and reinforced or discouraged and punished.
  b. Inhibition: refraining from a behavior, even when motivated to do so, because of each reinforcement.
  c. Substitution: replacement of one behavior by another to provide the same gratification.
  d. Imitation: acquisition of knowledge, skills, or behaviors from members of a social or cultural group.
  e. Identification: internalization of beliefs, behaviors, and values of a role model into the person's unique, overt expression.
14. b (931)
15. (934):
  a. Health-illness transition
  b. Developmental transition
  c. Situational transition
16. Lack of congruent or compatible role expectations (934)
17. (934):
  a. 2
  b. 3
  c. 4
  d. 1
18. Role ambiguity (935)
19. d (935)
20. Role strain (935)
21. **a.** 4 (939)
  b. 1 (937)
  c. 6 (939)
  d. 2 (938)
  e. 8 (940)
  f. 5 (939)
  g. 7 (940)
  h. 3 (938)
22. b (938)
23. True (940)
24. All three (943):
  a. Whatever the client communicates is normal and acceptable.
  b. The communication is not threatening or frightening to the nurse.
  c. The nurse will not reject or isolate the client because of anything communicated.

25. All five (949):
   a. Relate to the client as an equal.
   b. Find a common interest or experience for initiating conversation.
   c. Establish a smooth, easy pattern of conversation.
   d. Convey a keen, sympathetic interest in the other person, give full attention, listen carefully, and indicate that there is time to listen.
   e. Adopt the client's terminology and conventions, and meet the client on the client's own ground to the extent possible.

26. (952):
   a. Increased self-awareness
   b. Self-exploration
   c. Self-evaluation
   d. Formulation of realistic goals
   e. Commitment to goals and achievement through action

27. The nurse should seek assistance from other appropriate professionals (952).

28. False (952)

29. True (953)

CHAPTER 32

1. Sexuality is a holistic concept involving biological, psychological, social, and ethical components constituting a person's sense of being female or male. Sex has a limited meaning describing the biological aspects of sexuality such as genital sexual activity (960).

2. Gender identity (960)

3. Gender role (960, 961)

4. Sexual orientation (961)

5. c (961)

6. All four (962):
   a. Biology
   b. Personality
   c. Religious beliefs
   d. Society

7. Whether their sexual attitudes, feelings, and actions are normal (962)

8. See the table to the right (963, 964):

9. (965, 966):
   a. Gonadotropin-releasing hormone
   b. Follicle-stimulating hormone (or luteinizing hormone)
   c. Luteinizing hormone (or follicle-stimulating hormone)
   d. Estrogen
   e. Progesterone

10. c (966)

11. d (966)

12. Any four (966):
   a. Lower abdominal pain and discomfort
   b. Breast fullness and tenderness
   c. Weight gain
   d. Fluid retention
   e. Irritability
   f. Depression

13. See the table below (967, 968):

Structure/Organ	Function(s)

Vulva
  Labia minora
  Labia majora
	Cover and protect vaginal and urinary opening; sensitive to touch, pressure, pain, and temperature

Clitoris	Sensitive to touch, pressure, temperature, and sexual arousal and pleasure
Vestibule	
Introitus	Vaginal opening
Bartholin's glands	Small amount of lubrication of introitus during sexual arousal
Hymen	Membranous fold partly covering the introitus
Vagina	Passageway for menstrual flow, childbirth, and sexual pleasure
Uterus	
Cervix	Contains glands that secrete mucus, providing a plug for the opening to the uterus
Body	
Myometrium	Protective environment for developing fetus; contractions expel fetus during labor and delivery
Endometrium	Vascular, cushioned environment for ovum implantation and maintenance
Fallopian tubes	Conduit for passage of ovum and sperm
Ovaries	Produce ovum; secrete female hormones
Breasts	Milk production, sexual arousal and pleasure

Structure/Organ	Function(s)
Penis	Transmission of urine and seminal fluid, sexual arousal and pleasure
Scrotum	Houses and protects testicles, epididymis, and portion of vas deferens
Testis	Produces sperm and androgenic hormones, primarily testosterone
Seminiferous tubules	Location of sperm production
Epididymis	Duct transporting sperm from outside the testicle to the vas deferens
Vas deferens	Tube transporting sperm out of the scrotum to the ampulla
Ampulla	Reservoir for sperm
Seminal vesicles	Secrete seminal plasma to dilute and carry sperm and provide nutrition for the sperm; buffer vaginal acidity to aid in fertility
Prostate glands	
Bulburethral (Cowper's) glands	Secrete clear, alkaline lubricating fluid during sexual arousal; may neutralize urethral acidity to create a more favorable environment for sperm

14. Circumcision (968)
15. b (969)
16. d (969)
17. Menarche (970)
18. True (971)
19. Any four (971):
  a. Dating issues
  b. Masturbation
  c. Emotional commitment in relationships
  d. Virginity versus premarital sexual behavior
  e. Contraception
  f. Teen pregnancy and related issues (abortion, adoption, and single parenting)
  g. Risks of sexually transmitted diseases (STDs)
20. True (972)
21. Any four (972):
  a. Monotony in sexual relationships
  b. Career and financial concerns
  c. Mental or physical fatigue
  d. Overindulgence in alcohol
  e. Illness, fear of failure
  f. Lack of sexual partners
22. (973):
  a. Excitement: gradual increase in sexual arousal.
  b. Plateau: heightened response caused by vaso-congestion and myotonia.
  c. Orgasm: sudden release of pooled blood and tension in the muscles at the climax of sexual excitement associated with highly pleasurable feelings of physiological and psychological release.
  d. Resolution: physiological and psychological return to an unaroused state.
23. c (974)
24. True (974)
25. To avoid placing uterine weight on the major blood vessels which could cause decreased maternal blood flow and therefore potential fetal hypoxia (975)
26. Both responses (975):
  a. Semen contains prostaglandins, which may stimulate uterine contractions.
  b. Breast stimulation induces the release of oxytocin, which may also stimulate uterine contractions.
27. b (975)
28. Any seven (975):
  a. How does the method work?
  b. What are the risks involved in using the method?
  c. Are there contraindications that rule out particular methods?
  d. How will it affect lovemaking?
  e. Does the partner object to it?
  f. Will it cause any discomfort?
  g. Is it readily available, affordable, and easy to use?
  h. Will either partner feel embarrassed using it?
  i. Is the risk of pregnancy acceptable?
  j. Are there alternatives?
29. (976-979):
  a. (1) Abstinence

  (2) Calendar (rhythm) method
  (3) Mucus method
  (4) Basal body temperature method.
  b. (1) Oral contraceptive pill
  (2) Spermicides.
  c. (1) Vaginal sponge.
  d. (1) Condom
  (2) Diaphragm
  (3) Cervical cap
  (4) Intrauterine device.
  e. (1) Vasectomy
  (2) Tubal ligation
30. Abstinence (976)
31. a (976)
32. Either of the following (977):
  a. Days 6 to 21 (24 − 18 = 6; 32 − 11 = 21)
  b. To icrease effectiveness, days 1 to 21
33. d (977)
34. Changes in cervical mucus correlates with ovulation. Just before ovulation, the amount of mucus increases. Women are most fertile when the cervical mucus is wet, abundant, slippery, stretchable, and clear (977).
35. b (978)
36. True (978)
37. False (979)
38. c (980)
39. False (980)
40. a. 4 (982)
  b. 3 (981, 982)
  c. 2 (981)
  d. 5 (982)
  e. 3 (981, 982)
  f. 1 (980, 981)
  g. 5 (982)
  h. 1 (980, 981)
  i. 2 (981)
  j. 4 (982)
41. All five (982):
  a. Knowing one's sex partner or partners
  b. Having a relationship with open communication, enabling discussion about health, disease exposure, and use of protective devices
  c. Limiting the number of sex partners
  d. Avoiding sexual contact with intravenous drug users
  e. Using condoms properly
42. d (982)
43. True (982)
44. (983):
  a. Nervous system
  b. Vascular system
  c. Hormonal system
45. True (983)
46. Any two (984):
  a. Acknowledging the openness of the setting
  b. Knocking or signaling before entering the client's space
  c. Using a do-not-disturb sign

47. d (984)
48. Any six (984):
  a. Lack of knowledge about sexuality
  b. Ignorance of sexual techniques
  c. General misinformation about sexuality
  d. Belief that sexual performance is inherently developed
  e. Guilt and anxiety associated with early sexual learning
  f. Fear of failure or rejection
  g. Poor communication
  h. Relationship problems
  i. Fear of pregnancy
  j. History of sexual abuse
49. c (985)
50. Any four (985):
  a. Diabetes mellitus
  b. Alcohol
  c. Neurological problems
  d. Hormonal imbalance
  e. Pelvic disorders
  f. Drugs (medications)
51. All four (988, 989):
  a. Physical factors: actual or anticipated pain or discomfort associated with sexual activity, illness, fatigue, and medications; altered body image associated with changes in body structure or function.
  b. Relationship factors: relationship issues may divert sexual desire, particularly when there are any interpersonal communication difficulties.
  c. Lifestyle factors: use or abuse of alcohol, lack of time to devote to the relationship because of work or family commitments.
  d. Self-esteem factors: reduced sense of personal value and lack of confidence in sexual skills negatively affects sexual relationships and factors lowering an individual's self-esteem.
52. Any two (989):
  a. How do you feel about the sexual part of your life?
  b. Have you noticed any changes in the way you feel about yourself as a man, woman, husband, or wife?
  c. How has your illness, medication, or impending surgery affected your sex life?
  d. It is not unusual for people with your condition to be experiencing some sexual problems; has that been a concern to you at all?
53. Any two (989):
  a. Have you noticed your child exploring his or her body, for example, touching genitals?
  b. Has your child begun to ask questions about where babies come from?
  c. Have you talked with your child about sex, pregnancy, or contraception?
54. Many adolescents have questions about sexually transmitted diseases or whether their bodies are developing at the right rate. Do they have any questions about sex or other things? (989)
55. c (989)
56. Any six (989):
  a. Allow adequate time to conduct an uninterrupted interview.
  b. Ensure confidentiality and privacy.
  c. Use a warm, empathetic approach.
  d. Assume that all clients are uncomfortable talking about their sexuality.
  e. Listen carefully, and notice nonverbal cues from the client.
  f. Adapt the interview to the client's lifestyle and attempt to overcome cultural and language barriers.
  g. Have a rationale for each question and be willing to share this with the client.
  h. Assume that all clients are sexually experienced unless they tell you otherwise.
  i. Avoid pressuring clients to respond to questions about their sexuality.
  j. Move through questions from least sensitive to more sensitive.
  k. Use open-ended questions that encourage more than a yes-or-no response.
  l. Focus attention on the client, not on documenting responses.
57. All five (989):
  a. What does the client see as sexual concerns?
  b. When did these sexual concerns begin and how have they changed?
  c. What does the client see as the cause of the concerns?
  d. What sort of treatment has the client sought to help alleviate this concern?
  e. How would the client like this concern to be resolved, and what are the client's goals for treatment?
58. True (990)
59. Contract the pubococcygeus muscle (the muscle that controls urinary stream) and hold this for 3 seconds. Release for 3 seconds. Repeat a series of 10 contractions five times a day (990).
60. Whether the client perceives the problems in achieving sexual satisfaction (sexual dysfunction) or expresses concern regarding sexuality (altered patterns of sexuality) (991)
61. All four (991):
  a. To obtain knowledge of sexual development and functioning of women and men.
  b. To attain or maintain biologically and emotionally healthy sexual practices.
  c. To establish or maintain sexual satisfaction for self and partner if appropriate.
  d. To attain, maintain, or enhance positive self-esteem with integration of cultural/religious/ethical beliefs, sexual practices, past and present; and situational realities.
62. Refer the client to a more appropriate expert. (995)

CHAPTER 33

1. A conscious awareness of a personal relationship with a source outside of self (supreme being); and an expression of life values, beliefs, and relationships with self and others (1002)
2. A way of relating to self, others, and a supreme being that integrates the individual's past, present, and future with the supreme being as center (1002)
3. True (1003)
4. Religion (1003)
5. False (1003)
6. c (1003)
7. (1003, 1004):
   a. 4
   b. 3
   c. 2
   d. 1
   e. 5
8. (1004, 1005):
   a. Fetus would be buried.
   b. Fetus would be baptized and buried.
   c. How far into the fourth month the pregnancy had progressed would need to be determined; if greater than 130 days, the fetus would be treated as a fully developed human; only family and friends may touch the body.
9. (1004, 1005):
   a. After death: priest ties thread around neck or wrist and pours water into mouth; only family touches and washes body before cremation.
   b. Before death: confessions of sins and asking forgiveness of family; after death: only family washes body, then turns toward Mecca; no autopsy is performed.
   c. Before death: Anointing of the sick (last rites); after death: other prescribed restrictions or rituals concerning burial.
   d. After death: oppose autopsy and cremation; occasionally, body must be cleansed by members of a ritual burial society; burial is carried out as soon as possible.
   e. After death: last rites optional.
   f. No special rituals before or after death.
10. (1005):
   a. May be vegetarian; prohibit meat and intoxicants.
   b. Pork prohibited; daylight fasting during month of Ramadan (around June and July).
   c. Kosher dietary laws prohibit eating pork and shellfish, prohibit eating meat with milk or milk products, and regulate food preparation.
   d. Prohibit use of alcohol, coffee, tea, and tobacco.
   e. Fast and abstain from meat on Ash Wednesday and Good Friday; abstain from meat on Fridays during Lent (older Catholics may continue to adhere to abstinence every Friday); fast for one hour before receiving Communion.
11. Any six (1006):
   a. Who is the client's god—a supreme being, governing principle, money, power, another human being?
   b. What is the client's relationship with a supreme being—one of fear or of love?
   c. How does the client express this spiritual relationship and are spiritual or religious practices part of this expression?
   d. Does the client view the self positively or negatively and worthy of the supreme being's love?
   e. Does the client act authentically and relate openly?
   f. Does the client assume responsibility for behavior and its consequences?
   g. How effectively does the client relate to family and friends?
   h. How effectively does the client relate to health care personnel, to other clients, and to strangers?
   i. Does the client see illness as a supreme being's punishment or as an indication of love?
   j. Does the client view illness as threatening?
   k. How have the diagnosis and therapy affected the client's self-concept, emotional state, will to live, and cooperation with rehabilitation?
12. Three for each classification (1006, 1007):
   Spiritual health
   a. Believes in a supreme being
   b. Views ultimate welfare and peace in terms of relationship to supreme being and world at large
   c. Is generally aware of personal limitations
   d. Strives to act in accordance with personal beliefs
   e. Assumes life's responsibilities with joy and cheerfulness.
   Spiritual distress
   a. Expresses anger with supreme being, spiritual care team, or nurse
   b. Questions meaning of life and suffering
   c. Verbalizes inner conflict of beliefs and required treatments
   d. Questions the reasons for existence or suffering
   e. Chooses not to participate in or is unable to choose usual religious practices
   f. Seeks spiritual assistance, questions moral and ethical implications of therapeutic regimen
13. To support and enhance the client's belief system, which sustains spirituality, or find someone able to do so (1009)
14. True (1009)
15. Any five (1010):
   a. Family and friends
   b. Clergy
   c. Spiritual advisor
   d. Privacy
   e. Pastoral care department
   f. Administration of sacraments or rites
   g. Religious objects
   h. Taped meditation or music
   i. Religious services (attending services or observing televised services)

16. Any five (1011):
  a. Is the client's belief system stronger?
  b. Do professed beliefs support and direct the client's actions and words?
  c. Does the client derive peace and strength from spiritual resources (such as prayer and minister's visits) to face the rigors of treatment, rehabilitation, or impending death?
  d. Does the client seem more in control and have a clearer self-concept?
  e. Is the client at ease in being alone and in having life's plans changed?
  f. Is the client's behavior appropriate to the occasion?
  g. Has reconciliation of differences, if any, taken place between the client and family members or other persons?
  h. Are mutual respect and love obvious in the client's relationships with others?

17. True (1011)

CHAPTER 34

1. Any five (1018-1019):
  a. Body image.
  b. Social practices
  c. Socioeconomic status
  d. Knowledge
  e. Cultural variables
  f. Personal preferences
  g. Physical condition

2. (1019)
  a. **(1)** Offering bedpan or urinal to client confined to bed.
  (2) Assisting client in washing face and hands and with oral hygiene.
  b. **(1)** Offering bedpan or urinal to client confined to bed.
  (2) Assisting with a bath or shower, oral hygiene, foot care, nail care, hair care.
  (3) Providing a back rub.
  (4) Changing client's pajamas.
  (5) Changing bed linens and straightening the bedside unit and room.
  c. **(1)** Offering a bedpan or urinal to client confined to bed.
  (2) Assisting client in washing face and hands, and providing oral hygiene.
  (3) Straightening bed linens.
  d. **(1)** Offering bedpan or urinal to client confined to bed.
  (2) Changing soiled bed linens, and pajamas.
  (3) Assisting the client in washing face and hands and with oral hygiene.
  (4) Providing a back rub.

3. At least two factors for each function (letter) (1020):
  a. **(1)** Epidermis is weakened by using dry razors, tape removal, and improper turning or positioning techniques.

(2) Excessive dryness causes breaks in the skin integrity that can allow bacteria to enter.
  (3) Emollients and moisturizers prevent drying and protect the skin.
  (4) Excessive exposure to moisture causes maceration, which promotes bacterial growth.
  (5) Misuse of soap, detergents, and other skin preparations may cause skin irritation, drying, and changes from an acid to an alkaline pH, which may damage the skin surface and predispose to infection.
  (6) Cleansing removes excess oil, sweat, dead skin cells, and dirt that can promote bacterial growth.
  b. **(1)** Friction should be used judiciously to avoid client discomfort.
  (2) Removal of rings from the nurse's fingers prevents accidental client injury.
  (3) Bath water temperature should be carefully checked.
  (4) Bed linens should be smooth to avoid mechanical irritation.
  c. **(1)** Wet bed linens interfere with convection and conduction.
  (2) Excess coverings can interfere with heat loss through radiation and conduction.
  (3) Coverings can promote heat conservation.
  d. **(1)** Perspiration and oil can harbor bacterial growth.
  (2) Bathing removes excess body secretions.
  (3) Excessive bathing and misuse of skin care products may cause excessive drying.

4. (1019-1020):
  a. 4
  b. 7
  c. 3
  d. 8
  e. 6
  f. 1
  g. 5
  h. 2
  i. 9

5. d (1021)

6. Two interventions for each skin problem listed:
  a. Acne (1022):
  (1) Wash hair and skin thoroughly each day.
  (2) Wash with hot water and soap.
  (3) Use cosmetics sparingly.
  (4) Implement dietary restrictions if food-associated problems are noted.
  (5) Limit exposure to sunshine or heat lamps.
  b. Abrasion (1023):
  (1) Prevent abrasions through nurses' maintenance of short nails and limited jewelry.
  (2) Wash with mild soap and water.
  (3) Observe dressings and bandages for retained moisture, increasing the risk of infection.

c. Hirsuitism (1022):
  (1) Depilatories are most hazardous.
  (2) Shaving is safest.
  (3) Electrolysis (permanent removal), tweezing (temporary), and bleaching (temporary) of hair may also be used.
d. Dry skin (1022):
  (1) Bathe less frequently.
  (2) Rinse body of all soap.
  (3) Add moisture to air through humidification.
  (4) Increase fluid intake.
  (5) Use moisturizing lotion.
  (6) Use creams to clean skin.
e. Rash (1022):
  (1) Wash area thoroughly.
  (2) Apply antiseptic spray or lotion.
  (3) Use warm or cold soaks.
f. Contact dermatitis (1023):
  (1) Identify causative agent.
  (2) Avoid causative agent.

7. (1021, 1023):
  a. Skin extremely thin, epidermis and dermis loosely bound together, poorly developed immune system.
  b. Active play and absence of established hygiene habits.
  c. Increased hormone levels, changes in skin texture, increased glandular activity (sebaceous, eccrine, and apocrine).
  d. Reduced skin resiliency and moisture, epithelium thins, shrinking of elastic collagen fibers.

8. Any six (1023):
  a. Balance
  b. Activity tolerance
  c. Muscle strength
  d. Coordination
  e. Vision
  f. Ability to sit without support
  f. Hand grasp
  g. Range of motion
  h. Cognitive function

9. (1023-1024):
  a. Immobilization
  b. Reduced sensation
  c. Nutrition and hydration alterations
  d. Secretions and excretions on the skin
  e. Vascular insufficiency
  f. External devices

10. c (1023-1024)

11. d (1024)

12. Any three (1023, 1027):
  a. Skin will remain intact and free of body odors.
  b. Range of motion is maintained.
  c. Client achieves a sense of comfort and well-being.
  d. Client participates in and understands methods of skin care.

13. (1026, 1028-1034):

Therapeutic Bath	Purpose	Safety Factors
Sitz bath	Cleanses and reduces inflammation of perineal and anal area	Water temperature of 43°-45° C (109.4°-113° F) (danger of burns). Cold Sitz baths more effective in relieving postpartum pain
Hot water tub bath	Relieves muscle soreness or spasm	Water temperature of 45°-46° C (113°-114° F) (danger of burns). Pulse and blood pressure may change (hypotension).
Warm water tub bath	Relieves muscle soreness	Water temperature of 43° C (109.4° F).
Cool water bath	Relieves tension, lower body temperature (especially in children)	Water temperature of 37° C (98.6° F). Chilling must be avoided. Pulse and blood pressure may change (dysrhythmias).
Soak	Remove dead tissue, soften crusted secretions, reduce pain and swelling	Aseptic technique if skin integrity impaired

14. True (1027)
15. d (1029)
16. False (1030)
17. Use plain warm water. Use different sections of the washcloth for each eye. Move the cloth from inner to outer canthus. Soak any crusting on eyelid for 2 or 3 minutes with damp cloth or cotton balls before attempting removal. Dry gently but thoroughly (1030).
18. d (1034)
19. Bathing only body parts that would cause discomfort or odor if left unbathed (for example, hands, face, perineal area, and axillae) (1027)
20. c (1034)
21. b (1028)
22. 37° C (98.6° F) (1026, 1028)
23. All four (1027):
  a. Provide privacy.
  b. Maintain safety.
  c. Maintain warmth.
  d. Promote client independence.
24. (1027):
  a. Temperature control mechanisms are inadequate; exposure causes rapid cooling.

b. Soaps are usually alkaline and alter skin pH, increasing bacterial growth and the risk of infection.

c. Lotions and oils create a medium for bacterial growth and may also alter the skin pH, increasing the risk of infection.

d. Sudden movement could cause applicator to damage eardrum and mucous membranes.

e. Alcohol dries the cord and reduces the chance of infection.

f. Skin is very delicate and should be dried gently to avoid abrasion; thorough drying prevents evaporative heat loss.

25. Vernix caseosa (1027)

26. a (1027, 1035)

27. d (1035-1038)

28. b (1036-1037)

29. b (1040)

30. d (1039-1040)

31. b (1039)

32. (1042-1043):
  a. 2
  b. 3
  c. 5
  d. 1
  e. 6
  f. 4

33. Diabetic clients develop vascular insufficiency and neuropathy, increasing the risk for injury to the feet. Any trauma can easily lead to infection.

34. False (1043)

35. Podiatrist (1045)

36. Any three (1045):
  a. Skin and nail surfaces will remain intact and smooth.
  b. Client achieves sense of comfort and cleanliness.
  c. Client will walk and bear weight normally.
  d. Client will understand and correctly perform methods for foot and nail care.

37. Any four (1044):
  a. Older adults
  b. Clients with diabetes
  c. Clients with heart disease (heart failure)
  d. Clients with renal disease
  e. Clients with cerebrovascular accident (stroke)

38. c (1044-1045)

39. Any seven (1046):
  a. Wash and soak the feet daily using lukewarm water. Thoroughly pat the feet dry, and dry well between the toes.
  b. Do not cut corns or calluses or use commercial removers. Consult a physician or podiatrist.
  c. If the feet tend to perspire, apply a bland foot powder.
  d. If dryness is noted along the feet or between the toes, apply lanolin, baby oil, or even corn oil and rub it gently into the skin.

  e. File the toenails straight across and square, and do not use scissors or clippers; consult a podiatrist as needed.
  f. Do not use over-the-counter preparations to treat athlete's foot or ingrown toenails; consult a physician or podiatrist.
  g. Avoid wearing elastic stockings, knee-high hose, or constricting garters and do not cross the legs; these impair circulation to the lower extremities.
  h. Inspect the feet daily, including tops and soles, heels, and the area between the toes.
  i. Wear clean socks or stockings daily. Socks should be free of holes and darns that might cause pressure.
  j. Do not walk barefoot.
  k. Wear proper-fitting shoes and ensure that they are sturdy, closed in, and not restrictive to the feet; the soles of shoes should be flexible and nonslipping, and lamb's wool can be used between toes that overlap.
  l. Exercise regularly to improve circulation to the lower extremities: Walk slowly, elevate; rotate, flex, and extend the feet at the ankle; dangle the feet over the side of the bed for 1 minute, extend both legs and hold them parallel to the bed while lying supine for 1 minute, and then rest for 1 minute.
  m. Avoid applying hot-water bottles or heating pads to the feet; use warm soaks or extra coverings instead.
  n. Wash minor cuts immediately, use only mild antiseptics (for example, neosporin ointment), and avoid iodine or Mercurochrome; contact a physician for treatment of cuts or lacerations.

40. a (1047)

41. Any six (1048):
  a. How often does the client brush teeth?
  b. What type of toothpaste or dentifrice does the client use?
  c. Does the client have dentures, and when and how does the client clean them?
  d. Does the client use mouthwash or lemon-glycerin preparations?
  e. Does the client floss and, if so, how often?
  f. When was the client's last dental visit, and what were the results?
  g. How often does the client visit a dentist?
  h. Is the client's water fluoridated?

42. **a.** 4 (1049)
  b. 2 (1048)
  c. 7 (1049)
  d. 1 (1048)
  e. 3 (1049)
  f. 6 (1049)
  g. 5 (1049)
  h. 8 (1049)

43. Regular flossing and brushing (1049)

44. (1048):
   a. Causes soreness, dysphagia, dryness, taste changes, and possible oral infections.
   b. Prone to dryness of mouth, gingivitis, periodontal disease, and tooth loss.
   c. Lacks upper extremity strength or dexterity needed to perform oral hygiene.
   d. Tissues easily traumatized with swelling, inflammation, break in integrity of membranes, possible bleeding, and ulcerations.
   e. Prone to dehydration and drying of mucous membranes; thick secretions develop on the tongue and gums; lips become cracked and reddened.
   f. Unable or unwilling to attend to personal hygiene needs.

45. Any three (1049):
   a. Any sore in the mouth that does not heal
   b. History of pipe smoking or use of chewing tobacco
   c. Lumps or ulcers in or around the mouth
   d. Lumps or ulcers at the base of the tongue

46. Any three (1049):
   a. Oral mucosa will be intact and well hydrated.
   b. Client will be able to independently perform correct oral hygiene.
   c. Client achieves sense of comfort.
   d. Client understands oral hygiene practices.

47. b (1051)

48. d (1051, 1054)

49. c (1051)

50. a (1052)

51. c (1052, 1053)

52. True (1052, 1053)

53. True (1054)

54. d (1055)

55. Place a drop of oil or ether on the tick or cover it with petroleum jelly before removal (1058).

56. (1058):
   a. Pediculosis pubis (crab lice)
   b. Pediculosis corporis (body lice)
   c. Pediculosis capitis (head lice)

57. Any two (1059):
   a. Hair and scalp will be clean and healthy.
   b. Client achieves a sense of comfort and self-esteem.
   c. Client will participate in health care practices.

58. False (1059)

59. d (1059, 1060)

60. Any two (1060):
   a. Clients receiving anticoagulant medications
   b. Clients taking high doses of aspirin
   c. Clients with bleeding disorders (hemophilia and leukemia)

61. Any two for each sensory aid listed (1061):
   a. Eyeglasses:
      (1) Purpose for wearing glasses
      (2) Methods used to clean glasses
      (3) Presence of symptoms (blurred vision, headaches, irritation)
   b. Artificial eye:
      (1) Method of inserting and removing the eye
      (2) Method of cleansing the eye
      (3) Presence of symptoms (drainage, inflammation, and pain involving the orbit)
   c. Hearing aid:
      (1) Type of aid worn
      (2) Methods used to cleanse aid
      (3) Client's ability to change battery and adjust hearing aid volume

62. Any four (1063):
   a. Type of lenses worn
   b. Frequency and duration of the time lenses are worn (include sleep time)
   c. Presence of symptoms (burning, excess tearing, redness, irritation, swelling, and sensitivity to light)
   d. Techniques used to cleanse, store, insert, and remove lenses
   e. Use of eye drops or ointments
   f. Use of emergency identification bracelet or card warning others to remove lenses in case of emergency.

63. Any two (1064):
   a. Absence of infection
   b. Normal sensory organ function
   c. Understanding of methods used for care of the eyes, ears, and nose

64. (1064):
   a. More frequent eye care is needed.
   b. Eye patch may be necessary over involved eye.
   c. Lubricating eye drops may be given (according to physician's orders).

65. a (1068, 1069)

66. d (1066)

67. Any three (1066):
   a. Becomes unconscious
   b. Restricted hand movement
   c. Loss of clear judgment because of psychiatric illness
   d. Temporary confusion
   e. Substance abuse

68. (1066, 1067):
   a. Retract the lower eyelid and exert slight pressure just below the eye (alternative: use small, rubber bulb syringe or medicine dropper bulb to create a suction effect directly over the artificial eye to lift it from the socket).
   b. Use warm normal saline for the prosthesis; use clean gauze soaked in warm saline or clean tap water for the edges of the eye socket and surrounding tissue.
   c. Retract the upper and lower lids and gently slip the eye into the socket, fitting it under the upper eyelid.
   d. Store in a labeled container filled with tap water or saline.

69. d (1067)

70. (1077):
   a. Head of bed elevated at least 45 degrees

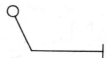

   b. Head of bed elevated approximately 30 degrees

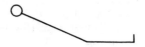

   c. Bed frame tilted head down

   d. Bed frame tilted foot down

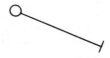

71. True (1077)
72. d (1078-1079)
73. d (1076, 1077)

CHAPTER 35

1. (1094):
   a. 3
   b. 5
   c. 2
   d. 6
   e. 4
   f. 1
2. All six:
   a. Water* (1095)
   b. Carbohydrates (1095)
   c. Proteins (1096)
   d. Lipids (1097)
   e. Vitamins (1097)
   f. Minerals (1099)
3. Both responses (1095):
   a. Infants
   b. Older adults
4. b (1097)
5. d (1095)
6. a. 4 kcal per gram × 20 grams = 80 kilocalories
   b. 9 kcal per gram × 15 grams = 135 kilocalories
   c. 4 kcal per gram × 50 grams = 200 kilocalories
7. Protein that contains all the essential amino acids in sufficient quantity to support growth and maintain nitrogen balance (also known as high biological value proteins) (1096)

8. Any three for each classification (1096):

Complete Proteins	Incomplete Proteins
Meat	Cereals
Fish	Legumes (beans, peas)
Poultry	
Milk	Vegetables
Eggs	

9. (1096):
   a. Condition in which intake and output of nitrogen are equal.
   b. Condition in which nitrogen loss exceeds nitrogen intake (associated with body tissue destruction).
   c. Condition in which body protein nitrogen is retained for building, repair, or replacement of body tissues (associated with period of growth).
10. b (1096, 1097)
11. (1097):
   a. Decreases blood cholesterol
   b. Minimal effect on blood cholesterol
   c. Increases blood cholesterol
12. a (1097)
13. Essential fatty acid = linoleic acid; any three (1097):
   a. Safflower oil
   b. Soybean oil
   c. Corn oil
   d. Cottonseed oil
   e. Peanut oil
14. a (1097)
15. b (1097)
16. c (1099)
17. Minerals serve as catalysts in biochemical reactions (1099).
18. Refer to Chapter 35, Tables 35-2, 35-3, 35-4, and 35-5 on pp. 1098-1101.
19. a. 2 ,4, and 9
   b. 1, 5, 6, 7, and 8
   c. 3
20. c (1102)
21. a (1102)
22. b (1103)
23. (1105):

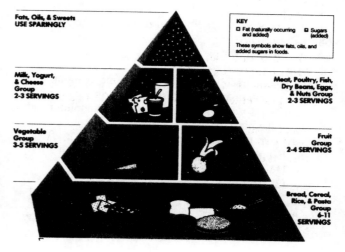

24. It is easily remembered and can be used as a buying and food preparation guide for individuals (1104).
25. The level of intake of essential nutrients considered in the judgment of the National Academy of Sciences to be adequate to meet nutritional needs of healthy people (1104)
26. Congressional legislation mandating nutritional labeling for most FDA regulated foods (1104,1105)
27. Any five (1105):
    a. Eat a variety of foods.
    b. Maintain healthy body weight.
    c. Choose a diet low in fat, saturated fat, and cholesterol.
    d. Choose a diet with plenty of vegetables, fruits, and grain products.
    e. Use sugar in moderation.
    f. Use salt in moderation.
    g. If you drink, do so in moderation.
28. (1106):
    a. 2
    b. 3
    c. 1
29. b (1107)
30. b (1107)
31. a (1107)
32. All four (1107):
    a. Vitamin C
    b. Vitamin D
    c. Fluoride
    d. Iron
33. 4 to 6 months (1109)
34. Any four (1109):
    a. Infant doubling birth weight.
    b. Ability to consume 8 ounces of formula and to become hungry in less than 4 hours.
    c. Ability to sit up.
    d. Ability to consume 32 ounces a day and want more.
    e. 6 months of age.
35. d (1108, 1109)
36. d (1110)
37. c (1110)
38. c (1111)
39. d (1114)
40. Any four (1114):
    a. Income*
    b. State of health
    c. Living arrangements (living alone)
    d. Diminished taste acuity
    e. Less efficient digestion (because of decreased gastric secretions)
    f. Dental (chewing) problems
41. All four (1115):
    a. Nursing history
    b. Observation (assessment)
    c. Anthropometry
    d. Laboratory data
42. All seven (1116):
    a. Health status
    b. Culture and religion
    c. Socioeconomic status
    d. Personal preference
    e. Psychological factors
    f. Alcohol and drugs
    g. Misinformation and food fads
43. Any three (1116):
    a. Money is spent on alcohol rather than more nutritional foods.
    b. Alcohol may replace part of the diet, reducing intake of nutrients.
    c. Alcohol can depress the appetite.
    d. Alcohol reduces the efficiency of digestion and nutrient absorption.
44. Refer to Chapter 35, Table 35-11, pp. 1117-1118.
45. All five (1118-1120):
    a. Weight
    b. Height
    c. Wrist circumference
    d. Mid-upper arm circumference (MAC)
    e. Triceps skin fold (TSF)
46. c (1120)
47. (1121):
    a. Anorexia nervosa
    b. Bulimia
48. Any two (1123):
    a. Client will return to within 10% of ideal body weight.
    b. Client will maintain fluid/electrolyte balance within normal limits.
    c. Client will not experience complications associated with nutritional therapies.
49. All five (1123):
    a. Glucose,
    b. Amino acids
    c. Lipids
    d. Minerals
    e. Vitamins
50. Any three (1124):
    a. Remove any reminders of treatments (completed or anticipated).
    b. Control odors.
    c. Provide mouth care.
    d. Position comfortably.
    e. Provide suitable alternatives when foods are refused.
51. d (1124)
52. (1124, 1125):
    a. Clear liquid
    b. Soft
    c. Low residue
    d. Regular
    e. Liberal bland
    f. Full liquid
    g. High fiber
53. Both responses (1128):
    a. Oral
    b. Tube feedings
54. a (1128)
55. c (1128)

56. (1129):
  a. Measure the total distance from the client's nose to ear to zyphoid.
  b. Add an additional 20 to 30 cm to the distance determined above.
57. Both responses (1131):
  a. Aspirate gastric secretions and check gastric residual.
  b. Measure pH of gastric aspirate.
58. False (1128, 1131, 1132)
59. The amount of a feeding remaining in the stomach (1132)
60. c (1132)
61. It is difficult to aspirate even small volumes of fluid through small-bore feeding tubes, making accurate determination of gastric residual impossible. Abdominal distention, nausea, and vomiting may indicate gastric retention and alert the nurse to the risk of regurgitation and possible aspiration of gastric contents (1128, 1131, 1132).
62. b (1133)
63. High Fowler's (1132)
64. **a.** Dilates the central veins and reduces the risk of air embolism (1136).
  b. Increases venous filling of the vein and reduces the risk of air embolism (1136).
  c. Confirms correct placement and identifies complications such as accidental puncture of the lung or parietal pleura (pneumothorax) (1136).
  d. Reduces risk of infection (1137).
  e. Maintains infusion at prescribed rate to avoid too rapid administration (hyperglycemia, osmotic diuresis, hypoglycemia, and fluid overload) (1137).
  f. Evaluates the presence of hyperglycemia or hypoglycemia (1136, 1137).
65. c (1137)
66. False (1136, 1137)

CHAPTER 36

1. State of decreased mental and physical activity leaving a person refreshed, rejuvenated, and ready to resume activities of the day (1146)
2. Recurrent state of altered consciousness occurring for sustained periods; restores energy and well-being (1146)
3. All three (1146):
  a. Physical comfort
  b. Freedom from worry
  c. Sufficient sleep
4. c (1147)
5. b (1147)
6. See the table at right (1147, 1148):
7. (1148-1150):
  a. 2
  b. 4
  c. 1
  d. 5
  e. 3
8. d (1150)

	Sleep Mechanism	Arousal Mechanism
Name	Bulbar synchronizing region (BSR)	Reticular activating system (RAS)
Anatomical location	Raphe sleep system; pons and medial forebrain	Upper brainstem
Neurotransmitter	Serotonin	Catecholamine (norepinephrine)

9. a (1151)
10. False (1153)
11. Any five:
  a. Physical illness: often associated with pain, discomfort, anxiety, or depression; creates problems falling asleep, staying asleep, sleeping in unaccustomed positions (1153).
  b. Drugs and substances: prescribed, over-the-counter, and illicit drugs can disrupt rest and sleep; although medications may be used to induce sleep, they provide only temporary effect and potentially create additional problems (1154).
  c. Lifestyle: routine patterns of daily living may influence sleep patterns; for example, rotating shifts, performing unaccustomed work, late-night social activities, and changing evening mealtimes (1154, 1155).
  d. Sleep patterns: duration of sleep and the time sleep begins influence succeeding attempts to fall asleep; problems with sleep patterns in turn influence an individual's performance of daily functions (1155).
  e. Emotional stress: stress, tension, and worry may alter sleep patterns and reduce the benefits of rest derived from time spent sleeping (1155).
  f. Environment: conditions in which the individual attempts to rest or sleep affect these patterns; factors in the environment include ventilation, position and condition of the bed, presence or absence of a bed partner, noise levels, light levels, and room temperature (1155, 1156).
  g. Exercise and fatigue: moderate fatigue promotes restful sleep, excessive fatigue may make falling asleep difficult; optimal time for exercise that promotes rest and sleep is at least 2 hours before bedtime (1156).
  h. Caloric intake: weight loss and gain influence sleep patterns; weight gain tends to lengthen sleep periods and reduce the frequency of cycle interruptions; weight loss tends to shorten and fragment sleep (1156).
12. L-Tryptophan (1154)
13. **a.** 6 (1157)
  b. 3 (1156)
  c. 7 (1158)
  d. 1 (1156)
  e. 5 (1156, 1157)
  f. 8 (1158)

g. 4 (1157)
h. 2 (1156)
14. Condition in which the individual experiences a decrease in the amount, quality, and consistency of sleep; results in changes in the normal sequence of sleep stages accompanied by alterations in the individual's behavior (1157, 1158)
15. Any four symptoms for each category (1157):

Physiological Symptoms	Psychological Symptoms
Hand tremors	Changes in mood
Decreased reflexes	Disorientation
Slower response time	Irritability
Reduction in word memory	Decreased motivation
Decreased reasoning, judgment	Fatigue
Cardiac dysrhythmias	Sleepiness
Decreased auditory/visual alertness	Hyperactivity
	Agitation

16. d (1158)
17. Any five:
    a. Description of client's sleeping problem (1160)
    b. Normal sleep pattern (1160, 1161);
    c. Physical illness (1161)
    c. Current life events (1161)
    d. Emotional and mental status (1161)
    e. Bedtime rituals and environment (1161, 1162)
    f. Sleep/wake log (1162)
    g. Sleep deprivation behaviors (1162)
18. Any three (1164, 1165):
    a. Client feels a sense of restfulness and renewed energy after sleep.
    b. Client identifies factors promoting or disrupting sleep.
    c. Client assumes self-care behaviors to control factors contributing to sleep deprivation.
    d. Client establishes a healthy sleep pattern.
19. Any six:
    a. Environmental control (1165)
    b. Promoting bedtime rituals (1166)
    c. Promoting comfort (1166)
    d. Establishing periods of rest and sleep (1166)
    e. Controlling physiological disturbances (1167)
    f. Stress reduction (1167)
    g. Bedtime snack (1167)
    h. Administration of sleeping medications (1167)
    i. Client teaching (1168)
20. a (1165)
21. d (1165)
22. b (1166)
23. Any four (1165):
    a. Avoid physical and mental stimulation before bedtime.
    b. Exercise 2 hours before bedtime.
    c. Engage in a relaxing activity before bedtime (for example, reading, watching television, or listening to music).
    d. Use bedroom only as bedroom, not as a work area.

e. Maintain a consistent bedtime.
f. Eat a light snack before bedtime.
g. Void before going to bed.
h. Practice relaxation techniques at bedtime (for example, relaxation exercises, guided imagery, praying, meditation, or yoga).
24. Any six (1166):
    a. Administer analgesics and/or sedatives about 30 minutes before bedtime.
    b. Encourage clients to wear loose-fitting clothing to bed.
    c. Remove any irritants against the client's skin (such as moist or wrinkled sheets or drainage tubes).
    d. Position and support body parts to protect pressure points and aid muscle relaxation.
    e. Offer a massage just before bedtime.
    f. Provide caps and socks for older clients and those prone to cold.
    g. Administer necessary hygiene measures.
    h. Keep bed linen clean and dry.
    i. Provide a comfortable mattress.
    j. Encourage client to void before bedtime.
25. False (1156)
26. c (1167)
27. d (1167)
28. b (1168)
29. d (1168)

CHAPTER 37

1. "An unpleasant, subjective sensory experience associated with actual or potential tissue damage, or described in terms of such damage" (IASP, 1979, cited p. 1176)
2. c (1176)
3. True (1176)
4. a (1176)
5. **a.** Reception: transmission of pain signals through special neuropathways to neuroreceptors (1177).
   b. Perception: the point at which pain is experienced; results from interaction of psychological and cognitive factors with neurophysiological factors (1178, 1180).
   c. Reaction: physiological and behavioral response to pain; occurs after pain perception (1181).
6. The point at which the pain stimulus is intense enough to create a nerve impulse and be perceived by the individual (1181)
7. (1179):

Type	A Fibers	C Fibers
Fiber size	Large	Small
Myelination status	Myelinated	Unmyelinated
Transmission speed	Rapid	Slow
Nature of pain message	Localize source; detect pain intensity	Diffuse response

8. (1180):
  a. 3
  b. 5
  c. 1
  d. 2
  e. 4
9. a (1178)
10. All three (1180):
  a. Sensory-discriminative
  b. Motivational-affective
  c. Cognitive-evaluative
11. False (1181)
12. (1181):
  a. S
  b. P
  c. P
  d. S
  e. S
  f. P
13. a. Anticipation phase: awareness that pain will occur; most important because it can affect the other phases; allows person to learn about pain and its relief (1181).
  b. Sensation phase: phase when pain is felt; involves physical and behavioral responses to the pain (1181, 1182).
  c. Aftermath phase: occurs when pain is reduced or stopped; does not terminate client's need for nursing care; may involve physical or behavioral responses requiring nursing intervention.
14. The point at which there is an unwillingness to accept pain of greater severity or duration (1182)
15. Pain impulses can be regulated or blocked by gating mechanisms located along the central nervous system. When gates are open, pain impulses flow freely. When gates are closed, pain impulses are blocked. Partial opening of the gates may also occur. The opening or closing of a gate depends on large and small fiber transmission, reticular formation activity, and cerebral cortex and thalamic mechanisms (1179).
16. b (1179-1181)
17. Any four (1183):
  a. Rapid onset
  b. Variable intensity (mild to severe)
  c. Brief duration (less than 6 months)
  d. Warns of impending injury or disease
  e. Self-limiting
18. c (1183)
19. Any four (1183):
  a. Absence of overt pain symptoms
  b. Fatigue
  c. Insomnia
  d. Anorexia
  e. Weight loss
  f. Depression
  g. Hopelessness
  h. Anger

20. b (1183)
21. Any seven (1184):
  a. Age
  b. Sex
  c. Culture
  d. Meaning of pain
  e. Attention
  f. Anxiety
  g. Fatigue
  h. Previous experience
  i. Coping style
  j. Family and social support
22. c (1189)
23. d (1190)
24. True (1191)
25. A symptom that often accompanies pain (such as nausea, headache, dizziness, urination, constipation, or restlessness) (1191)
26. Two examples for each behavioral indicator (1191):
  a. Vocalizations:
    (1) Moaning
    (2) Crying
    (3) Screaming
    (4) Gasping
    (5) Grunting.
  b. Facial expressions:
    (1) Grimace
    (2) Clenched teeth
    (3) Wrinkled forehead
    (4) Tightly closed or widely open eyes or mouth
    (5) Lip biting
    (6) Tightened jaw.
  c. Body movement:
    (1) Restlessness
    (2) Immobilization
    (3) Muscle tension
    (4) Increased hand and finger movements
    (5) Rhythmic or rubbing motions
    (6) Pacing activities
    (7) Protective movement of body parts.
  d. Social interaction:
    (1) Avoidance of conversation
    (2) Focus only on activities for pain relief
    (3) Avoidance of social contacts
    (4) Reduced attention span
27. b (1195)
28. Any three (1195):
  a. Obtain a sense of well-being and comfort.
  b. Maintain the ability to perform self-care.
  c. Maintain existing physical and psychosocial function.
  d. Explain factors contributing to the pain experience.
29. c (1195, 1196)
30. Any eight (1196):
  a. Establish a relationship of mutual trust.
  b. Provide pain relief measures before pain becomes severe.
  c. Use different types of pain-relief measures.

d. Consider the client's ability or willingness to participate in pain-relief measures.

e. Choose pain-relief measures on the basis of the client's behavior reflecting the severity of pain.

f. Use measures the client believes are effective.

g. If a therapy is ineffective at first, encourage the client to try it again before abandoning it.

h. Keep an open mind about what may relieve pain.

i. Keep trying.

j. Protect the client.

k. Educate the client about pain.

31. True (1196)

32. **a.** 3 (1200)
b. 2 (1197)
c. 1 (1197)
d. 2 (1200)
e. 1 (1197)
f. 2 (1197)
g. 3 (1200, 1202)

33. Transcutaneous electric nerve stimulation: stimulates cutaneous skin over or near the pain site; believed to increase release of endorphins or activate large-diameter sensory fibers to block transmission of painful impulses from small-diameter fibers (1199)

34. c (1200)

35. a (1201)

36. True (1200)

37. d (1196, 1200)

38. Any five (1202):
a. Occurrence, onset, and expected duration of pain
b. Quality, severity, and location of pain
c. Information on how the client's safety is ensured
d. Cause of pain
e. Methods nurse and client take for pain relief
f. Expectations of the client during a procedure

39. Any six (1203):
a. Rapid onset
b. Effective action over a prolonged time
c. Availability for all ages
d. Oral and parenteral use
e. Lack of severe side effects
f. Nonaddicting
g. Inexpensive

40. All four (1204):
a. Know the client's previous response to analgesics.
b. Select the proper medication when more than one is ordered.
c. Know the accurate dosage.
d. Assess the right time and interval for administration.

41. d (1202, 1204)

42. Patient-controlled analgesia: portable computerized pump with a chamber for a syringe allowing clients to administer pain medications when they want or need them (1204)

43. Any three (1205):
a. Clients have control over their pain.

b. Pain relief does not depend on nurse availability.
c. Clients tend to take less medication.
d. Small doses of nalgesics delivered at short intervals stabilize serum drug concentrations for sustained pain relief.

44. b (1205, 1206)

45. Four goals and one related action for each goal (1207):
a. Prevent catheter displacement
(1) Limit client's activity.
(2) Secure catheter (if not connected to implanted reservoir) carefully to outside skin.
b. Maintain catheter function
(1) Check external dressing around catheter site for dampness or discharge (leak of cerebrospinal fluid may develop).
c. Prevent infection
(1) Use strict aseptic technique when caring for catheter
(2) Change tubing every 24 hours.
d. Prevent undesirable complications
(1) Monitor vital signs (hypotension, respiratory depression, and bradycardia indicate systemic absorption)
(2) Assess for blurred vision, ringing in ears, pruritis (itching), and nausea and vomiting.
e. Maintain urinary and bowel function
(1) Monitor intake and output
(2) Assess for bladder and bowel distention.

46. Any treatment that produces an effect because of its intent rather than its physical or chemical properties (1207)

47. False (1207)

48. d (1207)

49. a (1206)

50. Posterior rhizotomy (1208)

51. False (1208)

52. False (1208)

53. (1208, 1209)

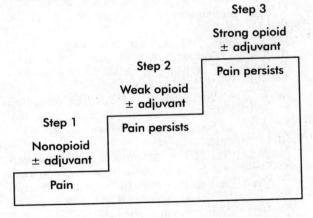

54. b (1208, 1209)

55. Any four (1209):
a. Observe for side effects, including sedation, hy-

potension, dizziness or fainting, nausea, vomiting, respiratory depression, and constipation.
  b. Be prepared to administer naloxone intramuscularly to reverse respiratory depression.
  c. Keep the central venous catheter patent; maintain minimum pump flow rate. and irrigate catheter routinely with heparin flush.
  d. Prevent air from entering central venous catheter; clamp catheter when infusion has stopped.
  e. Prevent infection at catheter site; keep site clean.
56. a (1211)

CHAPTER 38

  1. Myocardial fibers have contractile properties enabling the fiber to stretch during filling. In the healthy heart, as the myocardium stretches, the strength of the subsequent contraction also increases (1218).
  2. c (1218)
  3. False (1218)
  4. **a.** 4
     b. 2
     c. 5
     d. 3
     e. 1 (1220)
  5. Refer to Fig. 38-3 on p. 1221 in your text.
  6. Refer to Fig. 38-4 in your text.
  7. The process by which gases are moved into and out of the lungs (1222)
  8. Phrenic nerve (1222)
  9. b (1222)
 10. (1222, 1223)
     a. 2
     b. 3
     c. 1
     d. 4
 11. Spirometer (1223)
 12. Blood flow, movement of blood to the tissues (1223, 1224)
 13. c (1223, 1224)
 14. Movement of molecules from an area of high concentration to an area of lower concentration (1225)
 15. All four (1225):
     a. Ventilation (oxygen entering the lungs)
     b. Perfusion (blood flow to the lungs and tissues)
     c. Diffusion (exchange of carbon dioxide and oxygen between alveoli and capillary)
     d. Capacity of blood to carry oxygen (dissolved oxygen in plasma, amount of hemoglobin, tendency of hemoglobin to bind with oxygen)
 16. Both responses (1225)
     a. Neural regulation: influence of the central nervous system in controlling respiratory rate, depth, and rhythm through cerebral cortex (intermittent voluntary control) and medulla oblongata (continuous automatic control).
     b. Chemical regulation: influence of chemicals such as carbon dioxide and hydrogen ions on the rate and depth of respiration through chemoreceptors

in the medulla and aortic and carotid bodies (serves as a short-term adaptive mechanism).
 17. (1226, 1227):
     a. 4
     b. 2
     c. 1
     d. 6
     e. 5
     f. 3
     g. 4 or 5
     h. 1
     i. 4
 18. All three (1226):
     a. Decreased hemoglobin production
     b. Increased red cell destruction
     c. Blood loss
 19. d (1226)
 20. One for each developmental level: (1226, 1227)
     a. Premature infant: surfactant deficiency.
     b. Infant and toddler: frequent exposure to other children; teething process, increasing nasal congestion; and airway obstruction from foreign objects of airway infections.
     c. School-age child and adolescent: exposure to others with infections, respiratory risk factors (for example, smoking, [active or passive]).
     d. Young adult: exposure to multiple cardiopulmonary risk factors.
     e. Older adult: decreased lung elasticity, alveolar enlargement, bronchodilation, osteoporotic changes in the thoracic cage.
 21. (1228):
     a. Nutrition: obesity decreases lung expansion; malnutrition and associated muscle wasting diminish respiratory excursion and ability to effectively cough; high-fat diet increases cholesterol and atherogenesis in coronary arteries; and obesity and malnourishment increase risk for anemia.
     b. Exercise: exercise increases metabolism and therefore oxygen requirements; exercise and physical conditioning can enhance oxygen consumption and use, decrease heart rate, decrease blood pressure, decrease cholesterol level, increase blood flow, and increase oxygen extraction.
     c. Cigarette smoking: associated with several disease states, including chronic obstructive pulmonary disease (COPD), lung cancer, and heart disease.
     d. Substance abuse: chronic substance abuse is often associated with poor nutritional intake and anemia; some substances can depress respiratory center in the central nervous system (CNS).
     e. Anxiety: severe anxiety increases oxygen requirements; although tolerated in normal individuals, the additional oxygen demand created by anxiety cannot be tolerated by individuals with certain illnesses.
 22. Dysrhythmia (1229)

23. (1229):
  a. 5
  b. 4
  c. 1
  d. 3
  e. 2
24. a (1229)
25. c (1229, 1232)
26. b (1232)
27. a. Angina pectoris can be aching, sharp, tingling, or burning or feel like pressure. Pain is located on the left side or is substernal with radiation to the left or both arms, jaw, neck, and back, Pain is precipitated by activities such as exercise, anxiety, and stress; lasts from 3 to 15 minutes; and is relieved with rest and coronary vasodilators (most commonly nitroglycerin) (1232).
  b. Myocardial infarction pain may be described as crushing, squeezing, or stabbing. The pain may be retrosternal and left precordial; it may radiate down left arm and to the neck, jaws, teeth, epigastric area, and back. Pain occurs at rest or exertion, lasts more than 30 minutes, and is unrelieved by rest, position change, or sublingual nitroglycerin administration (1232).
28. State of ventilation in excess of that required to maintain normal carbon dioxide levels; excreting excess carbon dioxide (1232)
29. False (1232)
30. Any six (1233):
  a. Tachycardia
  b. Shortness of breath
  c. Chest pain
  d. Dizziness
  e. Light-headedness
  f. Decreased concentration
  g. Paresthesia
  h. Numbness (extremities, circumoral)
  i. Tinnitus
  j. Blurred vision
  k. Disorientation
  l. Tetany (carpopedal spasm)
31. c (1223)
32. Both responses (1233):
  Atelectasis and inappropriate administration of oxygen
33. Because client with COPD have adapted to a high carbon dioxide level, their respiratory drive is hypoxia. Administration of high concentration of oxygen (greater than 24% to 28% [1 to 3 liters]) will eliminate the hypoxic drive, depress breathing, and in some cases precipitate respiratory arrest (1233).
34. Any five (1233):
  a. Dizziness
  b. Headache
  c. Lethargy
  d. Disorientation
  e. Decreased ability to follow instructions
  f. Cardiac dysrhythmias (arrhythmias)

  g. Electrolyte imbalances
  h. Convulsions
  i. Coma
  j. Cardiac arrest
35. Inadequate cellular oxygenation that results from a deficiency in oxygen delivery at the cellular level (1233)
36. Any four (1233):
  a. Decreased hemoglobin level
  b. Diminished oxygen concentration in inspired air
  c. Inability of the tissues to extract oxygen from the blood
  d. Decreased diffusion of oxygen from the alveoli to the blood
  e. Poor tissue perfusion
  f. Impaired ventilation
37. Any seven (1234):
  a. Restlessness
  b. Apprehension and anxiety
  c. Decreased ability to concentrate
  d. Decreased level of consciousness
  e. Increased fatigue
  f. Dizziness
  g. Behavioral changes
  h. Increased pulse rate
  i. Increased rate and depth of respiration
  j. Elevated blood pressure
  k. Cardiac dysrhythmias
  l. Pallor
  m. Cyanosis
  n. Clubbing
  o. Dyspnea
38. d
39. Shortness of breath or difficulty breathing (pathological when it is not associated with short-term response to exercise or excitement) (1234)
40. Any eight (1234, 1236):
  a. Cough
  b. Dyspnea
  c. Wheezing
  d. Pain
  e. Environmental or geographic exposures
  f. Frequency of respiratory tract infection
  g. Risk factors
  h. Past respiratory problems
  i. Fatigue
  j. Medications
41. Any five (1235):
  a. Color or change in color
  b. Consistency and quality
  c. Quantity
  d. Taste
  e. Odor
  f. Presence of blood
42. d (1235)
43. Orthopnea (1235)
44. A form of rhonchus characterized by a high-pitched, musical quality that does not clear with coughing (1236)

45. (1237):
  a. Vasoconstriction and diminished peripheral blood flow
  b. Heart failure (right sided and left sided)
  c. Heart failure (right sided)
  d. Increased work of breathing and dyspnea;
  e. Anemia
  f. In young and middle adults: hyperlipidemia; in older adults: normal
  g. Decreased oxygenation (hypoxia)
  h. Chronic hypoxemia
  i. Hyperlipidemia

46. (1238):
  a. 3
  b. 6
  c. 2
  d. 5
  e. 4
  f. 1

47. Asynchronous breathing with the chest contracting during inspiration and expanding during expiration (1238)

48. a (1238)

49. a (1239)

50. Oximetry (1240)

51. Information about diffusion of gases across the alveolar capillary membrane and adequacy of tissue oxygenation (hydrogen ion concentration, partial pressure of carbon dioxide, oxygen concentration, and oxyhemoglobin saturation) (1239)

52. The importance of holding breath, not coughing, and not moving (1242)

53. Any four (1243):
  a. Ineffective airway clearance
  b. Impaired gas exchange
  c. Ineffective breathing pattern
  d. Decreased cardiac output
  e. Activity intolerance
  f. High risk for infection

54. Any five (1243):
  a. Improved activity tolerance
  b. Maintenance and promotion of lung expansion
  c. Mobilization of pulmonary secretions
  d. Maintenance of a patent airway
  e. Maintenance of promotion of tissue oxygenation
  f. Restoration of cardiopulmonary function

55. See the table at right (1244-1249):

56. b (1248)

57. Pneumothorax (1248)

58. d (1248, 1249)

59. d (1250)

60. True (1249)

61. All three (1251):
  a. Percussion: striking the chest wall over the area being drained using a cupped hand.
  b. Vibration: fine, shaking pressure applied to the chest wall during exhalation.

Nursing Intervention	Purpose
Positioning the client	Increase chest wall expansion
	Prevent stasis of pulmonary secretions
Pursed-lip breathing	Decrease work of breathing
	Slow respiratory rate
	Increase tidal volume
	Decrease dead space ventilation
Diaphragmatic breathing	Decrease work of breathing
	Decrease air trapping
	Promote relaxation
	Control pain
Flow-oriented incentive spirometer	Encourage voluntary deep breathing
	Prevent or treat atelectasis
Blow bottles	Encourage voluntary deep breathing
Maintaining hydration	Maintain normal mucociliary action
Inserting an oral airway	Prevent obstruction of trachea by displacement of tongue
	Facilitate orotracheal suctioning

  c. Postural drainage: use of positioning techniques that draw secretions from specific segments of the lungs and bronchi into the trachea for easier expectoration

62. d (1251)

63. a (1252)

64. b (1252)

65. c (1249)

66. b (1253)

67. All three (1252):
  a. Coughing techniques
  b. Suctioning
  c. Artificial airway

68. See table at right (1252):

69. Any two (1252):
  a. Sputum expectoration
  b. Client's report of swallowed sputum
  c. Clearing of adventitious sounds on auscultation

70. c (1254)

71. b (1259)

72. All five:
  a. Right client
  b. Right drug (oxygen)
  c. Right dose (liter flow/percentage)
  d. Right route (delivery method)
  e. Right time (continuous, prn)

73. Any three (1260):
  a. Post "no smoking" signs on client door and over bed.
  b. Inform clients, visitors, and roommates that smoking is prohibited in the area in which oxygen is in use.
  c. Ensure that electrical equipment is functioning correctly and properly grounded.

Cough	Technique	Action/Benefits
Controlled cough	Take two slow, deep breaths (inhaling through nose, exhaling through mouth) Inhale deeply the third time and hold breath to count of 3 Cough fully for two to three consecutive coughs without inhaling between coughs Instruct to "push all air out of lungs" Splint any painful areas while coughing	Clears secretions from upper and lower airways
Cascade cough	Take a slow, deep breath and hold it for 2 seconds while contracting expiratory muscles Open mouth and perform a series of coughs throughout the breath	Promotes airway clearance and patent airway in clients with large volumes of sputum
Huff cough	While exhaling, say the word "huff"	Stimulates natural cough Generally only effective in clearing central airways Useful as initial technique in clients unable to perform cascade cough
Quad cough	Client or nurse pushes in and up on abdominal muscles toward diaphragm while client breathes with maximal expiratory effort	Used for clients without abdominal muscle control (for example, clients with spinal cord injuries)

d. Know the institution's fire procedures.

e. Know the location of the closest fire extinguisher.

74. All three (1263):

a. Absence of respirations

b. Absence of pulse

c. Dilated pupils

75. (1263):

a. Establish an airway (A).

b. Initiate breathing (B).

c. Maintain circulation (C).

CHAPTER 39

1. b (1267)

2. An element or compound that when melted or dissolved in water or another solvent dissociates into ions and is able to carry an electric current (1276)

3. All four:

a. Diffusion: process by which solid particulate matter such as sugar in fluid moves from an area of higher concentration to an area of lower concentration resulting in an even distribution of particles in the fluid or across the cell membrane permeable to that substance (1277).

b. Osmosis: movement of pure solvent such as water through a semipermeable membrane from a solution that has a lower solute concentration to one that has a higher solute concentration (membrane is permeable to solvent but it is impermeable to the solute) (1277).

(1) Osmotic pressure: the "drawing power" for water, dependent on the activity of solutes separated by a semipermeable membrane causing water to be pulled through the membrane.

c. Active transport: movement of materials across the cell membrane by chemical activity or energy expenditure allowing the cell to admit larger molecules than it would otherwise be able to admit or to move molecules from areas of lesser concentration to areas of greater concentration (1278).

d. Filtration: process by which water and diffusible substances move together in response to fluid pressure (1277).

(1) Hydrostatic pressure: the pressure exerted by a liquid, pushing it from one compartment to another.

4. c (1278)

5. a (1277)

6. (1277):

a. Isotonic

b. Hypotonic

c. Hypertonic

7. Increased plasma osmolarity or decreased blood volume stimulates the thirst center located in the hypothalamus. Osmoreceptors are receptor cells that continually monitor osmotic pressure so that when too much fluid is lost, the osmoreceptors detect the loss and activate the thirst center (1278).

8. All four (1279):

a. Kidneys

b. Lungs

c. Skin

d. Gastrointestinal tract

9. 55 ml (1 ml/kg/hr: $1 \times g$) (1279)

10. Water loss that is continuous and is not perceived by the person or measurable in usual clinical situations (1279)

11. (1279, 1280):

Hormone	Stimuli	Action
ADH	Increased blood osmolarity reflecting water deficit	Increases reabsorption of water by kidney tubules, decreasing production of urine
Aldosterone	Fluid deficits	Causes kidney tubules to excrete potassium and reabsorb sodium Sodium reabsorption causes water reabsorption
Glucocorticoids	Normally present without significant influence on fluid or electroltes, but when other conditions cause increased or decreased release, imbalances may occur	With excess: Sodium and water retention Potassium loss (exchanged for sodium in tubule)

12. c (1280)
13. a. Sodium (135 to 145 mEq/L) (1280).
  (1) Function: maintains water balance, transmits nerve impulses, facilitates muscle contraction.
  (2) Regulatory mechanisms: salt intake, aldosterone, urinary output.
b. Potassium (3.5 to 5.3 mEq/L) (1280).
  (1) Function: regulates neuromuscular excitability and muscle contraction, assists in maintaining acid-base balance.
  (2) Regulatory mechanisms: kidney is primary regulatory mechanisms, aldosterone stimulates K^+ excretion, also exchanges with sodium ion in the tubule (Na^{++} excreted, K^+ retained; Na^{++} retained, K^+ excreted).
c. Calcium (ionized): 4.0 to 5.0 mEq/L; nonionized: 5 mg/100 ml) (1280).
  (1) Function: cell membrane integrity and structure, cardiac conduction, blood coagulation, bone growth and formation, and muscle relaxation.
  (2) Regulatory mechanisms: parathyroid hormone (PTH) controls balance among bone Ca^{++}, gastrointestinal absorption, and kidney excretion; thyrocalcitonin from the thyroid inhibits bone release of Ca^{++}.
d. Magnesium (1.5 to 2.5 mEq/L) (1280).
  (1) Function: enzyme activities, neurochemical activities, and muscular excitability.
  (2) Regulatory mechanisms: renal excretion.
e. Chloride (100 to 106 mEq/L) (1281).
  (1) Function: balances cations within the extracellular fluid to maintain electroneutrality in extracelluar fluid.
  (2) Regulatory mechanisms: dietary intake and renal excretion.
f. Bicarbonate (22 to 26 mEq/L arterial; 24 to 30 mEq/L venous) (1281).
  (1) Function: major chemical base buffer.
  (2) Regulatory mechanisms: renal regulation in response to pH of extracellular fluid.
g. Phosphate (2.5 to 4.5 mg/100 ml) (1281).
  (1) Function: development and maintenance of bones and teeth, promotes normal neuromuscular action, participates in carbohydrate metabolism, and assists in acid-base regulation.
  (2) Regulatory mechanisms: regulated by kidneys, parathyroid hormone, activated by vitamin D, absorbed through GI tract, and serum levels inversely proportional to Ca^{++}

14. d (1281)
15. 7.35 to 7.45 (1281)
16. (1281,1282):
a. Primarily involves the carbonic acid and bicarbonate buffer system, which is the first buffering system to react to changes in the pH. Process of accepting or donating hydrogen ions to buffer a strong acid or base to maintain a relatively constant pH. Secondary chemical buffering, which is limited, involves plasma proteins that can bind with or release hydrogen ions.
b. Involves cellular release or absorption of hydrogen ions. The positively charged ion must be exchanged with another positively charged ion, frequently potassium. Hyperkalemia (with acidosis) and hypokalemia (with alkalosis) may result. Another biological buffer is in the hemoglobin-oxyhemoglobin system, in which chloride and bicarbonate may exchange between the blood cell and the plasma.
c. Involves lungs and kidneys. Lungs provide rapid response through changes in respiratory rate and depth (influencing retention or release of carbon dioxide, which combines with water to create carbonic acid for chemical regulation). Kidneys are the slowest to respond, influencing hydrogen ion concentration through bicarbonate regulation, combining phosphate ions with hydrogen to form phosphoric acid and converting ammonia to ammonium by attaching a hydrogen ion to ammonia.
17. d (1282)
18. Refer to *16c.*
19. Both responses (1282, 1283):
a. Isotonic imbalances: created by water and electrolytes being gained or lost in equal proportions.
b. Osmolar imbalances: created by losses or excesses of only water.

20. (1282, 1283):
   a. 5
   b. 1
   c. 4
   d. 2
   e. 3
21. Any six (1283):
   a. Postural hypotension
   b. Tachycardia
   c. Weak pulse
   d. Dry skin and mucous membranes
   e. Poor skin turgor
   f. Collapsed veins
   g. Lethargy
   h. Oliguria
   i. Rapid weight loss
22. Any five (1283):
   a. Hypertension
   b. Edema (especially in dependent areas)
   c. Rapid weight gain
   d. Polyuria
   e. Neck vein distention
   f. Increased venous pressure
   g. Crackles in lungs
23. Refer to Table 39-3, pp. 1285-1286.
24. d (1287)
25. c (1287)
26. b (1287)
27. All five:
   a. Age (1287)
   b. Body size (1289, 1290)
   c. Environmental temperature (1290)
   d. Lifestyle (1290)
   e. Level of health (1290, 1291)
28. a. Inadequate nutritional intake can cause breakdown of glycogen and fat stores to preserve protein stores; when these resources are depleted, body begins to destroy protein stores; and if serum protein levels fall and hypoalbuminemia occurs, serum colloid osmotic pressure decreases and fluids shift from circulation to interstitial spaces creating edema. Generally, electrolyte status may also be influenced by normal diet (1290).
   b. Stress increases release of aldosterone and glucocorticoids causing sodium and water retention; ADH secretion increases, causing water retention and decreasing urinary output (1290).
   c. Exercise increases sensible water loss from the skin through sweat (1290).
29. a. Stress response causes postoperative fluid imbalance from increased secretion of aldosterone, glucocorticoids, and ADH. Response typically occurs during the second to fifth day after surgery and helps maintain circulating blood volume and blood pressure after surgery. When hormone levels return to normal, excess sodium and water are excreted (1290, 1291).
   b. Water is lost through one of five routes: plasma to interstitial shift, loss of serum proteins from

extracellular fluids, plasma and interstitial fluids lost as burn exudate, water vapor and heat loss because there is no skin barrier, and blood leakage from damaged capillaries. Sodium and water also shift into the cells, further depleting extracellular fluid volume (1291).
   c. Decreased cardiac output associated with a failing heart results in decreased renal perfusion and decreased urinary output. In an effort to increase perfusion, sodium and water are retained, contributing to circulatory overload (producing more peripheral and pulmonary edema) (1291).
   d. Renal failure produces an abnormal retention of sodium, chloride, potassium, and water in the extracellular fluid. Plasma levels of metabolic wastes are also elevated because the kidneys are unable to filter and excrete toxic waste products.
   e. Cancer causes a variety of fluid-electrolyte imbalances depending on the type and progression of the cancer. Electrolyte imbalances can occur and are caused by anatomical distortion and functional impairment from tumor growth and tumor-caused metabolic endocrine abnormalities (1291).
30. Any six (1292):
   a. Age
   b. Chronic diseases
   c. Trauma
   d. Burns
   e. Therapies (diuretics, steroids
   f. IV fluids, and TPN)
   g. Gastrointestinal losses
   h. Gastroenteritis
   i. Nasogastric suctioning
   j. Fistulas
31. (1293, 1294):
   a. Moderate fluid volume deficit.
   b. Metabolic or respiratory alkalosis, hyperosmolar imbalance, hypernatremia, and hypokalemia.
   c. Metabolic acidosis or alkalosis, respiratory acidosis, and hypercalcemia.
   d. Fluid volume excess in the infant.
   e. Fluid volume excess.
   f. Fluid volume deficit and hypernatremia.
   g. Hypocalcemia and hypomagnesemia.
   h. Fluid volume excess.
   i. Metabolic acidosis, respiratory alkalosis and acidosis; potassium imbalance (hyperkalemia or hypokalemia), and hypomagnesemia.
   j. Fluid volume deficit and hypokalemia.
   k. Fluid volume deficit, hyponatremia, hyperkalemia, and hypermangesemia.
   l. Fluid volume excess (in the adult).
   m. Fluid volume excess, respiratory alkalosis, and metabolic acidosis.
   n. Fluid volume excess.
   o. Metabolic acidosis.
   p. Metabolic acidosis.
   q. Fluid volume deficit.

r. Fluid volume deficit or excess.

s. Fluid volume deficit.

t. Hypocalcemia and metabolic or respiratory alkalosis.

u. Hypocalcemia, hypomagnesemia, and metabolic alkalosis.

v. Hypercalcemia, hypermagnesemia.

w. Hypernatremia, hyperosmolar imbalance, and metabolic acidosis.

x. Third space syndrome.

y. Fluid volume deficit.

z. Fluid volume excess.

32. d (1295)

33. False (1295, 1296)

34. Refer to the table below (1298):

35. b (1299)

36. 1.003 to 1.030 (1299)

37. Any two (1301):

  a. Restore and maintain fluid, electrolyte, and acid-base balance.

  b. Identify and correct the causes of the imbalance.

  c. Prevent complications from therapies needed to restore balance.

38. (1299):

  a. 120 ml

  b. 0 ml

  c. 0 ml

  d. 240 ml

  e. 240 ml

  f. 15 ml

  g. 615 ml

39. True (1302)

40. a (1302)

41. d (1302)

42. (1303):

  a. 500 ml

  b. 400 ml

  c. 100 ml

43. To correct or prevent fluid and electrolyte disturbances (1304).

44. c (1304)

45. b (1304)

46. Any three (1305):

  a. Very young clients

  b. Very old clients

  c. Obese clients

  d. Thin, emaciated clients

  e. Individuals who have had multiple venipunctures

f. Severely dehydrated clients or clients with decreased extracellular fluid volume

47. (1305, 1311):

Peripheral lines are located in the hands, arms, feet, or legs; catheter size is small; and peripheral lines are used for any fluid replacement except delivery of extremely large volumes or total parenteral nutrition. (Nurses may insert peripheral venous access devices.) Central lines are located in large, central veins, such as the subclavian vein; catheter size is large; and central lines are used to monitor central venous pressures (CVP) and to deliver large volumes of fluid or total parenteral nutrition. (Physicians insert central venous lines.)

48. (1312, 1313):

  a. $83 \dfrac{1000}{12} = 83$

  b. $21 \dfrac{100 \times 10}{480} = 21$

  c. $21 \dfrac{500 \times 15}{360} = 21$

  d. $100 \dfrac{50 \times 60}{30} = 100$

  e. $14 \dfrac{1000 \times 10}{720} = 14$

49. Any four (1311):

  a. Patency of the IV needle or catheter

  b. Infiltration

  c. Knot or kink in the tubing

  d. Height of the solution

  e. Position of the client's extremity

  f. Viscosity of solution

  g. Lumen of cannula

50. Both responses (1311):

  a. Deliver a measured amount of fluid over a specific period.

  b. Monitor IV fluids based on flow rate or drops per minute.

51. c (1315)

52. a (1311)

53. (1315):

  a. 4

  b. 1

  c. 6

  d. 3

  e. 5

  f. 2

Laboratory Value	Metabolic Alkalosis	Metabolic Acidosis	Respiratory alkalosis	Respiratory Acidosis
pH	Increased	Decreased	Increased	Decreased
P_{CO_2}	Unchanged (increased with compensation)	Unchanged (decreased with compensation)		
HCO_3	Increased	Decreased	Unchanged	Unchanged (early)
K^+	Decreased	Increased	Decreased	Increased

54. Place the pole next to the involved arm. Hold the pole with the involved hand. Push the pole with the involved hand. Report any blood in the tubing, stoppage in flow, or increased discomfort (1315).

55. b (1315)

56. See the table at the bottom of the page (1315, 1319):

57. All four (1319):
 a. Use vigorous hand-washing techniques before applying gloves for venipuncture.
 b. Change all IV solutions at least every 24 hours.
 c. Replace all peripheral venous catheters at least every 72 hours (and preferably every 48 hours).
 d. Maintain sterility of the system when changing tubing, solutions, and dressings.

58. True (1319)

59. 1 to 2 minutes (unless client has a bleeding disorder or is receiving anticoagulant medications) (1319)

60. All three (1320):
 a. To increase circulating blood volume after surgery, trauma, or hemorrhage
 b. To increase the number of red blood cells and to maintain hemoglobin levels in clients with severe anemia
 c. To provide selected cellular components as replacement therapy (for example, plasma-clotting factors to help control bleeding in clients with hemophilia)

61. (1320):

	Blood Type			
	A	B	O	AB
Antigens present	A	B	None	AB
Antibodies produced	Anti-B	Anti-A	Anti-A and anti-B	None

62. (1320):
 a. Type O
 b. Type AB

63. The collection, anticoagulation, filtration, and reinfusion of blood from an active bleeding site; or an individual's elective donation of his or her own blood for storage and later autotransfusion (during intraoperative or postoperative periods) (1320)

64. False (1320)

65. (1320, 1323):
 a. Large catheter promotes flow because blood and its components are large than the molecules of usual IV fluids; larger catheter prevents hemolysis of cells.
 b. Other solutions, such as D_5W, are hypotonic when compared with blood and cause the red blood cells to hemolyze.
 c. Risk for subsequent transfusions is not increased; however, the client may be anxious and require increased support.
 d. Changes in vital signs can indicate a transfusion reaction.
 e. Client is at risk for reaction, particularly during the first 15 minutes.

66. a (1324)

67. Any five (1323):
 a. Fever (with or without chills)
 b. Headache
 c. Nausea and vomiting
 d. Nonproductive cough
 e. Dyspnea
 f. Hypotension (and increased heart rate)
 g. Chest pain

68. c (1323, 1326)

69. 5 minutes (longer for client with bleeding disorders or receiving anticoagulant medication) (1326)

CHAPTER 40

1. (1334):
 a. Kidneys: filter and remove wastes from the blood and forms urine.
 b. Ureters: transport urine from kidneys to bladder.
 c. Bladder: holds urine.
 d. Urethra: transports urine from bladder to outside of body.

2. Nephron (1334)

3. a (1334)

4. False (1334)

5. d (1134)

6. Nocturia (1339)

7. d (1337)

8. (1337, 1338):
 a. 2

Complication	Assessment Finding	Nursing Action
Infiltration	Swelling, pallor at site, decreased or stopped flow, pain	Discontinue infusion; elevate extremity in warm towel for 20 minutes; restart if indicated.
Phlebitis	Pain, increased skin temperature over vein; may have red line along vein path	Discontinue infusion; apply warm, moist heat; restart if indicated.
Fluid overload	Signs of fluid volume excess	Slow infusion rate; notify physician; prepare for additional treatment (e.g., diuretics)
Bleeding	Bleeding around venipuncture site; most common in clients with bleeding disorders or clients receiving anticoagulant therapy	Application of pressure dressing over site

b. 5
c. 4
d. 6
e. 3
f. 7
g. 1
9. d (1338)
10. a (1339)
11. a. Sense or urgency and increased frequency of urination; may be unable to urinate completely (urinary retention) (1339).
   b. Weakens abdominal and pelvic floor muscles, impairing bladder contraction and control of external urethral sphincter (1339).
   c. Loss of bladder tone; muscle atrophy (1339).
   d. With normal cardiac and renal function: ingested fluids increase volume of circulating plasma and therefore increase glomerular filtration and volume of urine produced and excreted (1339).
   e. Diabetic neuropathy decreases bladder tone, decreases sensation of fullness, and causes difficulty controlling urination (1339, 1340).
   f. Slows glomerular filtration rate, decreases sensation of bladder fullness, and decreases ability to initiate and inhibit micturition (1340).
12. Retention (urinary retention) (1341)
13. Accumulated urine in the bladder causes pressure to rise. Pressure increases to a point that the external urethral sphincter is unable to hold back the urine, and it temporarily opens to allow a small volume of urine to escape. When urine exits, bladder pressure falls enough to allow the sphincter to regain control and close (1342).
14. Any three (1342):
   a. Urethral obstruction
   b. Surgical trauma
   c. Alterations in motor and sensory innervation of the bladder
   d. Medication side effects
   e. Anxiety
15. c (1342)
16. Hematuria (1342)
17. Any six (1342):
   a. Dysuria
   b. Fever
   c. Chills
   d. Nausea and vomiting
   e. Malaise
   g. Frequency
   h. Urgency
   i. Hematuria
   j. Concentrated, cloudy urine
      If infection spreads to the kidneys (pyelonephritis), flank pain and tenderness.
18. Urinary incontinence (1342)
19. Repeated involuntary urination in children who have reached the age when voluntary control is possible (usually 5 years of age) (1344)
20. (1320):

a. 4
b. 5
c. 2
d. 1
e. 3
21. Temporary or permanent changes in the route of urine flow, from the kidneys directly to the abdominal surface (1344)
22. d (1344)
23. All three (1345):
   a. Patterns of urination
   b. Symptoms of urinary alterations
   c. Factors affecting urination
24. (1346):
   a. 3
   b. 7
   c. 4
   d. 6
   e. 2
   f. 1
   g. 5
25. c (1346)
26. Use of fist percussion over the costovertebral angle (angle formed by the spine and twelfth rib) (1346)
27. Hypospadias (1347)
28. False (1347)
29. False (1347)
30. False (1348)
31. a (1347,1348)
32. c (1351)
33. d (1348)
34. Collection begins after the client urinates. The nurse indicates the starting time as the time of urination and discards the first sample. The client then collects all urine voided in the designated time (1351).
35. a (1352)
36. True (1353)
37. c (1355)
38. Any four (1355):
   a. Instruct client to remain in bed as ordered.
   b. Assess for signs of urinary retention and first voiding.
   c. Observe characteristics of urine, noting hematuria or cloudy urine.
   d. Encourage increased fluid intake and monitor intake and output.
   e. Observe for fever, dysuria, or hypotension.
   f. Administer medications to alleviate bladder spasms and/or lower back pain.
39. Any four (1358):
   a. Understanding normal urinary elimination
   b. Promoting normal micturition
   c. Achieving complete bladder emptying
   d. Preventing infection
   e. Maintaining skin integrity
   f. Gaining a sense of comfort
40. Any five (1360):
   a. Assist to a normal position for voiding.
   b. Provide sound of running water.

c. Stroke inner aspect of client's thigh.
d. Place client's hand in a pan of warm water.
e. Warm bedpan.
f. Pour warm water over the client's perineum.
g. Offer client a drink.

41. Any two (1361, 1362):
    a. Have client try to stop flow of urine during urination and then restart it.
    b. Instruct client to tighten muscles around anus without tensing leg, buttock, or abdominal muscles.
    c. Instruct client to tighten the posterior muscles and slowly contract anterior muscles while counting slowly to four, and then relax muscles completely.
    d. Have client do sit-ups.
42. c (1361)
43. c (1362)
44. To restore a normal pattern of voiding by inhibiting or stimulating voiding (1362)
45. (1353):
    a. 1
    b. 2
    c. 1
    d. 2
46. (1365):
    a. No. 8 to No. 10 French
    b. No. 14 to No. 16 French
    c. No. 16 to No. 18 French
47. c (1369)
48. b (1369)
49. True (1365)
50. a (1376)
51. Both responses (1373):
    a. Promote normal bladder function.
    b. Prevent trauma to the urethra
52. True (1373)
53. Surgical placement of a catheter through the abdominal wall above the symphysis pubis directly into the urinary bladder (1375).
54. Any two (1375):
    a. Provide thorough cleansing of the urethral meatus and penis.
    b. Caution not to secure the band tightly.
    c. Do not use standard adhesive tape to secure the condom catheter.
    d. Change a condom catheter daily to check for skin irritation.
55. Any three (1376):
    a. Good hand washing
    b. Perineal hygiene
    c. Oral intake between 2000 and 3000 ml every 24 hours
    d. Acidifying urine
56. Any six (1377):
    a. Follow good hand-washing techniques.
    b. Do not allow the spigot on the drainage bag to touch a contaminated surface.

c. Do not open the drainage system at connection points to obtain specimens or measure urine.
d. If the drainage tubing becomes disconnected, do not touch the ends of the catheter or tubing. Wipe the ends of the tube with antimicrobial solution before reconnecting.
e. Use a separate receptacle for measuring urine for each client.
f. Prevent pooling of urine and reflux of urine into the bladder.
g. Avoid prolonged clamping or kinking of the tubing (except during conditioning).
h. Empty the drainage bag at least every 8 hours.
i. Secure the catheter in place with tape or Velcro leg band.
j. Provide routine perineal hygiene.
k. Remove the catheter as soon as possible (after conferring with the physician).
57. a (1376)
58. True (1376)
59. Treatment for renal failure including peritoneal dialysis, hemodialysis, and organ transplantation (1340)
60. Washing with mild soap and water (1377)
61. c (1377)

CHAPTER 41

1. All three (1388):
   a. Absorb fluid and nutrients
   b. Prepare food for absorption and use by body cells
   c. Provide temporary storage of feces
2. a (1388)
3. b (1390)
4. All four (1391):
   a. Absorption: absorbs large amounts of water, sodium, and chloride through haustral contractions
   b. Protection: releases supply of mucus to lubricate the colon, preventing trauma to the inner walls (particularly important near the distal end of the colon, where contents become drier and harder)
   c. Secretion: aids in electrolyte balance; bicarbonate secreted in exchange for chloride; and potassium released
   d. Elimination: removes waste products and gas
5. Flatus (1391)
6. Feces (1391)
7. Hemorrhoids (1391)
8. (1391, 1392):
   a. 4
   b. 3
   c. 2
   d. 5
   e. 1
9. Voluntary contraction of abdominal muscles during forced expiration with a closed glottis (holding one's breath while straining) (1391)
10. Any six (1392):
    a. Loss of teeth and thus ability to chew
    b. Decreased digestive enzymes in saliva

c. Decreased volume of gastric acid
d. Decreased lipase
e. Decreased peristalsis
f. Slowed esophageal emptying
g. Changes in absorptive properties of intestinal mucosa
h. Decreased muscle tone of perineal floor and anal sphincter
i. Decreased awareness of the need to defecate

11. Fiber provides bulk in fecal material. Bulk-forming foods absorb fluids and increase stool mass, stretching the bowel walls, creating peristalsis, and initiating the defecation reflex (1392).

12. Any four (1392):
    a. Raw fruits
    b. Cooked fruits
    c. Greens
    d. Raw vegetables
    e. Whole grains

13. Lactose intolerance (1393)

14. d (1393)

15. False (1394)

16. (1394):
    a. Lubricant: decreases fat-soluble vitamin absorption
    b. Suppresses peristalsis: common treatment of diarrhea
    c. Decrease peristalsis
    d. Decrease acid secretion: depress gastric motility, increase constipation
    e. Disrupt normal GI flora, causing diarrhea (1394)

17. True (1394)

18. Increased fluids (if not contraindicated), laxatives (if ordered), and enemas (if unresponsive to fluids and laxatives) (1394)

19. d (1394, 1395)

20. Any four (1395):
    a. Irregular bowel habits: when normal defecation reflexes are ignored, they tend to become weakened; changes in routine can disrupt normal defecation patterns
    b. Inadequate diet: low-fiber diet high in animal fats and refined sugars can cause constipation; low fluid intake impairs peristalsis
    c. Lack of exercise: decreased mobility and lack of regular exercise cause constipation
    d. Medications: frequent use of laxatives causes loss of intestinal muscle tone with loss of normal defecation reflexes; tranquilizers, opiates, anticholinergics, and iron cause constipation
    e. Age: slowed peristalsis and loss of abdominal muscle elasticity associated with aging increase frequency of constipation; decreased intestinal secretion of mucus reduces lubrication; many older adults live alone and eat improper diets that are low in fiber
    f. Diseases: abnormalities of the GI tract may cause constipation; spinal cord injury or tumor may also cause altered GI function

21. Any three (1395):
    a. After recent abdominal or rectal surgery
    b. Cardiovascular disease
    c. Increased intraocular pressure (glaucoma)
    d. Increased intracranial pressure

22. Exhaling through the mouth during straining (1395)

23. A collection of hardened feces, wedged in the rectum, that cannot be expelled (1395)

24. Any four (1395):
    a. Inability to pass a stool for several days despite a repeated urge to defecate
    b. Continuous oozing of diarrheal stool that develops suddenly
    c. Anorexia
    d. Abdominal distention
    e. Cramping
    f. Rectal pain
    g. Palpable rectal mass

25. An increase in the number of stools and the passage of liquid, unformed feces (1395)

26. Both responses (1395):
    a. Fluid and electrolyte imbalance
    b. Skin breakdown

27. b (1396)

28. Stoma (1397)

29. Ileostomy (1397)

30. Colostomy (1397)

31. b (1398)

32. Any eight (1399, 1400):
    a. Determination of the usual elimination pattern
    b. Identification of routines followed to promote normal elimination
    c. Description of any recent change in elimination pattern
    d. Client description of usual characteristics of stool
    e. Diet history
    f. Description of daily fluid intake
    g. History of exercise
    h. Assessment of the use of artificial aids at home
    i. History of surgery or illnesses affecting the GI tract
    j. Presence and status of bowel diversions
    k. Medication history
    l. Emotional state
    m. Social history

33. c (see Chapter 20)

34. (1400):
    a. Abdominal distention
    b. Paralytic ileus
    c. Small intestine obstruction and inflammatory disorders
    d. Gas or flatulence
    e. Masses, tumors, and fluid

35. a (1400)

36. (1401):
    a. Absence of bile
    b. Iron ingestion or upper GI bleeding
    c. Lower GI bleeding and hemorrhoids

   d. Diarrhea and reduced absorption
   e. Obstruction and rapid peristalsis
37. True (1401)
38. b (1401)
39. (1403):
   a. Any three:
      (1) Age over 50 years
      (2) Family history of colon polyps or colorectal cancer
      (3) History of inflammatory bowel disease (colitis or Crohn's disease)
      (4) Living in urban area
      (5) Diet high in fats and low in fiber
   b. Both responses (1403):
      (1) Change in bowel habits
      (2) Rectal bleeding
40. c (1403-1405)
41. Any four (1404):
   a. Instruct client to avoid eating or drinking until the gag reflex returns (2 to 4 hours)
   b. Check the gag reflex before providing food or fluids
   c. Explain that hoarseness and a sore throat are normal for several days
   d. Provide cool fluids and normal saline gargling to relieve soreness
   e. Observe for bleeding, fever, abdominal pain, difficulty swallowing, and difficulty breathing
42. Any five (1406, 1407):
   a. Understanding normal elimination
   b. Attaining regular defecation habits
   c. Understanding and maintaining proper fluid and food intake
   d. Maintaining a regular exercise program
   e. Achieving comfort
   f. Maintaining skin integrity
   g. Maintaining self-concept
43. Any three (1407):
   a. Take time for defecation
   b. Begin establishing a routine during a time when defecation is most likely to occur
   c. Make certain that treatment routines do not interfere with the client's schedule
   d. Provide privacy
44. a (1408)
45. Shortly before the client's usual time to defecate or immediately after a meal (1409)
46. (1410)
   a. 4
   b. 3
   c. 1
   d. 5
   e. 2
47. b (1409)
48. a (1411)
49. b (1411)
50. Enemas are repeated until the client passes fluid that is clear and contains no fecal material (1411).
51. False (1411)

52. c (1413)
53. True (1411)
54. Vagal stimulation from rectal pressure could cause reflex slowing of the heart (1411)
55. Any five (1415):
   a. Type of ostomy
   b. Size and contour of the abdomen
   c. Condition of the skin around the stoma
   d. Physical activities of the client
   e. Client's personal preference
   f. Cost of equipment
56. Enterostomal therapist (ET) (1415)
57. Any six (1415):
   a. Ascending colostomies
   b. Temporary colostomies
   c. Disease in remaining colon
   d. Infant or child
   e. Physical limitations
   f. Mental limitations
   g. Inadequate sanitary facilities
   h. Stomal abnormalities
58. Both responses (1422):
   a. While lying supine, tighten the abdominal muscles as though they were being pushed to the floor; hold the muscles tight to a count of three and then relax; repeat 5 to 10 times as tolerated
   b. Flex and contract the thigh muscles by raising the knees one at a time slowly toward the chest (repeat each leg at least five times; increase as tolerated)
59. b (1422)
60. d (1423)
61. False (1423)
62. Any four (1424):
   a. Give client an opportunity to discuss concerns or fears about elimination problems
   b. Provide client and family with information to understand and manage elimination problems
   c. Give positive feedback when the client attempts self-care measures
   d. Help client with ostomy to manage condition, but do not expect client to like it
   e. Provide client privacy during care
   f. Show acceptance and understanding
63. c (1415, 1419, 1422-1423)

CHAPTER 42

1. All five (1432):
   a. Basic needs are achievable
   b. Physical hazards are reduced
   c. Transmission of pathogens and parasites is reduced
   d. Sanitation is maintained
   e. Pollution is controlled
2. a (1432, 1433)
3. Any three (1433, 1434):
   a. Ensure adequate lighting
   b. Decrease obstacles
   c. Control bathroom hazards

    d. Secure the home

4. Any microorganisms capable of producing an illness (1434)

5. An organisms living in or on another organism and obtaining nourishment from it (1434)

6. Immunization (1434)

7. d (1434, 1435)

8. Any four (1435):
    a. Disruption of processing ability and problem solving
    b. Increased anxiety
    c. Paranoia
    d. Hallucinations
    e. Depression
    f. Unrealistic feelings

9. All five (1434):
    a. Developmental stage
    b. Lifestyle habits
    c. Mobility status
    d. Sensory impairments
    e. Safety awareness

10. a (1435)

11. True (1435)

12. b (1435)

13. True (1437)

14. True (1437)

15. Any eight (1437):
    a. Arthritic changes affecting ROM, balance, and weight bearing
    b. Decreased circulation in the brain, causing dizziness and fainting
    c. Mechanical obstruction of vertebral arteries to the brain caused by crushed osteoporotic vertebrae
    d. F9 Decreased auditory acuity
    e. Decreased night vision, color vision, or visual acuity
    f. Orthostatic hypotension
    g. Loss of sense of position
    h. Diminished space perception
    i. Decreased muscle mass, strength, and coordination
    j. Decreased ability to balance
    k. Osteoporosis and increased stress on weight-bearing areas, resulting in unsteady gait and susceptibility to fractures
    l. Decreased muscle activity necessary for adequate venous return
    m. Decreased capacity of blood vessels
    n. Slowed nervous system response
    o. Changes in metabolism, affecting the rate of drug metabolism and systemic effects of medication

16. All four (1438):
    a. Falls
    b. Client-inherent accidents
    c. Procedure-related accidents
    d. Equipment-related accidents

17. d (1439)

18. b (1439)

19. Any six (1440):
    a. Loose control knobs
    b. Ungrounded equipment
    c. Frayed cords or cords improperly taped to floor
    d. Circuits overloaded by too many appliances in one area
    e. Improperly functioning equipment
    f. Use of extension cords
    g. Tangled or cluttered cords
    h. Use of electrical appliances near sink, bathtub, shower, or other wet or damp areas

20. d (1439)

21. All four (1443):
    a. Change in appetite
    b. Change in sleep
    c. Change in activity levels
    d. Apathy

22. d (1443, 1444)

23. Any five (1443):
    a. Enroll in a driver's education course
    b. Wear seat belts
    c. Do not drive after using a psychoactive substance, alcohol, or other drugs (or ride when the driver has used such substances)
    d. Contract to drive any teenager who has been drinking with no questions asked
    e. Develop safe eating, sleeping, and relaxation habits
    f. Develop awareness of safe-sex decisions and practices
    g. Recognize changes in behavior and mood
    h. Listen to adolescents
    i. Do not try to be a buddy, remain a parent

24. All three (1446):
    a. Falls
    b. Automobile accidents
    c. Burns

25. Any eight (1447):
    a. Identify clients at risk for falls
    b. Assign clients at risk rooms near the nurse's station
    c. Alert all health care personnel to the client's increased risk of falling
    d. Use a night light in room
    e. Reinforce to client or family the need for assistance when client is ambulating or getting up
    f. Keep side rails up
    g. Have call light easily accessible; promptly answer call light
    h. Keep client's personal items within easy reach
    i. Maintain a scheduled toileting routine
    j. Reassess client's risk of falling each shift
    k. Frequently observe client
    l. Use restraints or sitters properly

26. b (1447)

27. All four (1448):
    a. To reduce the risk of falling out of bed or from chair or wheelchair

b. To prevent interruption of therapy such as traction, IV infusions, nasogastric tube feedings, or Foley catheter

c. To prevent the confused or combative client from removing life-support equipment

d. To reduce the risk of injury to other persons by the client

28. c (1449)

29. c (1449)

30. c (1450, 1451)

31. b (1450, 1451)

32. d (1430, 1431)

33. Side rails up and application of a jacket restraint (1452)

34. Any six (1452):

a. Know the phone number for reporting a fire, and be sure the number is attached to all telephones

b. Know the agency's or unit's fire drill or fire evacuation routine

c. Know location of fire alarms

d. Post accurate, easy-to-follow routes to fire exits

e. Know the location of fire extinguishers, how to use them, and which type of extinguishers to use for specific types of fires

f. Report a fire before attempting to extinguish it, regardless of its size

g. Keep hallways free of unnecessary equipment or furniture

h. Periodically check the efficiency of fire extinguishers

i. Post signs on the outside of elevators warning persons to take the stairs in the event of fire

35. All three (1452):

a. To protect clients from injury*

b. To report the location of the fire

c. To contain the fire

36. d (1452)

37. R = Rescue
A = Alarm
C = Confine
E = Extinguish

38. Syrup of Ipecac (1454)

39. b (1453)

40. a (1454)

CHAPTER 43

1. The coordinated effort of the musculoskeletal and nervous systems to maintain balance, posture, and body alignment during lifting, bending, moving, and performing activities of daily living (ADLs) (1462)

2. a (1462)

3. A force that occurs in a direction to oppose movement (1462)

4. Both responses (1462):

a. Base of support is widened by separating feet to a comfortable distance

b. Balance is increased when the center of gravity is moved over and closer to the base of support

5. All three (1462, 1463):

a. Skeletal system

b. Muscle system (skeletal muscles)

c. Nervous system

6. All four (1463):

a. Movement

b. Protection of vital organs

c. Regulation of calcium balance

d. Production and storage of red blood cells (RBCs)

7. Pathological fractures (1463)

8. **a.** 4 (1463)

b. 3 (1463)

c. 7 (1463)

d. 6 (1464)

e. 2 (1563)

f. 5 (1463)

g. 1 (1463)

9. Isotonic (1465)

10. Isometric (1465)

11. True (1466)

12. c (1466)

13. b (1466)

14. Proprioception (1466)

15. d (1467)

16. True (1467)

17. c (1467)

18. (1468):

a. 6

b. 5

c. 2

d. 4

e. 1

f. 3

g. 7

19. a (1469)

20. Fracture (1469)

21. All four (1469, 1470):

a. Physical inactivity (bedrest)

b. Physical restriction or limitation (cast or traction)

c. Restriction in body position changes and posture

d. Sensory deprivation

22. Any three (1470):

a. Reducing physical activity and oxygen needs of the body

b. Reducing pain, including postoperative pain, and the need for larger doses of analgesics

c. Allowing ill or debilitated clients to rest and regain strength

d. Allowing exhausted clients the opportunity for uninterrupted rest

23. False (1470)

24. c (1470)

25. Two for each classification:

a. Metabolic (1470)

(1) Decreased BMR

(2) Decreased glucose tolerance

(3) Negative nitrogen balance

(4) Increased fat stores

(5) Increased bone resorption

b. Respiratory (1471)
   (1) Decreased lung volume
   (2) Decreased hemoglobin levels
   (3) Weakened respiratory muscles
   (4) Increased work of breathing
   (5) Decreased ability to cough productively
   (6) Mucous accumulation in airways (hypostatic pneumonia)
c. Cardiovascular (1471)
   (1) Orthostatic hypotension
   (2) Increased cardiac workload
   (3) Thrombus formation
d. Muscular (1472)
   (1) Permanently impaired mobility
   (2) Decreased endurance
   (3) Decreased muscle mass
   (4) Muscle atrophy
   (5) Decreased stability
e. Skeletal (1473)
   (1) Impaired calcium metabolism
   (2) Joint abnormalities
   (3) Contractures
   (4) Footdrop
f. Integumentary (1474)
   (1) Decreased healing
   (2) Increased risk of pressure ulcers
g. Elimination (1474)
   (1) Urinary stasis
   (2) Urinary infection
   (3) Urinary calculi
   (4) Constipation

26. d (1474)
27. (1475):
    a. 4
    b. 5
    c. 6
    d. 1
    e. 2
    f. 3
28. All four:
    a. ROM—maximum amount of movement at the joint in one of three planes of the body (sagittal, frontal, and transverse) (1476)
    b. Gait—manner or style of walking, including cadence, rhythm, and speed (1476)
    c. Exercise and activity tolerance—kind and amount of exercise or work a person is able to perform (1476, 1477)
    d. Body alignment: relationship of body parts within the three planes (sagittal, frontal, and transverse), center of gravity, and line of gravity (1481, 1482)
29. False (1481)
30. Any five (1481):
    a. Determine normal physiological changes in body alignment resulting from growth and development
    b. Identify deviations in body alignment caused by poor posture

c. Provide an opportunity for the client to observe own posture
d. Identify learning needs of the client for maintaining correct body alignment
e. Identify the presence of trauma, muscle damage, or nerve dysfunction
f. Obtain information about other factors contributing to poor alignment

31. Any 10 (1487):
    a. Maintaining proper body alignment
    b. Regaining proper body alignment or optimal level of body alignment
    c. Reducing injuries to the skin and musculoskeletal system resulting from improper body mechanics or alignment
    d. Achieving full or optimal ROM
    e. Preventing contractures
    f. Maintaining patent airway
    g. Achieving optimal lung expansion and gas exchange
    h. Mobilizing airway secretions
    i. Maintaining cardiovascular function
    j. Increasing activity tolerance
    k. Achieving normal elimination patterns
    l. Maintaining normal sleep-wake patterns
    m. Achieving socialization
    n. Achieving independent completion of self-care activities
    o. Achieving physical and mental stimulation
32. All four (1488):
    a. Position of weight
    b. Height of object
    c. Body position
    d. Maximal weight
33. 35% of body weight (1488)
34. a (1488)
35. See table at right (1489):
36. False (1490)
37. All three (1490):
    a. Joints should be supported
    b. Position of the joints should be slightly flexed
    c. Pressure points should be removed or minimized
38. a. Fowlers-sacrum and heels (1494)
    b. Supine-occiput region of head, lumbar vertebrae, elbows, and heels (1495)
    c. Prone-chin, elbows, hips, knees, and toes (1495)
    d. Side-lying-ear, ilium, knees, and ankles
    e. Sims-ilium, humorous, clavicle, knees, ankles
39. Any five (1490):
    a. Raising the rail on the side of the bed opposite the nurse to prevent the client from falling out of bed
    b. Elevating the level of the bed to a comfortable height
    c. Assessing the client's mobility and strength to determine what assistance the client can offer during transfer
    d. Determining the need for assistance

Device	Uses
Pillow	Supports body or extremity, elevates body part, splints incisional arae to reduce post-operative pain during activity or coughing and deep breathing
Footboard or posey footguard	Maintains feet in dorsiflexion
Trochanter roll	Prevents external rotation of legs in supine position
Sandbag	Provides support and shape to body contours, immobilizes extremity, maintains specific body alignment
Hand-wrist	Maintains proper functional alignment of thumb and splint fingers, maintains wrist in slight dorsiflexion
Trapeze bar	Enables client to raise trunk from bed, transfer from bed to wheelchair, perform exercises to strengthen upper arms
Side rail	Allows weak client to roll from side to side or sit up in bed
Bed board	Provides additional support to the mattress and improves vertebral alignment

    e. Explaining the procedure and describing what is expected of the client

    f. Assessing for correct body alignment and pressure areas after each transfer

40. a (1496)

41. Any four (1495, 1496):

    a. If the client's illness prohibits exertion

    b. If the client understands what is expected

    c. Level of the client's comfort

    d. Nurse's own strength and knowledge of the procedure

    e. Determiniation whether the client is too heavy or immobile for the nurse to work alone

42. b (1496)

43. True (1496)

44. d (1496, 1497)

45. c (1503)

46. All five (1504):

    a. Assess the client's activity tolerance, strength, presence of pain, coordination, and balance to determine assistance needed

    b. Explain how far the client should try to walk, who is going to help, when the walk will take place, and why walking is important

    c. Check the environment to be sure there are no obstacles in the client's path

    d. Establish rest points in case the activity tolerance is less than estimated or the client becomes dizzy

    e. Assist the client to a position of sitting followed by stationary standing before attempting to walk

47. d (1504)

48. b (1504)

49. b (1504)

50. Measure includes three areas (1506):

    a. Client height—3 to 4 finger widths from axilla to point 6 inches (15 cm) lateral to client's heel will determine crutch length

    b. Angle of elbow flexion—20 to 25 degrees

    c. Distance between the crutch pad and axilla—3 to 4 fingerwidths

51. Any four (1506):

    a. Clients must not use crutches that fit improperly or lean on crutches to support their weight

    b. Crutch tips should be inspected routinely; worn tips should be replaced

    c. Crutch tips should remain dry and should be dried immediately if they become wet

    d. Structure of crutches should be inspected routinely

    e. Client should be provided with a list of medical suppliers in the community to obtain any repairs or replacement parts for crutches

52. (1507, 1508):

    a. 1

    b. 3

    c. 5

    d. 4

    e. 2

53. a. 3

    b. 2

    c. 4

    d. 1

54. False (1508)

55. a (1504)

56. a. Improve nutrition (1510):
High protein, high calories, and increased B vitamins and vitamin C

    b. Promote lung expansion (1510):
Postural changes at least every 2 hours, cough and deep breathe every 1 to 2 hours, cough and deep breath at peak of analgesic administration, and remove abdominal binders or rib supports every two hours (if not contraindicated)

    c. Prevent stasis of pulmonary secretions (1511):
Change position every 2 hours, cough and deep breath every 1 to 2 hours, and use chest physiotherapy

    d. Maintain patent airway (1511):
Cough and deep breathe every 1 to 2 hours, and suction (nasotracheal, orotracheal, endotracheal, or tracheal)

    e. Decrease orthostatic hypotension (1511):
Out of bed as soon as possible, change positions gradually, and monitor vital signs during position changes

    f. Decrease cardiac workload (1511):
Minimize Valsalva maneuver

    g. Prevent thrombus formation (1503):
Therapeutic elastic stockings, positioning techniques (to avoid pressure over veins in lower extremeties), and ROM

h. Maintain muscle strength and joint mobility (1514):
ROM, progressive exercise program

i. Maintain normal patterns of elimination (1514): Maintain adequate hydration (2000 to 3000 ml in 24 hours); increase fruit, vegetables, and bulk in the diet

j. Minimize psychosocial effects (1515):
Minimize night disruptions, involve client in care, maintain body image, and provide meaningful environmental stimuli

57. d (1516, 1517)
58. b (1471)
59. True (1516)
60. True (1513)

CHAPTER 44

1. A localized area of tissue necrosis (death) that tends to develop when soft tissue is compressed between a bony prominence and an external surface for a prolonged period (1524)
2. True (1524)
3. Either scale (1254):
  a. Norton Scale: physical condition, mental condition, activity, mobility, and continence.
  b. Braden Scale: sensory perception, activity, moisture, friction, and nutrition.
4. A localized absence of blood or major reduction in flow resulting from mechanical obstruction (1525)
5. Reactive hyperemia (1525)
6. Induration (1525)
7. True (1525)
8. (1626):
  a. Impaired sensory input
  b. Impaired motor function
  c. Altered level of consciousness
  d. Casts and traction
9. Each of the following (1527-1528):
  a. Shearing force—skin and subcutaneous layers adhere to bed surface and layers of muscle and bones slide in the direction of body movement; underlying tissue capillaries are compressed and severed, causing bleeding and deep tissue necrosis.
  b. Moisture—decreases skin resistance to other physical factors.
  c. Poor nutrition—decreases muscle mass and subcutaneous tissue, creating less padding between skin and bones; fluid and electrolyte imbalances increase edema formation, further compromising capillary blood flow.
  d. Anemia—decreases oxygen available to tissues and alters cellular metabolism.
  e. Infection—usually associated with fever that increases the metabolic needs of the body, making already hypoxic tissue more susceptible to ischemic injury.
  f. Fever—increases metabolic needs of the body making already hypoxic tissue more susceptible to ischemic injury; fever results in diaphoresis and increased skin moisture, further predisposing skin to breakdown.
  g. Impaired peripheral circulation—decreased circulation causes tissue hypoxia with greater susceptibility to ischemic damage than other tissue.
  h. Obesity—adipose tissue is poorly vascularized, and the adipose and underlying tissues are more susceptible to ischemic damage.
  i. Cachexia—a cachexic client has lost the adipose tissue necessary to protect bony prominences from pressure.
  j. Age—ulcer development is more prominent in clients over age 75.
10. (1529):
  a. 4
  b. 2
  c. 1
  d. 3
11. True (1529)
12. Any two (1533):
  a. Low serum albumin
  b. Low serum total protein
  c. Less than 90% ideal body weight
  d. Greater than 10% ideal body weight
13. Any four (1535):
  a. Maintain vitality of the skin through hygiene and topical care.
  b. Reduce and prevent injuries to the skin and musculoskeletal system from pressure, friction, and shearing force.
  c. Improve nutritional intake.
  d. Improve mobility and activity.
  e. Improve or maintain body alignment.
14. At least two interventions for each risk factor (1536):
  a. Immobility—establish individualized turning schedule, provide pressure-relief surface, and reduce shear and friction.
  b. Inactivity—provide assistive devices to increase activity.
  c. Incontinence—assess need for incontinence management, and clean and dry skin after soiling.
  d. Malnutrition—provide adequate nutritional and fluid intake; consult dietitian for nutritional evaluation.
  e. Diminished sensation, decreased mental status: assess client's and family's ability to provide care, educate care giver about pressure ulcer prevention.
  f. Impaired skin integrity: avoid pressure, do not use donut-shaped cushions, lubricate skin, do not massage red areas, and do not use heat lamps.
15. False (1538)
16. False (1528)
17. a (1545)
18. c (1545)
19. All three (1547):
  a. Prevent injury to skin and tissues
  b. Reduce injury to skin and underlying tissues
  c. Restore skin integrity

CHAPTER 45

1. All three (1554):
   a. Reception
   b. Perception
   c. Reaction
2. a (1554)
3. Any seven (1555):
   a. Age
   b. Medications
   c. Environment
   d. Comfort level
   e. Preexisting illnesses
   f. Smoking
   g. Noise levels
   h. Endotracheal intubation
4. A defect in the normal function of sensory reception and perception (1555)
5. Sensory deprivation (1556)
6. All three (1556):
   a. Reduced sensory input (for example, hearing or visual loss)
   b. Elimination of order or meaning from input (for example, a strange environment)
   c. Restriction of the environment producing monotony and boredom (for example, bed rest)
7. Sensory overload (1556)
8. Two for each category (1556):
   a. Reduced capacity to learn, inability to problem solve, poor task performance, disorientation, and bizarre thinking.
   b. Boredom, restlessness, increased anxiety, emotional lability, amd increased need for physical stimulation and socialization.
   c. Reduced attention span, disorganized visual and motor coordination, temporary loss of color perception, disorientation, and confusion of sleeping and waking states.
9. Any three (1557):
   a. Older adults
   b. Immobilized clients
   c. Clients isolated (in home or hospital)
   d. Clients with known sensory deficit
10. Refer to Table 45-1, p. 1558.
11. c (1559)
12. Aphasia (1559)
13. a (1559)
14. Any five (1561):
   a. Maintain optimal functioning of existing senses.
   b. Control the environment to create meaningful sensory stimuli.
   c. Establish a safe environment.
   d. Prevent additional sensory loss.
   e. Communicate effectively with existing sensory alterations.
   f. Understand the nature and implications of sensory loss.
   g. Achieve self-care.

15. All four (1563):
   a. Strengthening visual stimuli
   b. Using other senses
   c. Using sharp visual contrasts
   d. Minimizing glare
16. Any four (1563):
   a. Telephone bell amplification
   b. Telephone speaker simplification
   c. Amplification of other environmental sounds (for example, smoke alarms)
   d. Reduction of background noise
   e. Proper fit and function of hearing aids
17. d (1564)
18. a (1564)
19. c (1565)
20. d (1566)
21. c (1567)
22. Any six (1567):
   a. Get client's attention.
   b. Face client, with face and lips illuminated.
   c. If client wears glasses, be sure they are clean.
   d. Speak slowly and articulate clearly, using normal tones of voice and inflections.
   e. Restate with different words when you are not understood.
   f. Do not shout.
   g. Talk toward the client's "best" or normal ear.
   h. Use visual aids and gestures to enhance the spoken word.
   i. Do not restrict use of the client's hands
23. False (1567)

CHAPTER 46

1. Any drug, chemical, or biological entity that can be self-administered (1574)
2. True (1574)
3. Drug use occurs when a drug is appropriately taken as it is prescribed (for intended psychological or physiological effects). Drug misuse occurs when the drug is taken indiscriminately or taken improperly (whether it is a prescribed or over-the-counter drug). Drug abuse occurs when the drug is regularly taken indiscriminately in excessive quantities that impair the person's physiological, psychological, or social functioning.
4. b (1574,1575)
5. Psychological dependence
6. Fetal alcohol syndrome (FAS): a permanent disorder characterized by retardation and physical abnormalities; caused by maternal alcoholism (1576).
7. d (1574, 1575)
8. (1577):
   a. 3
   b. 2
   c. 4
   d. 1
9. True (1579)
10. b (1577, 1578)

11. (1587-1588):

Substance	Psychological Effect
Alcohol	Euphoria followed by depression Decreased inhibitions Impaired judgment
Sedatives- hypnotics	Relaxation or sedation Drowsiness Euphorial followed by depression
Benzodiazepines (tranquilizers)	Fatigue Decreased attentiveness Confusion Emotional bluntness Lethargy, smnolence Feeling of tranquility Increased self-confidence
CNS sympathomimetics	Euphoria, elation Initially increased interllectual function Grandiosity Feeling of power Hyperalertness Anorexia Insomnia Hypomanic behaviors With progressive abuse: dysphoria, psychomotor agitation, sadness, depression, apathy, seclusiveness
Hallucinogens	Distorted perception Feelings of power, strength, invulnerability Disorientation with "blank stare" Euphoria Disordered thought processes Depresonalization Hallucinations Paranoid behavior Self-destruction
Marijuana	Relaxation Distorted perceptions of time and space Moments of excitement or hilarity Impaired decision making Fear, panic, or paranoia
Inhalants	Excitatory phase: euphoria, excitation, exhilaration, "drunkenness," feelings of omnipotence, distortion of visual and spatial perceptions, dizziness CNS depression phase: glazed eyes and vacant stare, ataxia, loss of self-control, somnolence

12. Both responses (1581, 1582):
  a. Pleasure seeking
  b. Escape mechanism
13. (1582):
  a. Primary disease: situation in which the abuse problem is seen as primary, with other problems (psychological or physical) viewed as secondary.
  b. Genetic: chemical dependency viewed as predisposed through heredity but influenced through environment.
  c. Psychological: variety of theories, including stress as contributing to the onset and continuation of addiction and substance use and continuation associated with a reward or reinforcement.
  d. Sociocultural: abuse viewed as part of person's socialization through the values, perceptions, norms, and beliefs passed from one generation to another.

14. Preoccupation with the acquisition of the chemical, compulsive use in the presence of negative consequences, and relapses or voluntary return to the substance (1583).

15. c (1583)

16. d (1584)

17. True (1584)
18. (1585):
   a. Nurse provides accurate information to the health care system and communities regarding chemical dependency.
   b. Nurse works as case finder in assisting parents, educators, and other health care professionals in identifying persons with actual or potential chemical abuse problems.
   c. Nurse cares for clients in chemical dependency treatment centers, acute care hospitals, home care settings, clinics, and long-term care facilities.
19. Any four (1590, 1591):
   a. Remain free from injury within the first 7 days of hospitalization.
   b. Experience increasing comfort and safety.
   c. Experience gradual weight gain during rehabilitation.
   d. Regain a balanced nutritional status.
   e. Promote and maintain psychosocial integrity of the client and family.
   f. Develop support systems.
   g. Develop stress-management techniques.
   h. Identify community resources to support client and family.
20. All three (1591):
   a. Recognize the disease and how it has affected the person's life.
   b. Learn about chemical dependency. Provide tools for changing behavior.
21. Detoxification (1591)
22. d (1591)
23. c (1593)
24. All seven (1593):
   a. Support during detoxification
   b. Acute care interventions
   c. Interventions for abusive behavior
   d. Teaching
   e. Counseling
   f. Family interventions
   g. Community resource and referral
25. All four (1593):
   a. Referral to the appropriate community agency or mental health clinic
   b. Education about drugs
   c. Promotion of effective coping mechanisms
   d. Provision of needed physical and psychosocial support
26. False (1593)

CHAPTER 47

1. The role of the nurse during the preoperative, intraoperative, and postoperative phases of a client's surgical experience (1603)
2. All three (1603):
   a. Seriousness
   b. Urgency
   c. Purpose

3. (1603):
   a. 6
   b. 4
   c. 9
   d. 5
   e. 3
   f. 11
   g. 2
   h. 1
   i. 7
   j. 10
   k. 8
4. Any four (1604):
   a. Assess the client's physical and emotional well-being.
   b. Recognize the degree of surgical risk.
   c. Coordinate diagnostic tests.
   d. Identify nursing diagnoses reflecting client's and family members' needs.
   e. Prepare the client physically and mentally for surgery.
   f. Communicate pertinent information to the surgical team.
5. (1605):
   a. Increases risk of hemorrhage intraoperatively and postoperatively.
   b. Impairs wound healing and increases risk of infection from altered glucose metabolism and associated circulatory impairment; blood sugar levels may cause CNS malfunction during anesthesia.
   c. Stress of surgery increases demands on myocardium to maintain cardiac output; general anesthesia further depresses cardiac function.
   d. Increases risk of other respiratory complications during anesthesia.
   e. Alters metabolism and elimination of drugs administered during surgery; impairs wound healing because of altered protein metabolism.
   f. Predisposes client to fluid and electrolyte imbalances; may indicate underlying infection.
   g. Reduces client's ability to compensate for acid-base alterations; anesthetic agents reduce respiratory function, increasing risk for severe hypoventilation.
   h. Increases risk of infection and delays postoperative wound healing.
6. False (1605)
7. Chronic smoker has increased amounts and thickness of mucous secretions already present in the lungs. General anesthetics increase airway irritation and stimulate pulmonary secretions, which are retained from reduced ciliary activity during anesthesia. The client who smokes has greater difficulty clearing the airway of mucous secretions.
8. False (1607)
9. d (1608, 1609)
10. Any three (1609):

a. Age—very young and elderly clients are surgical risks as a result of immature or declining physiological status.

b. Nutrition—normal tissue repair and resistance to infection depend on adequate nutrients, and these needs are intensified by surgery; malnourishment predisposes to improper wound healing, reduced energy, and infection; obese clients are often malnourished and also have reduced ventilatory and cardiac function; further, the structure of fatty tissue, which contain a poor blood supply, inhibits wound healing.

c. Radiotherapy—used preoperatively to reduce the size of the cancerous tumor, causes excess thinning of skin layers, destruction of collagen, and impaired vascularization of tissues; impairing wound healing.

d. Fluid-electrolyte balance—surgery is a form of trauma that precipitates the adrenocortical stress response (sodium and water retention and potassium loss); fluid imbalance or electrolyte disturbance poses significant risks intraoperatively and postoperatively.

11. d (1609)
12. a (1610)
13. c (1611)
14. a (1611)
15. Any six (1613):
  a. Understanding physiological and psychological responses to surgery
  b. Understanding intraoperative and postoperative events
  c. Acquiring emotional comfort
  d. Gaining a return of normal physiological function postoperatively
  e. Maintaining a normal fluid and electrolyte balance intraoperatively and postoperatively
  f. Achieving comfort and rest
  g. Remaining free of postoperative surgical wound infection
  h. Remaining safe from harm intraoperatively
16. False (1613)
17. c (1613)
18. a (1614)
19. All four (1614):
  a. Improved ventilatory function
  b. Optimal recovery of physical functional capacity
  c. Improved sense of well-being
  d. Shortened length of hospital stay
20. c (1614)
21. Any six (1615, 1619-1621):
  a. Client cites reasons for each of the preoperative instructions and exercises.
  b. Client states the time surgery is scheduled.
  c. Client states the unit to which he or she will return after surgery and the location of family during the intraoperative and immediate recovery periods.

d. Client discusses anticipated monitoring and therapeutic devices or materials likely to be used postoperatively.
e. Client describes, in general terms, the surgical procedure and subsequent treatment plan.
f. Client describes anticipated steps in postoperative activity resumption.
g. Client verbalizes expectations about pain relief and measures likely to be taken to alleviate pain.
h. Client expresses feelings regarding surgical intervention and its expected outcomes.
22. a. Improve circulation and prevent stasis mobilize secretions, and promote lung expansion (1618).
  b. Assist in removing retained mucus in airways (1617).
  c. Improve lung expansion and oxygen delivery without using excess energy, clear anesthetic gases remaining in airway (1616).
  d. Improve blood flow to lower extremities and reduce stasis (1618).
23. (1621-1623):
  a. Decrease risk of vomiting and aspiration; prevent complications associated with slowing of gastrointestinal peristalsis.
  b. Decrease incidence of postoperative wound infections.
  c. Reduce incidence of postoperative constipation.
  d. Promote effective rest and sleep before surgery.
24. False (1621)
25. True (1623)
26. To provide the nurse with a guideline for ensuring completion of all required nursing interventions before the client's surgery (1623, 1624)
27. All eleven (1623, 1624, 1629, 1630):
  a. Check medical record and complete required recording.
  b. Check vital signs.
  c. Provide hygiene.
  d. Check hair and cosmetics.
  e. Remove prosthetics.
  f. Prepare bowel and bladder.
  g. Apply antiembolic stockings.
  h. Promote client dignity.
  i. Perform special procedures.
  j. Safeguard client valuables.
  k. Administer preoperative medications.
28. (1629, 1630):
  a. 2
  b. 3
  c. 4
  d. 1
29. d (1629)
30. a (1630)
31. Any nine (1631):
  a. Sphygmomanometer, stethoscope, and thermometer
  b. Emesis basin
  c. Clean gown

d. Washcloth, towel, and facial tissues
e. Intravenous pole
f. Suction equipment
g. Oxygen equipment
h. Extra pillows for positioning the client comfortably
i. Bed pads to protect bed linen from drainage
j. Bed raised to stretcher height with bed linens pulled back
32. c (1632)
33. b (1633)
34. d (1633)
35. d (1635)
36. d (1636)
37. All six (1636):
a. Respiratory rate
b. Respiratory rhythm
c. Depth of ventilation
d. Symmetry of chest wall movement
e. Breath sounds
f. Color of mucous membranes
38. All three (1636):
a. Aspiration of emesis
b. Accumulation of mucous secretions in the pharynx
c. Swelling or spasm of the larynx
39. c (1636)
40. True (1636)
41. a (1636)
42. All four (1636, 1637):
a. Nail bed and skin color
b. Peripheral pulses
c. Heart rate and rhythm
d. Blood pressure
43. (1637):

Area of Assessment	Characteristic Finding
Blood pressure	Decreased
Heart rate	Increased
Respiratory rate	Increased
Pulse volume	Weak thready
Skin	Cool, clammy, pale
Client behavior	Restless

44. d (1637)
45. b (1637)
46. False (1637)
47. c (1637)
48. b (1637)
49. By noting the number of saturated gauze sponges and drawing a circle around the outer perimeter of the drainage (1637)
50. True (1638)
51. 140 ml per hour (formula: 2 ml/kg/hr):
Step 1: 154 ÷ 2.2 = 70 kg
Step 2: 2 ml × 70 kg = 140 ml

52. c (1638)
53. False (1638)
54. True (1638)
55. d (1638)
56. b (1638)
57. All five (1639):
a. Physician's office phone number
b. Surgery center's phone number
c. Follow-up appointment, date, and time
d. Review of prescribed medications
e. Guidelines related to specific surgery (for example, activity restrictions, wound care, and warning signs of complications)
58. All nine (1639):
a. Vital signs stable
b. Body temperature controlled
c. Good ventilatory function
d. Orientation to surroundings
e. Absence of complications
f. Minimal pain and nausea
g. Controlled wound drainage
h. Adequate urine output
i. Fluid-electrolyte balance
59. Obtain a complete set of vital signs and compare them to those obtained in the recovery room (1639).
60. False (1639)
61. Any four (1641):
a. Gaining a return of normal physiological function
b. Remaining free of postoperative surgical wound infection
c. Achieving rest and comfort
d. Maintaining self-concept
e. Returning to a functional state of health within limitations posed by surgery
62. c (1642)
63. See table on p. 308 for three interventions for each area (1641, 1643-1645):
64. b (1643)
65. c (1642)
66. c (1645)
67. Any five (1646):
a. Provide privacy during dressing changes or inspection of the wound.
b. Maintain client's hygiene.
c. Prevent drainage sets from overflowing.
d. Maintain a pleasant environment.
e. Offer opportunities for client to discuss feelings about appearance.
f. Provide family with opportunities to discuss ways to promote the client's self-concept.

CHAPTER 48

1. (1655, 1656):
a. 3;6
c. 9
d. 2
e. 14

Area of Need	Nursing Intervention
Maintaining respiratory function	Encourage diaphragmatic breathing and coughing at least every 2 hours.
	Instruct client to use incentive spirometer.
	Encourage early ambulation.
	Turn every 1 to 2 hours.
	Provide oral hygiene.
	Provide orotracheal or nasotracheal suction as indicated.
Preventing circulatory stasis	Encourage performance of leg exercises at least every hour while awake.
	Apply elastic antiembolism stockings as ordered.
	Apply pneumatic antiembolism stockings as ordered.
	Encourage early ambulation.
	Avoid positioning with pressure on popliteal vessels or sitting with legs crossed.
	Elevate legs on footstool when out of bed in chair.
	Give anticoagulants as ordered.
	Provide adequate fluid intake.
Promoting normal bowel elimination	Assess return of peristalsis.
	Maintain gradual progression in dietary intake.
	Promote ambulation and exercise.
	Maintain adequate fluid intake.
	Administer cathartics, laxatives, enemas, suppositories, and rectal tubes as ordered.
Promoting adequate nutrition	Remove sources of noxious odors.
	Assist to comfortable position during meals (sit up if possible).
	Provide small serivings of food.
	Provide frequent oral hygiene.
	Provide meals when client is rested and pain-free.
Promoting normal urinary elimination	Assist to normal positions during voiding.
	Check frequently for need to void.
	Assess for bladder distention; obtain catheterization order if needed.
	Monitor intake and output.

f. 15
g. 4
h. 10
i. 1
j. 8
k. 5
l. 11
m. 7
n. 12
o. 13
2. a (1654)
3. d (1654)
4. (1656, 1657):
   a. Inflammatory phase: Reparative processes beginning within minutes and lasting up to 3 days; controls bleeding (hemostasis), delivers blood and cells to the injured area (inflammation), forms epithelial cells at the injury site (epithelialization).
   b. Destructive phase: Occurs between days 2 through 5; macrophages continue clearing wound of debris and stimulate formation of fibroblasts (cells that will synthesize collagen).
   c. Proliferative phase: Occurs between days 3 through 24; appearance of new blood vessels, wound closes with new tissue, tensile strength of wound increases.
   d. Maturation phase: Final phase may take more than 1 year depending on the depth and extent of the wound.
5. b (1656, 1657)
6. Any four (1656):
   a. Amino acids
   b. Oxygen
   c. Vitamin B
   d. Vitamin C
   e. Growth hormone
7. b (1657)
8. Hematoma (1658)
9. a (1658)
10. b (1658)
11. Any four (1658):
    a. Fever
    b. Tenderness and pain at the wound site
    c. Elevated white blood cell count
    d. Wound edges inflamed
    e. Purulent, odorous yellow, green, or brown drainage (if present)
12. b (1658)
13. Place sterile towels soaked in sterile saline over the

extruding tissues, stay with client, monitor vital signs, and call physician immediately (1658).
14. Fistula (1658)
15. c (1659)
16. Delayed wound closure; deliberate attempt by the surgeon to allow drainage of a clean-contaminated or contaminated wound. Wound remains open until all edema and wound debris are removed. Occlusive dressing prevents bacterial contamination, then closed by primary intention.
17. All five (1657):
   a. Protein: collagen formation
   b. Vitamin C: synthesis of collagen
   c. Vitamin A: reduced negative effects of steroids on wound healing
   d. Zinc: epithelialization, collagen synthesis
   e. Copper: collagen fiber linking
18. (1660, 1661):
   a. Age: Alters all phases of wound healing; vascular changes impair circulation to wound site; reduced liver function alters synthesis of clotting factors, inflammatory response is depressed; reduced formation of antibodies and lymphocytes; collagen tissue less pliable; scar tissue less elastic.
   b. Malnutrition: all phases of healing impaired; stress increases nutritional requirement.
   c. Obesity: fatty tissue lacks adequate blood supply to resist bacterial infection and deliver nutrients and cellular elements for healing.
   d. Impaired oxygenation: alters synthesis of collagen and formation of epithelial cells; tissues fail to receive needed oxygen; decreased hemoglobin reduces oxygen in capillaries and interferes with tissue repair.
   e. Smoking: Reduces amount of functional hemoglobin in blood, decreasing tissue oxygenation; increases platelet aggregation and causes hypercoaguability; interferes with normal cellular mechanisms that facilitate oxygen release to tissues.
   f. Steroids: reduce inflammatory response and slow collagen synthesis; suppress protein syntheses, wound contraction, and epithelialization.
   g. Antibiotics: May increase risk of superinfection.
   h. Chemotherapeutic drugs: depress bone marrow function, lower number of leukocytes, and impair inflammatory response.
   i. Diabetes: causes small blood vessel disease impairing tissue perfusion; causes hemoglobin to have greater affinity for oxygen, so it fails to release oxygen to tissues; alters ability of leukocytes to perform phagocytosis and supports overgrowth of fungal and yeast infection.
   j. Radiation: fibrosis and vascular scarring increase tissue fragility and reduce oxygenation.
   k. Wound stress: vomiting, abdominal distention,

and respiratory effort may stress suture line and disrupt wound layer; sudden, unexpected tension on incision inhibits formation of endothelial cell and collagen networks.
19. All six (1661-1663):
   a. Appearance
   b. Character of drainage: amount, color, odor, and consistency
   c. Presence of drains
   d. Wound closure: staples, sutures, and wound closures
   e. Palpation with sterile gloves: localized tenderness, and drainage collection
   f. Pain; cultures (if purulent or unusual drainage)
20. d (1661, 1662)
21. (1662):
   a. Purulent
   b. Serous
   c. Serosanguineous
   d. Sanguineous
22. True (1663)
23. Aerobic: use a sterile swab from a Culturette tube, gently swabbing wound to collect deeper secretions; return swab to Culturette tube and activate inner ampule containing the medium for organism growth. Anaerobic: use a syringe without a needle; gently place syringe tip in the inner wound and aspirate; on removal apply a sterile needle, expel air from syringe and needle, and inject into special vacuum container or cork the needle (1663).
24. Any six (1665):
   a. Promoting wound hemostasis
   b. Preventing infection
   c. Preventing further tissue injury
   d. Promoting wound healing
   e. Maintaining skin integrity
   f. Regaining normal function
   g. Gaining comfort
25. (1665):
   a. Stabilizing cardiopulmonary function
   b. Promoting hemostasis
   c. Cleansing the wound
   d. Protecting the wound from further injury
26. a (1665)
27. d (1663)
28. (1666):
   a. 4
   b. 2
   c. 1
   d. 3
   e. 5
29. Any six (1667):
   a. Protect a wound from microorganisms contamination.
   b. Aid in hemostasis.
   c. Promote healing by absorbing drainage and debriding a wound.
   d. Support or splint the wound site.

e. Protect the client from seeing the wound (if perceived as unpleasant).
f. Promote thermal insulation to the wound surface.
g. Provide maintenance of high humidity between the wound and dressing.

30. (1667):
  a. Contact or primary dressing: covers the incision and part of the adjacent skin
  b. Absorbent dressing: serves as a reservoir for additional secretions, wicking action pulls excess drainage into the dressing and away from the wound
  c. Outer protective later: helps prevent bacteria and other external contaminants from reaching the wound surface; supports or immobilizes to minimize movement or underlying incision and injured tissues; insulates and keeps wound surface well hydrated

31. c (1667)
32. d (1667)
33. The nurse may add dressings without removing the original one (1668).
34. All four (1668):
  a. The nurse should perform thorough hand washing before and after wound care.
  b. Personnel should not touch an open or fresh wound directly without wearing sterile glove.
  c. If a wound is sealed, dressings may be changed without gloves.
  d. Dressings over closed wounds should be removed or changed when they become wet or if the client has signs or symptoms of infection.
35. All four (1668):
  a. Administer required analgesics so that peak effects occur during the dressing change.
  b. Describe steps of the procedure to lessen anxiety.
  c. Describe normal signs of healing.
  d. Answer questions about the procedure or wound.
36. c (1669)
37. a (1673)
38. d (1673, 1674)
39. All three (1674):
  a. Clean wound
  b. Apply heat
  c. Apply medications.
40. True (1674)
41. d (1674, 1675)
42. True (1657)
43. Sutures (1674)
44. A portable unit that connects to tubular drains lying within a wound bed and exerts a safe, constant, low-pressure vacuum to remove and collect drainage (for example, Hemovac, Jackson-Pratt) (1678)
45. Skin barriers (1677)
46. Any five (1678, 1679):
  a. Create pressure over a body part.
  b. Immobilize a body part.
  c. Support a wound.

  d. Reduce or prevent edema.
  e. Secure a splint.
  f. Secure a dressing.
47. All four (1679):
  a. Inspect the skin for abrasions, edema, discoloration, or exposed wound edges.
  b. Cover exposed wounds or open abrasions with a sterile dressing.
  c. Assess the condition of underlying dressings and change them if soiled.
  d. Assess the skin of underlying body parts and parts that will be distal to the bandage for signs of circulatory impairment.
48. True (1679)
49. b (1669)
50. (1686):
  a. H
  b. C
  c. H
  d. C
  e. H
  f. C
51. Any five (1685):
  a. Very old or very young
  b. Open wounds, broken skin, stomas
  c. Areas of edema or scar formation
  d. Peripheral vascular disease (for example, diabetes, arteriosclerosis)
  e. Confusion or unconsciousness
  f. Spinal cord injury
  g. Abscessed tooth or appendix
52. All six (1686):
  a. Duration of application
  b. Body part
  c. Damage to body surface
  d. Prior skin temperature
  e. Body surface area
  f. Age and physical condition
53. All four (1687):
  a. Presence of any contraindicating conditions
  b. Client's response to assessment stimuli
  c. Client's level of consciousness
  d. Condition of equipment to be used
54. Three for each category:
Do's:
  a. Explain sensations to be felt during the procedure
  b. Instruct client to report changes in sensation or discomfort immediately
  c. Provide a time, clock, or watch so the client can help time the application
  d. Keep the call light within client reach
  d. Refer to the institution's policy and procedure manual for safe temperatures.
Don'ts:
  a. Allow the client to adjust temperature settings
  b. Allow the client to move an application or place hands on the wound site

   c. Place the client in a position that prevents movement away from the temperature source

   d. Leave client unattended who is unable to sense temperature changes or move from the temperature source

55. True (1687)

56. c (1687)

57. **a.** Cold compress (1692)

   b. Warm soak (1688)

   c. Sitz bath (1688)

   d. Heat lamp (1692)

58. **a.** 59° F (15°> C) (1692)

   b. 110° to 115°>(43° to 46° C) (1689)

   c. 105° to 110° F (40.5°> to 43°> C) (1688)

   d. 110° to 115° F (43°> to 46°> C) (1691)

59. a (1686)

60. False (1684)